2nd Edition

Care Coordination *and* Transition Management

Core Curriculum

For RN Practice Across Settings

Editors
Sheila A. Haas, PhD, RN, FAAN
Beth Ann Swan, PhD, CRNP, FAAN
Traci S. Haynes, MSN, BA, RN, CEN, CCCTM®

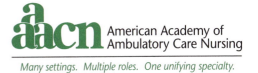

Care Coordination and Transition Management Core Curriculum (2nd Edition)
For RN Practice Across Settings

Editors
Sheila A. Haas, PhD, RN, FAAN
Beth Ann Swan, PhD, CRNP, FAAN
Traci S. Haynes, MSN, BA, RN, CEN, CCCTM®

Vice President, Jannetti Publications, Inc.: Kenneth J. Thomas
Director of Editorial Services: Carol M. Ford
Managing Editor: Kaytlyn N. Mroz
Director of Creative Design and Production: Jack M. Bryant
Layout Design and Production: Darin Peters

Chief Executive Officer: Linda Alexander
Director of Association Services: Jennifer Stranix
Association Services Coordinator: Nicole Livezey
Association Services Coordinator: Stephanie McDonald
Education Director: Michele Boyd, MSN, RN-BC

Publication Management
Anthony J. Jannetti, Inc.
East Holly Avenue, Box 56, Pitman, NJ 08071-0056
Phone: 856-256-2300; Fax: 856-589-7463; www.ajj.com
Published in Pitman, NJ.

SECOND EDITION
ISBN: 978-1-940325-58-3

Copyright © 2019
American Academy of Ambulatory Care Nursing (AAACN)
East Holly Avenue, Box 56, Pitman, NJ 08071-0056
800-AMB-NURS; FAX 856-589-7463; Email: aaacn@aaacn.org; www.aaacn.org

This publication is based on and includes information previously published by the American Academy of Ambulatory Care Nursing in the *Care Coordination and Transition Management Core Curriculum* (1st edition).

All rights reserved. No part of this publication may be reproduced or transmitted in any form or by any means, electronic or mechanical, including photocopying, recording, or any information storage and retrieval system without the written permission of the American Academy of Ambulatory Care Nursing.

Printed in the United States of America

Suggested Citation
Haas, S.A., Swan, B.A., & Haynes, T.S. (Eds.). (2019). *Care coordination and transition management core curriculum, 2nd Edition*. Pitman, NJ: American Academy of Ambulatory Care Nursing.

Notice: Care has been taken to confirm the accuracy of information presented and to ensure that treatments, practices, and procedures are accurate and conform to standards accepted at the time of publication. Constant changes in information resulting from continuing research and clinical experience, reasonable differences in opinions among authorities, unique aspects of individual clinical situations, and the possibility of human error in preparing such a publication require that the reader exercise individual judgment when making a clinical decision and, if necessary, consult and compare information from other authorities, professionals, and/or sources. Any procedure or practice described in this book should be applied by the health care practitioner under appropriate supervision in accordance with professional standards of care used with regard to the unique circumstances that apply in each practice situation.

Every effort has been made to ensure drug selections and dosages are in accordance with current recommendations and practice. Because of ongoing research, changes in government regulations, and the constant flow of information on drug therapy, reactions, and interactions, the reader is cautioned to check the package insert for each drug for indications, dosages, warnings, and precautions, particularly if the drug is new or infrequently used.

The authors, reviewers, editors, and publishers cannot accept any responsibility for errors or omissions or for any consequences from application of the information in this book and make no warranty, expressed or implied, with respect to the contents of the book.

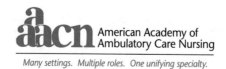

Endorsements

The American Academy of Ambulatory Care Nursing (AAACN) extends its gratitude to the following organizations that have endorsed the *Care Coordination and Transition Management Core Curriculum, 2nd Edition.*

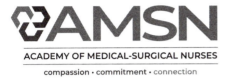
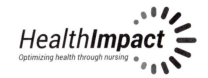
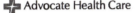
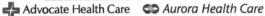
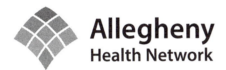
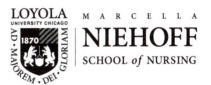
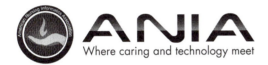
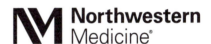
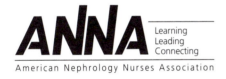
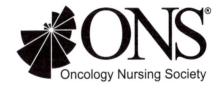
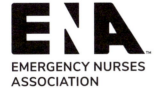
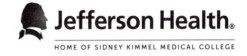
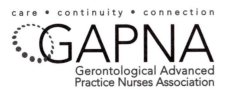
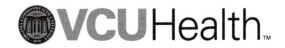

Table of Contents

Foreword vii

Preface ix

Contributors xii

Reviewers xiv

Expert Panels xv

Acknowledgments xvi

Chapter 1 1
Introduction

Chapter 2 19
Advocacy

Chapter 3 49
Education and Engagement of Individuals and Families

Chapter 4 75
Coaching and Counseling of Individuals and Families

Chapter 5 91
Person-Centered Care Planning

Chapter 6 121
Support for Self-Management

Chapter 7 137
Nursing Process

Chapter 8 159
Teamwork and Collaboration

Chapter 9 175
Cross Setting Communications and Care Transitions

Chapter 10 197
Population Health Management

Chapter 11 235
Care Coordination and Transition Management Between Acute Care and Ambulatory Care

Chapter 12 265
Informatics Competencies to Support Nursing Practice

Chapter 13 287
Telehealth Nursing Practice

Glossary 315

Resources 329

Applications 331

Index 333

Foreword

A Competency Model to Improve Quality and Safety, Care Coordination, and Transitions

Health care delivery involves a complex combination of processes, technologies, and human interactions, with an inevitable risk of adverse events. Despite rigorous efforts to improve health care quality and safety, preventable harm continues to be a global concern (National Academies of Sciences, Engineering, and Medicine [NASEM], 2018). Culture changes, organizational commitment, and redesign of education and training are necessary to develop health care teams with the competencies to design and lead high-reliability organizations – those with a focus on evidence-based care standards to improve safety.

The second edition of the *Care Coordination and Transition Management Core Curriculum* provides an update in the continuing efforts to improve patient care outcomes by defining a competency model integrating the Quality and Safety Education for Nurses (QSEN) competencies with standards from the American Academy of Ambulatory Care Nursing (AAACN). This book integrates the QSEN competencies (person-centered care, teamwork and collaboration, evidence-based practice, quality improvement, safety, and informatics) (Cronenwett et al., 2007) with the nine Care Coordination and Transition Management Registered Nurse (CCTM RN®) dimensions: self-management, individual/family education and engagement, communication and transition, population health management, coaching and counseling individuals and families, nursing process, teamwork and collaboration, person-centered care planning, decision-support and information systems, and advocacy.

As health care continues to evolve, both in delivery and economic forces, more attention is focused on improving outcomes. As patients transition across care settings, whether between acute and primary care, ineffective collaboration between care team members contributes to fragmented care. In primary and ambulatory care, the relationship between the clinician and the individual is a key to high-quality, safe, and effective health care (Agency for Healthcare Research [AHRQ], 2017) by implementing evidence-based strategies to improve patient outcomes by engaging individuals and families in their care.

By practicing to their fullest educational preparation, nurses are uniquely positioned to provide key leadership in improving care management across a myriad of care delivery settings (Institute of Medicine [IOM], 2010), but need guidelines that address specific settings and populations. Competency-based nursing education and professional practice models utilize the knowledge, skills, and education defining what nurses need to know, what they need to be able to do, and the values and beliefs that guide their actions. Standardized care objectives guide nursing actions, and address quality and safety concerns, which were first described in 2000 (IOM, 2000), as well as the subsequent quality goals (IOM, 2001) from STEEEP, an acronym for making sure all care is Safe, Timely, Equitable, Efficient, Effective, and Patient-centered (IOM, 2002). Still, however, the 2018 global quality report, "Crossing the Global Quality Chasm: Improving Health Care Worldwide" (NASEM, 2018), discloses continuing gaps in care reliability.

Three care coordination and transition management experts who are each Past Presidents of AAACN guided development with a futuristic perspective that provides a critical step in improving quality and safety of care by helping nurses understand better how to incorporate the QSEN and CCTM RN competencies in practice. Person-centered care is at the heart of safety; CCTM standards describe specific, evidence-based standards for accurate and personalized assessment as the basis for person-centered care. Safety awareness is even more important in considering unique practice settings that include advanced practice nurses, who may be in independent or group practice; nurses who must communicate and share care goals among interprofessional colleagues; those who manage small care teams; or nurses who supervise unlicensed personnel. Recognizing breakdowns in processes is the first step to develop quality improvement initiatives that can close gaps between ideal and actual performance measures. Competency in informatics provides a key strategy for communication, decision support, and documentation.

The power of this book is making care standards readily accessible to nurses. Standardization in care is a major component of safe care. Evidence-based standards share best practices based on the latest evidence gathered from the literature and documented experiences. Standardized handover processes and communication can assure care management without interruption. Nurses are the constant care providers who spend the most time with individuals; therefore, nurses have key information for making reliable care decisions. Sharing accurate and timely information between providers can reduce errors during transitions in care. Knowing when and how to speak up is critical for improving care outcomes, and knowing the essential standards can inspire confidence.

Competency models also provide measurement criteria for assessing competency achievement and clinical judgment. Reflection is a key component of competency models when thinking about how to improve one's work and developing awareness of the context of practice (Tanner, 2006). Competency development is more than achieving skills or completing tasks; a competency-based practice model guides organization of tasks within a person-centered perspective to address needs in a particular care delivery setting, such as nursing in an ambulatory care center or a specific patient population. Competency statements identifying the knowledge, skills, and attitudes are essential guides for educational curricula or specific training, licensure and certification requirements, position descriptions, personnel recruitment, and/or employee performance review.

The comprehensive nature of these competencies can leverage improvements across all settings and providers, and can be applied in multiple ways from orientation to evaluation. These evidence-based competencies are about empowering nurses to address unmet needs of the delivery system to give them tools to empower individuals applying the change model of *Will, Ideas, and Execution* (Philips, 2017). We know that nurses have the *will* to improve care when they have the *ideas* and the resources for *execution*. The *Care Coordination and Transition Management Core Curriculum, 2nd Edition,* is a vital resource for all nurses who fit the current practice arena and has the capacity to improve care for all. This second edition helps nurses navigate the ever-evolving health care delivery system, and economic provisions, diversity and the social determinants of health, and increasing comorbidities in complex ambulatory care settings. Finally, this second edition provides an updated roadmap to improve health care quality and safety, particularly in transitions across all care settings and providers.

Gwen Sherwood, PhD, RN, FAAN
Professor Emeritus
University of North Carolina at Chapel Hill
School of Nursing
Chapel Hill, NC

References

Agency for Healthcare Research and Quality (AHRQ, 2018). *The guide to improving patient safety in primary care settings by engaging patients and families.* Retrieved from https://www.ahrq.gov/professionals/quality-patient-safety/patient-family-engagement/pfeprimarycare/index.html

Cronenwett, L., Sherwood, G., Barnsteiner, J., Disch, J., Johnson, J., Mitchell, P., ... Warren, J. (2007). Quality and safety education for nurses. *Nursing Outlook, 55*(3), 122-131.

Institute of Medicine (IOM). (2001). *Crossing the quality chasm: A new health system for the 21st century.* Retrieved from http://www.nationalacademies.org/hmd/~/media/Files/Report%20Files/2001/Crossing-the-Quality-Chasm/Quality%20Chasm%202001%20%20report%20brief.pdf

Institute of Medicine (2010). *The future of nursing: Leading change, advancing health.* Retrieved from http://nacns.org/wp-content/uploads/2016/11/5-IOM-Report.pdf

National Academies of Sciences, Engineering, and Medicine (NASEM). (2018). *Crossing the global quality chasm: Improving health care worldwide.* Washington, DC: The National Academies Press. doi:10.17226

Philips. (2017). *Leading change: Impacting so many people.* Retrieved from https://www.philips.com/a-w/about/news/archive/blogs/innovation-matters/leading-change-impacting-so-many-people.html

Tanner, C. A. (2006). Thinking like a nurse: A research based model of clinical judgment in nursing. *Journal of Nursing Education, 45*(6), 204-211.

Additional Readings

Institute of Medicine (IOM). (1999). *To err is human: Building a safer health system.* Washington, DC: National Academies Press. Retrieved from http://www.nationalacademies.org/hmd/~/media/Files/Report%20Files/1999/To-Err-is-Human/To%20Err%20is%20Human%201999%20%20report%20brief.pdf

Pittman, P (2019). *Activating nursing to address unmet needs in the 21st century* [Position Paper]. Princeton, NJ: Robert Wood Johnson Foundation.

Preface

United States health care and health care systems have evolved in the five years since the publication of the *Care Coordination and Transition Management Core Curriculum, 1st Edition* (Haas, Swan, & Haynes, 2014). Yet the current U.S. health care system continues to be both ineffective and inefficient. The Commonwealth Fund rankings (Schneider, Sarnak, Squires, Shah, & Doty, 2017) of 11 industrialized countries found the United States in 2014 and 2017 ranked #11 overall on measures of access, efficiency, equity, and health care outcomes. With such poor outcomes, the U.S. health care system is also the most expensive, with per capita expenditures of more than $8,000. What is needed is a new vision for the role of registered nurses (RNs), one that is consistent with the Institute of Medicine (IOM) *Future of Nursing* vision (Altman, Butler, & Shern, 2015; IOM, 2010), and one that allows RNs to fully contribute to quality care and outcomes. The Care Coordination and Transition Management Registered Nurse (CCTM RN®) Model was developed with this purpose in mind.

Citizens in the United States are living longer, but often with chronic disease or multiple chronic conditions (MCCs). Although the Affordable Care Act is currently available, many persons do not have access to health care. Even if they can access care, challenges include access to providers and settings that exist in silos, and the continuing focus on acute care, with little attention to primary care, wellness care, disease prevention, and early detection. Persons with MCCs in the United States often require care from multiple health care providers in multiple settings. The problem of MCCs among Americans is a major issue; it is associated with suboptimal health outcomes and rising health care expenses (Parekh, Goodman, Gordon, & Koh, 2011). Poor outcomes include polypharmacy, redundant testing, readmission in less than 28 days post-discharge from acute care, and the inability to develop, maintain, and use a plan of care by individuals, families, and providers. Health care providers and systems are often reimbursed for care only if they can meet quality requirements of pay for performance. Readmission in less than 28 days post-discharge from acute care is a Centers for Medicare and Medicaid Services (CMS) "never event," and readmission is not reimbursed.

Chronic diseases are responsible for 7 of 10 deaths each year, and treating people with chronic diseases accounts for 86% of our nation's health care costs (Centers for Disease Control and Prevention [CDC], 2018). Eighty-eight percent of U.S. health care dollars are spent on medical care that only accounts for approximately 10% of a person's health. Many persons struggle with multiple illnesses combined with social complexities, such as mental health and substance abuse, extreme medical frailty, and a host of social needs, such as social isolation and homelessness (Humowiecki et al., 2018). Other determinants of health are lifestyle and behavior choices, genetics, human biology, social determinants, and environmental determinants – accounting for approximately 90% of their health outcomes (Lobelo, Trotter, & Heather 2016).

Traditionally, little attention was given to social determinants, which often play a part in a person's ability to participate in a plan of care for an active disease or condition. Delivery of health care services continues to employ outmoded "siloed" approaches that focus on individual chronic diseases (Parekh et al., 2011). An individual with MCCs presents to the health care system with unique needs, disabilities, and/or functional limitations. The literature on how to best support self-management efforts in those with MCCs is in early stages of development (Grady & Gough, 2014).

When the MCC population transitions between health care providers and settings, many gaps and errors can and do occur. Incomplete transfer of information is a major factor in such gaps and errors. Effective care transition communication is an expectation of quality and safe care. Adverse events and risk exposures occur due to ineffective or poor communication during transitions of care. Poor communication among health care providers and the lack of shared information about individuals result in under-treatment, suboptimal therapy, adverse drug events, and hospital admissions or re-admissions (IOM, 2013). Up to 49% of individuals experience at least one medical error after discharge, and one in five persons discharged from the hospital suffers an adverse event. Improved communication among providers could prevent up to half or more of these events (Society of Hospital Medicine, 2010). One in five individuals with Medicare who are discharged from hospitals are readmitted within 30 days, and 34% within 90 days (Brown, 2018; Robert Wood Johnson Foundation [RWFJ], 2013a, b).

Health care providers do not talk to each other enough. Members of the care team – physicians, nurses, social workers, and even caregivers – do not spend enough time communicating with each other about the individual's needs, and no one from the care team spends enough time communicating with the individual and his/her family. On average, a Medicare recipient has seven providers across four care settings involved in their care – five specialty providers and two primary care providers (IOM, 2013). Four out of five individuals are discharged

Preface

from hospitals without direct communication with their primary care provider (RWFJ, 2013a, b).

Exchange of information occurs informally and formally between members of the health care team who say communication is critical in health care (Lancaster, Kolakowsky-Hayner, Kovacich, & Greer-Williams, 2015). Communication is a vital component of the post-hospital discharge.

The CCTM RN Model has the potential to enhance care and outcomes of all individuals in all health care settings, and in particular, our most vulnerable patients – the MCC population. Development of the CCTM RN Model is described in an article by Haas, Swan, and Haynes (2013). The second edition of the *Care Coordination and Transition Management Core Curriculum* text provides essential content on each of the nine CCTM dimensions and competencies of CCTM. This edition has been updated and expanded to provide evidence-based assessments, interventions, evaluation, and outcomes within each dimension, as well as adding areas of RN practice where coordinating care and managing transitions are foundational and critical. New content areas in the second edition include *behavioral health, pediatrics, palliative care, end-of-life care, opioid addiction education and engagement, geriatric care,* and *interprofessional collaboration*. The chapter on population health management has been expanded to include big data, along with the chapter on informatics. All chapters contain case studies. In addition, there is an exemplar in the Advocacy chapter and a care plan in the Nursing Process chapter. There is also an appendix offering apps (applications) that may be useful for nurses or persons being cared for. CCTM RN evidence-based dimensions and competency specifications align with the American Association of Colleges of Nursing (AACN) (2018) recommendations for preparation of an entry level "generalist for practice across the life span and continuum of care in four spheres of practice: disease prevention/promotion of health, chronic disease care, regenerative or restorative, and hospice/palliative/supportive care" (p. 12). The *Care Coordination and Transition Management Core Curriculum, 2nd Edition* continues to employ the Quality and Safety Education in Nursing (QSEN) Competency framework (Cronenwett et al., 2007) to summarize knowledge, skills, and attitudes (KSAs) critical to RN practice in each of the nine CCTM dimensions. The unique KSA tables included in each chapter provide a rich resource by summarizing chapter content and enhancing understanding of the breadth and depth of each dimension. The tables categorize requisite skills and attitudes needed in addition to knowledge of content for each CCTM dimension.

The *Care Coordination and Transition Management Core Curriculum, 2nd Edition* is designed to be an educational resource for practicing nurses or health care organization educators responsible for continuing development of nurses in acute, subacute, primary care or specialty care clinics, ambulatory, home care or any health care setting. For practicing nurses, the Certified in Care Coordination and Transition Management (CCCTM®) certification is offered by the Medical-Surgical Nursing Certification Board (MSNCB). Online modules for each dimension and certification review resources are available to assist RNs taking the examination. Passage of the nationally recognized CCCTM examination provides evidence of expertise in CCTM. The CCCTM certification program received accreditation by the Accreditation Board for Specialty Nursing Certification (ABSNC) in Fall 2018 and is a recognized national certification currently included in the Magnet Demographic Data Collection Tool®.

The *Care Coordination and Transition Management Core Curriculum 2nd Edition* can guide development and implementation of CCTM courses for faculty teaching in prelicensure nursing education programs. We are proud to provide this rich evidence-based text to prelicensure faculty, educators in health services organizations, and RNs who want to grow in knowledge, skills, and competencies to coordinate care and manage transitions to better serve our most vulnerable populations.

Sheila A. Haas, PhD, RN, FAAN
Lead Editor

Beth Ann Swan, PhD, CRNP, FAAN
Co-Editor

Traci S. Haynes, MSN, BA, RN, CEN, CCCTM®
Co-Editor and Project Manager

References

Altman, S.H., Butler, A.S., & Shem, L. (Eds.). (2015). *Assessing progress on the Institute of Medicine Report 'The Future of Nursing.'* Washington, DC: The National Academies Press. Retrieved from https://www.ncbi.nlm.nih.gov/books/NBK 350166/

American Association of Colleges of Nursing (AACN). (2018). *Vision for nursing education.* Washington, D.C.: Author.

Brown, M.M. (2018). Transitions of care. In T.P. Daaleman & M.R. Helton (Eds.), *Chronic illness care* (pp. 369-373). Chapel Hill, NC: Springer International Publishing.

Centers for Disease Control and Prevention (CDC). (2018). *About chronic health.* Retrieved from https://www.cdc.gov/chronicdisease

Cronenwett, L., Sherwood, G., Barnsteiner, J., Disch, J., Johnson, J., Mitchell, P., ... Warrren, J. (2007). Quality and safety education for nurses. *Nursing Outlook, 55*(3), 122-131.

Grady, P.A., & Gough, L. (2014). Self-management: A comprehensive approach to management of chronic conditions. *American Journal of Public Health, 104*(8), e25-e31.

Haas, S., Swan, B.A., & Haynes, T. (2013). Developing ambulatory care registered nurse competencies for care coordination and transition management. *Nursing Economic$, 31*(1), 44-49, 43. Retrieved from https://www.aaacn.org/sites/default/files/documents/NursingEcArticleJan_Feb2013_DevelopingAmbulatoryCare.pdf

Haas, S., Swan, B.A., & Haynes, T. (Eds.). (2014). *Care coordination and transition management core curriculum* (1st ed.). Pitman, NJ: American Academy of Ambulatory Care Nursing.

Humowiecki, M., Kuruna, T., Sax, R., Hawthorne, M., Hamblin, A., Turner, S., ... Cullen, K. (2018). *Blueprint for complex care: Advancing the field of care for individuals with complex health and social needs.* Retrieved from https://www.nationalcomplex.care/wp-content/uploads/2018/12/Blueprint-for-Complex-Care_FINAL_120318.pdf

Institute of Medicine (IOM). (2010). *The future of nursing: Leading change, advancing health.* Washington, D.C.: National Academies Press.

Institute of Medicine (IOM). (2013). *Partnering with patients to drive shared decisions, better value, and care improvement: Workshop proceedings.* Washington, D.C.: National Academies Press.

Lancaster, G., Kolakowsky-Hayner, S., Kovacich, J., & Greer-Williams, N. (2015). Interdisciplinary communication and collaboration among physicians, nurses, and unlicensed assistive personnel. *Journal of Nursing Scholarship. 47*(3), 275-284.

Lobelo, F., Trotter, P., & Heather, A.J. (2016). *Chronic disease is healthcare's rising risk.* Retrieved from http://www.exerciseismedicine.org/assets/page_documents/Whitepaper%20Final%20for%20Publishing%20(002)%20Chronic%20diseases.pdf

Parekh, A.K., Goodman, R.A., Gordon, C., & Koh, H.K. (2011). Managing multiple chronic conditions: A strategic framework for improving health outcomes and quality of life. *Public Health Reports, 126*(4), 460-471.

Robert Wood Johnson Foundation (RWJF). (2013a). *Reducing avoidable readmissions through better care transitions.* Retrieved from http://www.rwjf.org/content/dam/farm/toolkits/toolkits/2013/rwjf404051

Robert Wood Johnson Foundation (RWJF). (2013b). *The revolving door: A report on U.S. hospital readmissions.* Princeton, NJ: Author.

Schneider, E.C., Sarnak, D.O., Squires, D., Shah, A., & Doty, M.M. (2017). *Mirror, mirror 2017: International comparison reflects flaws and opportunities for better U.S. health care.* Retrieved from http://www.commonwealthfund.org/publications/fund-reports/2017/jul/mirror-mirror-international-comparisons-2017

Society of Hospital Medicine. (2017). *Advancing successful care transitions to improve outcomes.* Retrieved from https://www.hospitalmedicine.org/clinical-topics/care-transitions/

Additional Readings

Centers for Disease Control and Prevention (CDC). (n.d.). *Making healthy living easier: National implementation and dissemination for chronic disease prevention.* Retrieved from https://www.cdc.gov/nccdphp/dch/pdfs/00-making-life-easier-nidcdp.pdf

Deland, E., Gordon, J.E., & Kelly, R.E. (2015). Let's talk about improving communication in healthcare. *Columbia Medical Review, 1*(1), 23-27. doi:10.7916/D8RF5T5D

Levit, L.A., Balogh, E.P., Nass, S.J., & Ganz, P.A. (Eds.). (2013). *Delivering high-quality cancer care: Charting a new course for a system in crisis.* Washington, D.C.: National Academies Press.

Contributors

Jacqueline Adams, MSN, RN, CORLN, CCCTM®
Clinical Specialist
Thomas Jefferson University Hospital
Philadelphia, PA

Karen Alexander, PhD, MSN, RN
Assistant Professor
Thomas Jefferson University
Philadelphia, PA

Robin Austin, PhD, DNP, RN-BC
Clinical Associate Professor
University of Minnesota School of Nursing
Minneapolis, MN

Sharon Bouyer-Ferullo, DNP, RN, MHA, CNOR
Perioperative Staff Specialist
Mass General Hospital
Boston, MA

Stefanie Coffey, DNP, MBA, MN, FNP-BC, RN-BC
Community Care Coordination Nurse Practitioner
VA Roseburg Health Care System
Roseburg, OR

Constance Dahlin, MSN, ANP-BC, ACHPN, FPCN, FAAN
Director of Professional Practice
Hospice and Palliative Nurses Association
Pittsburgh, PA
Palliative Nurse Practitioner
North Shore Medical Center
Salem, MA
Consultant
Center to Advance Palliative Care
New York, NY

Judy Dawson-Jones, MPH, BSN, RN
Executive Director of Nursing, Children's Services
Sidra Medicine
Doha, Qatar

Vanessa DeBiase, MSN, MEd, RN
Clinical Nurse Educator
Northwestern Medical Group
Chicago, IL

Anne M. Delengowski, MSN, RN, AOCN, CCCTM®
Director Oncology Nursing Education/Clinical Nurse Specialist
Thomas Jefferson University Hospital
Philadelphia, PA

William Duffy, RN, MJ, CNOR, FAAN
Director, Nursing & Healthcare Administration Program
Marcella Niehoff School of Nursing Loyola University
Chicago, IL

Eileen M. Esposito, DNP, MPA, RN-BC, CPHQ
Vice President, Ambulatory Clinical Practice
Catholic Health Services of Long Island
Garden City NY

Dawn M. Gerz, MSN, MBA, RN, NEA-BC, RN-BC
Vice President Ambulatory Nursing
Allegheny Health Network
Pittsburgh, PA

Sheila A. Haas, PhD, RN, FAAN
Dean and Professor Emeritus
Marcella Niehoff School of Nursing Loyola University Chicago
Maywood, IL

Traci S. Haynes, MSN, BA, RN, CEN, CCCTM®
Director of Clinical Services
LVM Systems, Inc.
Mesa, AZ

Mary Clare Houlihan, MS, RN, CCRN
Clinical Registered Nurse, Medical Intensive Care Unit
Northwestern Memorial Hospital
Chicago, IL

Anne T. Jessie, DNP, RN
Managing Director
Evolent Health
Arlington, VA

Sheila Johnson, MBA, RN
Vice President, Population Health Clinical Operations
Trinity Health
Livonia, MI

Rosemary Kennedy, PhD, RN, MBA, FAAN
CEO
eCare Informatics, LLC
Frazer, PA

Maribeth Kelly, MSN, RN, PCCN, CCCTM®
Clinical Nurse Specialist
Thomas Jefferson University Hospital
Philadelphia, PA

Kathryn Koehne, DNP, RN-BC, C-TNP
Director of Nursing & Operations
Crescent Cove
Brooklyn Center, MN
Adjunct Faculty
Viterbo University
La Crosse, WI

Cheryl Lovlien, MS, RN-BC
Nursing Education Supervisor
Mayo Clinic
Rochester, MN

Contributors

Kristine Meagher, MSN, RN, ACNS-BC, CCCTM®
Clinical Nurse Specialist
Jefferson Health
Philadelphia, PA

Naomi Mercier, DNP, MSN, RN-BC
Clinical Content Nurse Lead
Partners HealthCare
Boston, MA

Cynthia Murray, BN, RN-BC
Nurse Manager Clinical Operations
Veterans Health Administration
Atlantic County, NJ

Carol A. Newman, DNP, MSED, MSN, RN, CPNP-PC
SVP, Medical Management Operations and Business Support
WellMed Medical Management
San Antonio, TX

Cynthia R. Niesen, DNP, MA, RN, NEA-BC
Registered Nurse Care Coordinator | Assistant Professor of Nursing
Mayo Clinic
Rochester, MN

Susan M. Paschke, MSN, RN-BC, NEA-BC
Part-Time Faculty
Kent State University
Kent, OH

Denise Rismeyer, MSN, RN, RN-BC
Nursing Education Specialist
Mayo Clinic
Rochester, MN

Bonnie Robertson, MSN, RN-BC, CRNP, CCCTM®
Clinical Nurse Specialist
Thomas Jefferson University Hospital
Philadelphia, PA

Jude Sell-Gutowski, MSN, BSN, RN-BC
Quality Clinical Documentation Improvement
Dignity Health Medical Foundation
Rancho Cordova, CA

Jayme M. Speight, MSN, RN-BC
Education Coordinator
Akron Children's Hospital
Akron, Ohio

Rachel Start, MSN, RN, NE-BC
Director, Ambulatory Nursing and Nursing Practice
Rush Oak Park Hospital
Oak Park, IL

Diane Storer-Brown, PhD, RN, CPHQ, FNAHQ, FAAN
Senior Scientist
CALNOC
Walnut Creek, CA

Beth Ann Swan, PhD, CRNP, FAAN
Professor
Jefferson College of Nursing, Thomas Jefferson University
Philadelphia, PA

Kathryn D. Swartwout, PhD, APRN, FNP-BC
Associate Professor
Rush University
Chicago, IL

Gina Tabone, MSN, RNC-TNP
Vice President of Strategic Clinical Solutions
TEAMHealth Medical Call Center
Cleveland/Akron, OH

Judith Toth-West, PhD, RN, CCTM, CCM, CPHQ
Consultant
Longview, WA

Barbara Trehearne, PhD, RN
Consultant
Seattle, WA

Tina Truong, MS, RN, CCCTM®
Transitional Care Nurse
Oregon Health and Science University
Portland, OR

Frances R. Vlasses, PhD, RN, ANEF, FAAN
Professor
Marcella Niehoff School of Nursing, Stritch School of Medicine, Department of Family Medicine
Loyola University
Chicago, IL
Co-Director
Institute for Transformative Interprofessional Education
Chicago, IL

Mary Hines Vinson, DNP, RN-BC
Consulting Associate (Adjunct Faculty)
Duke University School of Nursing
Durham, NC

Suzanne Wells, MSN, RN
Adjunct Faculty
Webster University School of Nursing
Webster Groves, MO

Lisa Wus, DNP, RN, FNP-BC, PCCN-CMC, CCCTM®
Clinical Nurse Specialist
Thomas Jefferson University Hospital
Philadelphia, PA

Pa Choua Xiong, MSN, RN, CCCTM®
VA Central California Health Care System
Primary Care Service
Clinical Nurse Manager
Fresno, CA

Reviewers

Julie J. Alban, DNP, MPH, RN-BC, CCCTM®
Nurse Manager Primary Care
The Villages VA Outpatient Clinic
The Villages, FL

Katherine K. Andersen, MSN, RN-BC, CCM
Registered Nurse Care Coordinator
VISN 20 Clinical Resource Hub
Boise, ID

Ida M. Androwich, PhD, RN-BC, FAAN
Professor Emeritus
Marcella Niehoff School of Nursing Loyola University
Chicago, IL

Diane R. Davis, DNP, MHA, RN
Director
Concord Hospital
Concord, NH

Sarah L. Flores, MSN, RN, NE-C
Assistant Professor
Biola University
La Mirada, CA

Vicki Grant, MS, RN-BC
Retired
Poulsbo, WA

Dwight Hampton, MBA, RN-BC, PCMH CCE
Ambulatory Field Surveyor
The Joint Commission
Accreditation & Certification Operations
Oakbrook Terrance, IL

Denise Hannagan, MSN, MHA, RN-BC, EDAC, CCHP
Senior Healthcare Consultant
HDR, Inc.
Omaha, NE

Kenneth S. Horseman, MSN, RN-BC, CEN CPEN, CCCTM®
Lead Home Telehealth Care Coordinator
Department of Veterans Affairs
Wilmington, DE

E. Mary Johnson, BSN, RN-BC, NE-BC
Consultant - Career Coach for Nurses
Self-Employed
Macedonia, OH

Amy Lipsett, MHA, BSN, RN, ONC, CCCTM®
Orthopedic Staff Development Nurse
Thomas Jefferson University Hospital
Philadelphia, PA

Nancy May, DNP, RN-BC, NEA-BC
Interim Chief Nursing Executive, Chief Nursing Officer for Ambulatory Care
University of Michigan
Ann Arbor, MI

Brenda Miller, MSN, RN-BC
Ambulatory Care Nurse Clinician
VCU Health System
Richmond, VA

Edtrina Moss, PhD, RN-BC, NE-BC
Patient Safety/Utilization Manager Registered Nurse
DeBakey VA Medical Center
Houston, TX

Cynthia Murray, BN, RN-BC
Nurse Manager Clinical Operations
Veterans Health Administration
Atlantic County, NJ

Carol Rutenberg, MNSc, RN-BC, C-TNP
President
Telephone Triage Consulting, Inc.
Hot Springs, AR

Pamela Ruzic, MSN, RN-BC, CCCTM®
Resident Clinic Nurse/Operations Manager
Baylor Scott & White Health – Health Texas Provider
Dallas, TX

Assanatu I. Savage, PhD, DNP, FNP-BC, RN-BC, CDR, NC, USN
Director, Phase II DNP Program/Assistant Clinical Professor
Uniformed Services University of Health Sciences
Bremerton, WA

Sandra L. Siedlecki, PhD, RN, APRN-CNS
Senior Nurse Scientist, Office of Nursing Research and Innovation
Cleveland Clinic Health System
Cleveland, OH

Cynthia A. Standish, MSN, RN-BC
Nurse Educator
Captain James A. Lovell Federal Health Care Center
North Chicago, IL

Mary Kate Sweeney, MSN, RN-BC, CCCTM®
CBOC Nurse Manager
Captain James A. Lovell Federal Health Care Center
North Chicago, IL

Laurie Friday Walsh, RN, MSN, ANP-BC, GNP
Nurse Practitioner
Kaiser Permanente Medical Group
Sacramento, CA

Stephanie G. Witwer, PhD, RN, NEA-BC
Nurse Administrator Primary Care
Mayo Clinic
Rochester, MN

Expert Panels

Phase 1 Expert Panel

Karen Alexander, MSN, RN***
Janine Allbritton, MSN, RN**
Jo Ann Appleyard, PhD, RN
Deborah E. Aylard, MSN, RN**
Jeff Bergen, MSN, RN, CIC
Deanna Blanchard, MSN, RN
Elizabeth Bradley, MSN, RN-BC
Stefanie Coffey, DNP, MBA, FNP-BC, RN-BC****
Patricia Grady, BSN, RN, CRNS, FABC
Denise Hannagan, MSN, MHA, RN-BC**
Clare Hastings, PhD, RN, FAAN
Anne Talbott Jessie, MSN, RN****
Sheila A. Johnson, MBA, RN**
Cmdr. Catherine McNeal Jones, MSN, MBA, NC, USN HCM, RN-BC
Cheryl Lovlien, MS, RN-BC**
Carol Mannone, MSN, RN, CH-GC**
Sylvia McKenzie, MSN, RN, CPHQ
Shirley Morrison, PhD, RN, OCN
Janet Moye, PhD, RN, NEA-BC
Donna Parker, MA, BSN, RN-BC
Deborah Smith, DNP, RN
Erin Taylor, MSN, RN, CNOR
Debra Toney, PhD, RN, FAAN
Linda Walton, MSN, RN, CENP

Phase 2 Expert Panel

Karen Alexander, MSN, RN***
Marc Altshuler, MD
Jill Arzouman, MS, RN, ACNS, BC, CMSRN
Stefanie Coffey, DNP, MBA, FNP-BC, RN-BC****
Sandy Fights, MS, RN, CMSRN, CNE
Janet Fuchs, MBA, MSN, RN, NEA-BC***
Jamie Green, MSN, RN
Anne Talbott Jessie, MSN, RN****
Diane Kelly, DrPH, MBA, RN
Lisa Kristosik, MSN, RN
Rosemarie Marmion, MSN, RN-BC, NE-BC***
Kathy Mertens, MN, MPH, RN***
Stephanie G. Witwer, PhD, RN, NEA-BC***

Phase 3 Expert Panel

Stefanie Coffey, DNP, MBA, FNP-BC, RN-BC****
Janet Fuchs, MBA, MSN, RN, NEA-BC***
Anne Talbott Jessie, MSN, RN****
Nancy May, MSN, RN-C, NEA-BC
Rosemarie Marmion, MSN, RN-BC, NE-BC***
Kathy Mertens, MN, MPH, RN***
Carol Rutenberg, MNSc, RN-BC, C-TNP**
Barbara Ellis Trehearne, PhD, RN**
Stephanie G. Witwer, PhD, RN, NEA-BC***

Phase 4 Expert Panel

Karen Alexander, MSN, RN***
Janine Allbritton, MSN, RN**
Ida M. Androwich, PhD, RN, BC-NI, FAAN
Deborah E. Aylard, MSN, RN**
Mary Anne Bord-Hoffman, MN, RN-BC
Stefanie Coffey, DNP, MBA, FNP-BC, RN-BC****
Mary Sue Dailey, APN-CNS
Judy Dawson-Jones, MPH, BSN, RN
Janet Fuchs, MBA, MSN, RN, NEA-BC***
Vicki Grant, MSN, RN
Kristene Grayem, MSN, CNP, RN
M. Elizabeth Greenberg, PhD, RN-BC, C-TNP
Denise Hannagan, MSN, MHA, RN-BC**
Kari J. Hite, MN, RN, CDE
Anne Talbott Jessie, MSN, RN****
Sheila A. Johnson, MBA, RN**
Rosemary Kennedy, PhD, MBA, RN, FAAN
Candia Baker Laughlin, MS, RN-BC
Cheryl Lovlien, MS, RN-BC**
Carol Mannone, MSN, RN, CH-GC**
Rosemarie Marmion, MSN, RN-BC, NE-BC***
Naomi Mercier, MSN, RN-BC
Kathy Mertens, MN, MPH, RN***
Carol Rutenberg, MNSc, RN-BC, C-TNP**
Kathryn B. Scheidt, MSN, MS, BSN, RN
Kathleen T. Sheehan, MS, BSN, RN-BC, CH-GCN
Judith M. Toth-Lewis, PhD, CRNP, FAAN
Barbara Ellis Trehearne, PhD, RN**
Mary Hines Vinson, DNP, RN-BC
Stephanie G. Witwer, PhD, RN, NEA-BC***

Experts Who Performed a More Recent Review of Literature Between Phases 3 & 4

Karen Alexander, MSN, RN
Janine Allbritton, MSN, RN
Jo Ann Appleyard, PhD, RN
Stefanie Coffey, DNP, MBA, FNP-BC, RN-BC
Clare Hastings, PhD, RN, FAAN
Denise Hannagan, MSN, MHA, RN-BC
Anne Talbott Jessie, MSN, RN

Sheila A. Johnson, MBA, RN
Cheryl Lovlien, MS, RN-BC
Carol Mannone, MSN, RN, CH-GC
Debralee Quinn, MSN, RN-BC, CNN
Kathleen T. Sheehan, MS, BSN, RN-BC CH-GCN
Linda Walton, MSN, RN, CENP

*Indicates number of Expert Panels beyond one.

Acknowledgments

Production of the second edition of the *Care Coordination and Transition Management Core Curriculum* has been an adventure. We could see that this edition was needed given the explosion of information in content areas critical to care coordination and transition management registered nurse (CCTM RN®) practice. We are very grateful to our expert chapter authors who went above and beyond to bring best current evidence to each chapter and to include new content areas such as pediatric and geriatric care, the opioid crisis, health literacy, palliative care, and end of life care. Our chapter authors also developed case studies for each chapter and listed apps that could be useful for CCTM RNs and the individuals and families they care for. Chapter authors and reviewers have been awesome in their willingness to collaborate, participate, produce, and meet deadlines so that this edition could be finalized. We would like to acknowledge also the support of Kathy Mertens, AAACN President; our Board Liaison, Wanda Richards; and other Board members in the production of the *CCTM Core Curriculum, 2nd Edition*.

None of our work as volunteers could have progressed without the dedicated support of AAACN and the Anthony J. Jannetti, Inc. staff, especially Linda Alexander, CEO; Carol Ford, Director, Editorial Services; and Kaytlyn Mroz, Managing Editor.

Traci Haynes

We continue to appreciate all that Traci has done, yet again, to manage this second edition—her expertise in project management is exceptional. She has kept all of us on time and on target with unfailing grace and tact.

Personal Notes

I would like to acknowledge my husband, Tim, for his unwavering support during production of this second edition and for being my sounding board. My thanks also to my children, Meg, and her husband, Andy, and my son, John, and his wife, Jamie, for their patience and support for my continuing work with projects in the profession that I love. I know that our work on CCTM will benefit nurses and those they care for. I also would like to thank my five grandchildren, Nick, Grace, Madeline, Wilson, and Harper, who are all respectful of my commitments and willing to wait at times for me to get to their games and events. I must also acknowledge my two collaborators, Beth Ann and Traci, who have become even more awesome colleagues the second time around with production of this edition. It continues to be a delight to work with our chapter authors who generously share their knowledge and expertise and have been so responsive to requests to enhancements on this second edition.

—*Sheila Haas*

I would like to acknowledge my husband, Eric, you are my inspiration, always; my daughters, Erica and E. Connor, who support me daily with laughter, joy, mantras, and positive affirmations; and my parents, Elizabeth and John H. Reck, who taught me many things, including that how you treat people ultimately tells all—integrity is everything. Sheila and Traci, I appreciate our steadfast partnership and the magic in our collaboration. I dedicate this 2nd Edition in memory of my colleagues and warrior cancer buddies, Lyn Sobolewski and Dr. Kellie Smith, who always kept swimming.

—*Beth Ann Swan*

I would like to acknowledge Sheila and Beth Ann for their passion and leadership of the nursing profession and their expertise in CCTM. Their vision in 2010 has evolved from an idea to a specialty area of nursing practice including certification for over 900 CCTM RNs. Their tenacity is laudable and I'm forever in awe. Many, many thanks to all the authors who have shared their expert knowledge for all our benefit; and to the staff at AJJ and the AAACN Board of Directors for their continued commitment to CCTM. Lastly, thank you to my dear husband, Greg, for his unwavering support; and to our children, Chad, Abigail, and Clinton, and their spouses and children, for their belief in me and my dedication to our profession throughout the years.

—*Traci Haynes*

Chapter 1

Instructions for Continuing Nursing Education Contact Hours

Continuing nursing education credit can be earned for completing the learning activity associated with this chapter. Instructions can be found at aaacn.org/CCTMCoreCNE

Introduction

Beth Ann Swan, PhD, CRNP, FAAN
Sheila A. Haas, PhD, RN, FAAN
Traci S. Haynes, MSN, BA, RN, CEN, CCCTM®
Cynthia Murray, BN, RN-BC

Learning Outcome Statement

After completing this learning activity, the learner will be able to describe the background and significance of the Care Coordination and Transition Management registered nurse (CCTM® RN) Model.

I. Purpose

In September 2017, the AAACN Board of Directors approved the revision/update of the *Care Coordination and Transition Management Core Curriculum* (2014) due to the rapidly changing evidence in care coordination and transition management. The *CCTM Core Curriculum* text serves as the foundational reference for Care Coordination and Transition Management Registered Nurse (CCTM® RN) practice in all settings across the health care continuum and is an educational resource for nursing education curriculum, as well as currently practicing registered nurses. In addition, the CCTM Core Curriculum text is a resource for the Certified in Care Coordination and Transition Management (CCCTM®) certification. AAACN materials include:

- *Scope and Standards of Practice for Registered Nurses in Care Coordination and Transition Management* (2016).
- *Care Coordination and Transition Management Review Questions* (2016).
- *The Role of the Registered Nurse in Ambulatory Care Position Paper* (2017).
- Care Coordination and Transition Management Online Courses (e.g., CCTM 1, CCTM 2); Care Transition Hand-Off Toolkit.
- Care Coordination and Transition Management Toolkit, which utilizes current evidence-based strategies and best practice exemplars to describe how to educate the CCTM RN to enhance the role, build CCTM services, and develop outcome measures in various practice settings. Additional information sources include the American Association of Colleges of Nursing's (AACN) Vision for Nursing Education (2018) and the AACN baccalaureate, masters, and doctoral essentials currently being updated.

II. History

During the summer of 2011, the AAACN Health Care Reform Advisory Team made a recommendation to the AAACN Board of Directors that there was a need for written competencies for the CCTM RN role. The Advisory Team developed a survey asking members if they had access to CCTM competencies, and if not, did they feel there was a need for them.

In July 2011, AAACN members were asked to complete the online survey tool. It was revealed that very few sites had access to CCTM competencies, and those that did had developed them internally. Most respondents also felt that competencies needed to be evidence-based and thorough to support the care provided to individuals and their families. One member wrote: "Competency would create standardization and ensure excellence in the care we are providing." Another wrote: "They are needed because our work needs to be validated, supported, and replicated, and it needs to be evidence-based so we can provide the best quality of care." Other responses included: "Measurable and defined competencies would support improvement in the delivery of care;" "Competencies help ensure that staff have the right level of training and knowledge, which ultimately, helps improve patient safety;" "From a quality perspective, competencies are always important to indicate performance and performance improvement opportunities;" "We need a system to help ensure consistency and standardization within an organization and amongst organizations;" "There is an increasing need for RN care coordination with the Medical Home initiative. This is not a skill that is taught in nursing schools or that is acquired while working in the hospital setting."

Based on feedback received from AAACN membership, the AAACN Board of Directors made the decision to move forward in the development of the CCTM competencies. Two of AAACN's Health Care Reform Advisory Team members, Dr. Sheila Haas and Dr. Beth Ann Swan, agreed to Co-Chair this initiative, while Ms. Traci Haynes served as the Board Liaison and Project Manager.

III. Vision for the Core Curriculum as the Foundation for the CCTM Model
   A. Vision.
      1. The CCTM RN Model standardizes the work of all health care providers in all settings, using evidence from interprofessional literature on CCTM.
      2. The CCTM RN Model.
         a. Specifies the dimensions of CCTM and the associated competencies needed to be performed within the CCTM RN Model.
         b. Defines the knowledge, skills, and attitudes needed for each dimension.
         c. Meets the needs of individuals with complex chronic illnesses (and their families) being cared for in their homes, patient-centered medical homes (PCMH), as well as traditional and non-traditional acute and outpatient settings.
         d. Meets the needs of care for individuals with complex health and social needs (Humowiecki et al., 2018).
         e. Recommends that RNs educated and prepared to work as a CCTM RN be recognized by a certification credential and reimbursed by the Centers for Medicare & Medicaid Services (CMS).
      3. Consistent with the Institute of Medicine's (IOM) report, *The Future of Nursing: Leading Change Advancing Health* (Altman, Butler, & Shern, 2015; IOM, 2010), the CCTM RN Model:
         a. Supports RNs practicing to the full extent of their education and training.
         b. Promotes RNs achieving higher levels of education, training, and licensure through an improved education system that promotes seamless academic progression.
         c. Advocates that RNs are full partners, with physicians and other health care professionals, in redesigning health care in the United States.
         d. Highlights that effective workforce planning and policy making require better data collection and an improved information infrastructure.
         e. Expands opportunities for nurses to lead and diffuse collaborative improvement efforts.
         f. Prepares and enables nurses to lead change to advance health.

IV. Definitions
   A. Competence and achievement of professional practice competencies have long been expected of professionals and long assumed to be present by consumers. It is interesting, however, that consistent definitions for both are not easy to find. In 2008, the American Nurses Association (ANA) issued a Position Statement on Competence. It included definitions and concepts in competence that state: "An individual who demonstrates 'competence' is performing successfully at an expected level. A 'competency' is an expected level of performance that integrates knowledge, skills, abilities, and judgment. The integration of knowledge, skills, abilities and judgment occurs in formal, informal, and reflective learning experiences" (ANA, 2008, p. 2). Arriving at consensus on a definition of competence is still a challenge.
   B. Care coordination.
      1. Agency for Healthcare Research and Quality (AHRQ) definition: "Care coordination is the deliberate organization of patient care activities between two or more participants (including the patient) involved in a patient's care to facilitate the appropriate delivery of health care services. Organizing care involves the marshaling of personnel and other resources needed to carry out all required patient care activities and is often managed by the exchange of information among participants responsible for different aspects of care" (McDonald et al., 2007; McDonald et al., 2011, p. 4).
      2. National Quality Forum (NQF) (2010) definition: "Care coordination is defined as an information-rich, patient-centric endeavor that seeks to deliver the right care (and only the right care) to the right patient at the right time… A function that helps ensure that the patient's needs and preferences for health services and information sharing across people, functions, and sites are met over time… Care coordination maximizes the value of services delivered to patients by facilitating beneficial efficient, safe, and high-quality patient experiences and improved health care outcomes" (p. 2).

3. NQF (2016) updated definition: Care coordination is "the deliberate synchronization of activities and information to improve health outcomes by ensuring that care recipients' and families' needs and preferences for health care and community services are met over time" (p. 13).
C. Transitional care versus transition management.
 1. "Transitional care is defined as a broad range of time-limited services designed to ensure health care continuity, avoid preventable poor outcomes among at-risk populations, and promote the safe and timely transfer of patients from one level of care to another or from one type of setting to another" (Naylor, Aiken, Kurtzman, Olds, & Hirschman, 2011, p. 747).
    a. Core features of transitional care as defined by Naylor and Sochalski (2010) include:
       (1) "Comprehensive assessment of an individual's health goals and preferences, physical, emotional, cognitive, and functional capacities and needs, and social and environmental considerations.
       (2) Implementation of an evidence-based plan of transitional care.
       (3) Care that is initiated at hospital admission, but extends beyond discharge through home and telephone visits.
       (4) Mechanisms to gather and share information across sites of care.
       (5) Engagement of individuals and family caregivers in planning and executing the plan of care.
       (6) Coordinated services during and following the hospitalization by a health care professional with special preparation in the care of chronically ill people, often a master's-prepared nurse" (p. 2).
 2. "Care transitions refer to the movement patients make between health care practitioners and settings as their condition and care needs change during the course of a chronic or acute illness. For example, in the course of an acute exacerbation of an illness, a patient might receive care from a primary care physician or specialist in an outpatient setting, then transition to a hospital physician and nursing team during an inpatient admission before moving on to yet another care team at a skilled nursing facility. Finally, the patient might return home, where he or she would receive care from a visiting nurse. Each of these shifts from care providers and settings is defined as a care transition" (Coleman & Boult, 2003, p. 556).
 3. "Transitional care is defined as a set of actions designed to ensure the coordination and continuity of health care as patients transfer between different locations or different levels of care within the same location. Representative locations include (but are not limited to) hospitals, sub-acute and post-acute nursing facilities, the patient's home, primary and specialty care offices, and long-term care facilities" (Coleman & Boult, 2003, p. 556).
    a. Transitional care is based on a comprehensive plan of care and the availability of health care practitioners who are well-trained in chronic care and have current information about the individual's goals, preferences, and clinical status.
    b. It includes logistical arrangements, education of the individual and family, and coordination among the health professionals involved in the transition.
    c. Transitional care, which encompasses both the sending and receiving aspects of the transfer, is essential for persons with complex care needs (Coleman & Boult, 2003).
 4. The authors expanded on these terms and definitions of transitional care and care transitions to the term *transition management*. The authors define transition management in the context of RN practice in multiple settings as the ongoing support of individuals and their families over time as they navigate care and relationships among more than one provider and/or more than one health care setting and/or more than one health care service. The need for transition management is not determined by age, time, place, or health care condition, but rather by individuals' and/or families' needs for support for ongoing, longitudinal evidence-based, individualized plans of care and follow-up plans of care within the context of health care delivery (Haas, Swan, & Haynes, 2014).
D. CCTM.
 1. In all practice settings across the health care continuum and the community,

CCTM are integrated functions that may occur simultaneously or separately, and are not time-limited as defined above. One provision of the 2010 Affordable Care Act (ACA) to support this expanded definition is the need for individualized evidence-based plans of care and follow-up plans of care that move with individuals longitudinally over time.
    2. Individualized evidence-based plans of care and follow-up plans of care serve as the basis for the CCTM RN model, an innovative person-centered interprofessional collaborative practice care delivery model that integrates the RN role as care coordinator and transition manager (Swan & Haas, 2011).
    3. CCTM RN model recognizes the care coordination and transitional care activities performed by RNs and interprofessional team members in all practice settings across the health care continuum and the community.
E. Confusion over differences between existing care models and the CCTM RN Model.
    1. Many health care professionals assume that case management and nurse navigator roles are the same as CCTM. Both models were developed in the past to meet regulatory and individual needs for guidance in an increasingly complex care system. The CCTM RN role includes activities in case management and navigation, but case management and navigation are singular interventions and do not encompass all CCTM RN Model dimensions and activities/interventions. CCTM was developed through a scientifically sound Translational Research project. The activities/competencies within each of the nine CCTM dimensions are evidence-based and comprehensive.
    2. *Case management* is defined as a collaborative process that assesses, plans, implements, coordinates, monitors, and evaluates the options and services required to meet the client's health and human service needs. It is characterized by advocacy, communication, and resource management, and promotes quality and cost-effective interventions and outcomes (Commission for Case Manager Certification, 2018).
        a. Focus in case management is the individual plan of care versus the CCTM focus on population health management and the use of evidence-based population guidelines, such as those for hypertension and heart failure, to guide the development of individual plans of care that are then modified to reflect individual goals, values, and preferences.
        b. Another focal area of case management is utilization review.
    3. "Oncology nurse navigator: An oncology nurse navigator (ONN) is a professional RN with oncology-specific clinical knowledge who offers individualized assistance to patients, families, and caregivers to help overcome healthcare system barriers. Using the nursing process, an ONN provides education and resources to facilitate informed decision making and timely access to quality health and psychosocial care throughout all phases of the cancer continuum" (Oncology Nursing Society, 2017, p. 4).
        a. The ONN role is focused on education and support of persons and families need for informed decision making and timely access in all phases of the cancer continuum. The competencies of an ONN are included within the nine CCTM RN dimensions. A CCTM RN who works with oncology patients would develop specific expertise with oncology populations as they would with other patient populations such as those with diabetes and heart failure.

V. **Background and Significance of the CCTM Model**

A. Rationale and need.
    1. Growing demand for care coordination and transition management.
        a. Health care spending in the United States is disproportionate, half of U.S. health care dollars are spent on 5% of the population (AHRQ, 2010; McDonald et al., 2011).
        b. Chronic diseases are responsible for seven out of 10 deaths each year, and treating people with chronic diseases accounts for 86% of our nation's health care costs (Centers for Disease Control and Prevention [CDC], 2018).
        c. Eighty-eight percent of U.S. health care dollars are spent on medical care that only accounts for approximately 10% of a person's health. Other determinants of health are lifestyle and behavior choices, genetics, human biology, social determinants, and

environmental determinants – accounting for approximately 90% of their health outcomes (Lobelo, Trotter, & Heather, 2016).
   d. A small percentage of individuals with complex chronic conditions consumes a high proportion of health care services and accounts for the bulk of health care spending; chronic conditions are expensive to treat and a major driver of increased health care spending (Thorpe, 2013).
   e. Many individuals struggle with multiple illnesses combined with social complexities, such as mental health and substance abuse, extreme medical frailty, and a host of social needs, such as social isolation and homelessness (Craig, Eby, & Whittington, 2011).
   f. Individuals with multiple needs are not able to navigate the complex and fragmented health care system (Swan, 2012).
   g. Care providers recognize the need for better coordinated care that leverages community resources and aligns social determinants, such as food, housing, and safe environments, but payment structures in the health care system do not allow such alignment (Kangovi et al., 2013; Humowiecki et al., 2018).
   h. Individuals with chronic diseases and multiple co-morbidities are a vulnerable population. Health care for these at-risk individuals can be fragmented, leading to non-beneficial or redundant testing services. Uneven quality of care for at-risk populations can lead to poor outcomes and increased use of limited health care resources. At-risk individuals are not well served by the traditional "rescue care" approach to health care delivery, such as frequent emergency room visits and hospitalizations, and would benefit from aggressive CCTM through the health care system to ensure smooth, seamless continuity of care.
   i. The need for CCTM supports the Institute for Healthcare Improvement's Triple Aim "improving the individual experience of care, improving the health of populations, and reducing the per capita cost of care for populations" (Berwick, Nolan, & Whittington, 2008, p. 760).
B. Background for CCTM RN Model.
   1. March 1, 2010: Invitational Conference on Ambulatory Care Registered Nurse Performance Measurement (Swan, Haas, & Chow, 2010).
      a. Purpose: Formulate a research agenda and develop a strategy to study the testable components of the RN role related to care coordination and care transitions, improving outcomes, decreasing health care costs, and promoting sustainable system change.
      b. Expert participants came from the fields of nursing, public health, managed care, research, practice, and policy.
      c. Results: Framework for RNs contribution to care quality and in the context of national policies.
         (1) Recognize care in all practice settings across the health care continuum and the community, depends on an interprofessional team that significantly influences outcomes of care, and RNs are integral team members.
         (2) Build on current assets in the areas of measure endorsement, public reporting, and performance-based payment programs, and seek opportunities to 'join up' with other professional organizations.
         (3) Describe and define RNs' contribution to 'value-driven health care.'
         (4) Examine new opportunities within the Patient Protection and ACA related to the medical home and improving outcomes, decreasing health care costs, and promoting sustainable system change.
         (5) Explore a set of care coordination and care transition measures reflected in CMS rulemaking (Swan et al., 2010).
   2. March 23, 2010: ACA.
   3. Provisions of Health Care Reform relate to CCTM (Swan & Haas, 2011).
   4. April 2011: AAACN Conference Presentation on Health Care Reform.
   5. Constitutionality of ACA challenged.
   6. June 2012: Supreme Court upholds ACA.
   7. *Health Affairs* article: "A Nurse Learns Firsthand That You May Fend for Yourself after a Hospital Stay" (Swan, 2012).
   8. *Nursing Economic$* article: "Developing Ambulatory Care Registered Nurse

Chapter 1

   Competencies for Care Coordination and Transition Management" (Haas, Swan, & Haynes, 2013).
9. May 2013: Evolution of the Registered Nurse Care Coordination and Transition Management Model to Enhance Chronic Care Management, Podium Presentation, International Council of Nurses ICN International Congress, Melbourne, Australia (Haas, Swan, and Haynes).
10. January 2014: Making a Difference: RN Care Coordination and Transition Management in Ambulatory Care Presentation, Baylor Health System Interprofessional Leadership, Dallas, TX (Haas, Swan, and Haynes).
11. *Nursing Economic$* article: "Developing the Value Proposition for Registered Nurse Care Coordination and Transition Management Role in Ambulatory Care Settings" (Haas & Swan, 2014a).
12. September 2014: Development of the Care Coordination and Transition Management Model Podium Presentation, Palmer Research Symposium, Rome, Italy (Haas, Swan, and Haynes).
13. Chapter in *Care Coordination: The Game Changer* (by G. Lamb, editor): "Emerging Care Coordination Models for Achieving Quality and Safety Outcomes for Patients and Families" (Haas & Swan, 2014b).
14. April 2015: Closing the Gap: Enhancing RN Care Coordination and Transition Management for High Risk Chronic Care Populations across the Continuum, Preconference, AONE National Conference, Phoenix, AZ (Haas, Swan, and Haynes).
15. May, 2015: Using QSEN Competencies Format to Structure RN Care Coordination and Transition Management Role Expectations, Education and Performance Evaluation, Quality and Safety Education for Nurses National Forum, San Diego, CA (Haas, Swan, and Haynes).
16. July 2015: AAACN/AONE Joint Statement: The Role of the Nurse Leader in Care Coordination and Transition Management Across the Health Care Continuum.
17. August 2016: The Critical Role of Health Care Informatics in Delivery, Tracking and Evaluation of Care Coordination and Transition Management by Registered Nurses, University of Maryland School of Nursing Faculty and Hospital Nursing Staff (Haas).
18. November 2016: Care Coordination for Changing Healthcare Delivery System, International Nursing Administration Research Conference, Orlando, FL (Haas, Swan, and Haynes).
19. *Nursing Economic$* article: "Developing Staffing Models to Support Population Health Management and Quality Outcomes in Ambulatory Care Settings" (Haas, Vlasses, & Harvey, 2016).
20. May 2018: Invitational Summit on Care Coordination and Transition Management, Orlando, FL (Haas & Swan, 2019).

C. Significance of CCTM RN Model in relation to ACA.
1. Majority of provisions are related to care coordination and care transitions, as well as health promotion and disease prevention (Naylor et al., 2011).
    a. Interventions associated with these provisions are part of RNs' independent scope of practice (ANA, 2012).
    b. RNs have an essential role in the care coordination process (ANA, 2012).
2. Defined the PCMH team with RNs as team members.
3. Focused on access to primary care versus enhanced use of specialists and acute care.
4. Fostered care coordination for complex chronically ill persons in ambulatory care settings.
5. Specified the need for individualized person-centered care planning.
6. Extant models of care for chronically ill in the community are staffed by RNs working with complex chronically ill individuals, including Boult's Guided Care Model (Boult, Karm, & Groves, 2008) and Coleman's Care Transitions Model (Coleman, Parry, Chalmers, Chugh, & Mahoney, 2007).
7. Authorized the Accountable Care Organization (ACO) program be administered by a new Innovation Center at CMS.
8. In 2011, launched the *Partnerships for Patients* program to achieve two goals:
    a. Making care safer.
    b. Improving care transitions.
9. In 2013, CMS finalized transitional care management codes. Currently, these codes can be reported/billed by advanced practice nurses (APNs) but not RNs.
10. Beginning in January 2015, one provision of the ACA, the value modifier, provided differential payment based on the quality of care provided compared to cost during a defined performance period (CMS, 2013).

Chapter 1

VI. **Selected Extant Care Coordination Initiatives**

A. Patient-Aligned Care Teams (PACT) Model (True et al., 2012); United States Department of Veterans Affairs.
 1. In FY 2010, the Veterans Health Administration (VHA) began implementation of the patient-centered medical home mode of care, known today as PACT.
 2. PACT has transformed the VA Health Care system's foundational focus from acute care to primary care, utilizing a patient-centric approach across the care continuum.
 3. PACT principles are being applied to all delivery systems to include specialty care, geriatrics (Sullivan, Eisenstein, Price, Solimeo, & Shay, 2018), and academic training programs.
 4. Sustaining goals:
    a. Expand real time access to primary care through face-to-face encounters and by virtual modalities meeting the patient and caregivers' preferences and needs.
    b. Seamless coordination and transition management of care between VHA providers and community health partners.
    c. Facilitate a continuous patient-centered culture through expanded team roles within primary care practices.
    d. Expansion of the RN care manager role, assuring each nurse is practicing to his or her fullest scope (Morgan et al., 2015).
 5. Focus of the PACT model of care:
    a. Health care partnership with patient, families and/or care givers.
    b. Access to care utilizing diverse care delivery methods.
    c. Coordinated care among team members.
    d. Team-based care with the patient at the center of all PACT activities.
 6. PACT purpose:
    a. Patients work together with health care professionals to plan for their whole-person care, life-long health, and wellness.
    b. Care team considers all aspects of patient health emphasizing prevention and health promotion.
    c. Care is coordinated through communication and collaboration among team members.
    d. Team members have clearly defined roles creating trusting personal relationships, resulting in coordinated care across the life span.
       (1) PACT uses a team-based approach by building ownership of the process and incorporating improvement strategies into the teams daily practice.
       (2) The patient is at the center of the care team, which includes family and/or caregivers and health care professionals (a primary care provider, nurse care manager, licensed practical/vocational nurse or health technician, and advanced medical support assistant).
       (3) The PACT coordinates all health care services required to meet the patient's health goals, preferences, and needs.
 7. Implementation of the PACT model:
    a. Fundamental change is required in the organization of care within the primary care unit moving from individual providers to interprofessional teams.
    b. Standardized team-based clinical education resulting in a transformative interprofessional health care delivery system (Harada et al., 2018).
       (1) VA PACT University established to provide on demand online education that engages PACT members in professional development. Patient-centered medical home principles are taught to all primary care staff, including leadership at all levels.
       (2) Evidence-based practice is supported through the formation of facility-approved care team protocols.
    c. PACT compass:
       (1) The compass is a series of metric indicators reflective of the principles and dimensions of PACT.
       (2) The metrics are based on the assignment of patients to a team and provider through the Primary Care Management Module (PCMM).
       (3) The compass provides staff, managers, and leadership statistical data on:

(a) PCMM.
(b) Utilization of non-traditional care modalities.
(c) Access to care.
(d) Continuity of care.
(e) Coordination of care.
(f) Quality indicators.
  d. Decision support tools are accessible within the electronic medical record and are focused on ambulatory care sensitive conditions (ACSC), which aid in team-based care planning and care coordination for optimum patient outcomes. The following are a few examples:
  (1) Primary Care Almanac (PCA) provides real-time access to health data across the care continuum that can be drilled down to individual PACT panels that are utilized to guide specific patient care strategies and population health management.
  (2) The Care Assessment Needs (CAN) Score utilizes predictive analytics and data from various sources, including VHA's electronic health record, the Computerized Patient Record System (CPRS), to identify patients at the highest risk for negative health outcomes.
  (3) Patient Care Access System (PCAS) is a care coordination tool used in managing the identified high-risk patients.
 8. Benchmarking for the future:
  a. Bidassie (2017) notes that the VHA PACT Model provides innovative examples, resources, and tools to aid and inspire health care teams to develop systematic approaches to data-driven decision-making in the transformation of quality health care delivery and should be considered when benchmarking for future PCMH model planning.

VII. Methodology for CCTM RN Model for Nursing Adapted from Information Published in *Nursing Economic$* (Haas, Swan, & Haynes, 2013)

A. Developing the RN competencies for CCTM required:
 1. Expertise of nurse leaders across all practice settings and the community.
 2. Cost-effective, expeditious approach to bring leaders together.
 3. Opportunities to dialogue and build on each individual leader's knowledge, skills, and experience.
 4. Evidentiary Review completed by Expert Panel 1.
  a. Members represented practice and education, along with public, private, military, and veterans' organizations.
  b. Fifteen states in east, west, north, south, and central United States and the District of Columbia.
  c. Following a search in MEDLINE, CINAHL Plus, and PsycINFO, 82 journal articles plus white papers available online from major organizations were selected for review. Expert Panel 1 worked in dyads and reviewed four to five articles, then abstracted data to a table of evidence, concluding their work in February 2012. A second literature search was completed in the summer of 2013. An additional 58 articles were reviewed and abstracted following the same methodology by members of the Expert Panel, and then added to the existing table of evidence.
  d. The 26-member panel worked in dyads and abstracted data to a table of evidence, including:
   (1) Authors of study column.
   (2) Study title column.
   (3) Research questions column.
   (4) Research design type column.
   (5) Setting and sample, inclusion/exclusion criteria column.
   (6) Methods, intervention and/or instruments.
   (7) Analyses column.
   (8) Key findings column.
   (9) Recommendations column.
   (10) Column listing dimension or dimensions identified with activity or activities that are supporting and/or contributing to CCTM.
 5. Use of data summary techniques to capture and share outcomes achieved by each Expert Panel.
 6. Focus group methods.
  a. Defined as a method of bringing together people from similar backgrounds or experiences to discuss a specific topic, guided by a facilitator who elicits responses from the group but does not influence responses.

b. For this project, Focus Group Method and online time was used to:
   (1) Clarify methods and outcome expectations.
   (2) Discuss issues with evidence evaluation, such as ambiguities and contradictions in evidence.
   (3) Absence of sufficient description in evidence materials.
   (4) Sharing of concerns.
   (5) Sharing of insights and expertise.

B. Identifying dimensions of CCTM.
   1. Defining dimensions.
      a. In the literature on care coordination, often, activities that are part of care coordination are listed, such as developing a plan of care or monitoring progression of established goals.
      b. These activities fit together within a broader construct or dimension, such as planning.
      c. When developing a role that reflects all major dimensions or constructs that make up the role, use of dimensions allows for the addition or subtraction of relevant activities under each dimension as the role evolves.
   2. Dimensions identified and defined by Expert Panel 2.
      a. This 16-member panel was charged with:
         (1) Defining the dimensions, identifying core competencies.
         (2) Describing activities linked with each competency for CCTM in settings across the continuum.
         (3) Using focus group methods online, the expert panel identified nine person-centered care dimensions and associated activities of CCTM.
      b. Nine evidence-based dimensions.
         (1) Support for self-management.
         (2) Education and engagement of patient and family.
         (3) Cross-setting communication and transition.
         (4) Coaching and counseling of patients and families.
         (5) Nursing process, including assessment, plan, implementation/intervention, and evaluation; a proxy for monitoring and intervening.
         (6) Teamwork and collaboration.
         (7) Patient-centered care planning.
         (8) Decision support and information systems.
         (9) Advocacy.
      c. The evidence-based dimensions and activities were validated using informal focus groups at the 2012 AAACN Annual Conference.
   3. Preliminary competencies identified by Expert Panel 2 using the Quality and Safety in Education in Nursing (QSEN) framework (Cronenwett et al., 2007) are:
      a. Knowledge.
      b. Skills.
      c. Attitudes.
   4. Work was also guided by Wagner's Chronic Care Model (Wagner, 1998) (see Figure 1-1).

C. Developing competencies for CCTM.
   1. Once dimensions were discovered in the translational research project, the named dimension became the competency. The original *CCTM Core Curriculum* is a first edition, and the implementation of the CCTM RN is a new role; therefore, the definition of each competency of the first page of each chapter offers several definitions of the competency taken from the evidence discovered in the literature. Users (organizations) are free to use the definitions offered to create a more abbreviated definition that is consonant with their setting and population served.
   2. Specify education and evaluation needed for successful practice within each dimension of the role.
   3. In 2003, the IOM's Health Professions Education Report recommended educators provide learning experiences so graduates were prepared to provide patient-centered care as collaborating members of an interprofessional team using evidence-based practice, quality improvement methods, and informatics. This was a stimulus for development of the QSEN initiative (Cronenwett et al., 2007). The six QSEN competencies, as well as their Knowledge, Skills, and Attitudes (KSA) tables of expected behaviors, have been embraced by nursing undergraduate and graduate educators. Of note is the QSEN specification of attitudes instead of abilities and judgment that were specified in the preliminary position statement (ANA, 2008). Attitudes are extremely relevant in specification of quality and safety competencies, and behavior or performance expectations. Often, health care provider attitudes override knowledge and skills expectations of performance. A

**Figure 1-1.
The Chronic Care Model**

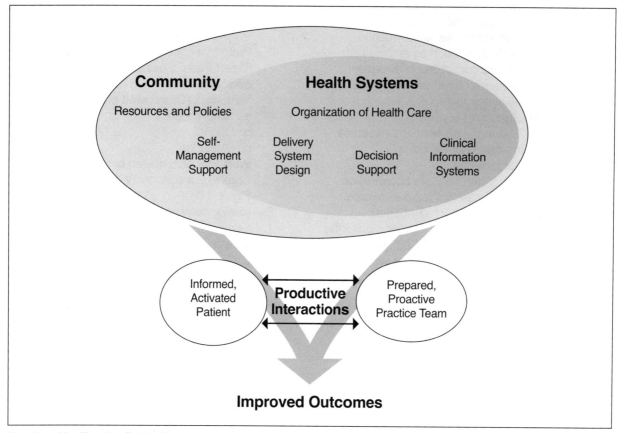

Developed by The MacColl Institute.
® ACP-ASIM Journals and Books. Reprinted with permission.

good example of this is hand hygiene. Providers have extensive knowledge of rationale for hand washing and skills to do it, but often, do not practice hand hygiene, letting attitudes about emergent needs take precedence. That is why hand hygiene compliance is about 60% in health care.
4. The QSEN format (Cronenwett et al., 2007) was used to identify KSA behavior for each CCTM competency or dimension.
D. Verifying dimensions and competencies.
1. In August 2012, using focus group methods online, Expert Panel 3 reviewed, confirmed, and created a table of dimensions, activities, and competencies, including knowledge, skills, and attitudes for the CCTM RN.
2. After much discussion, Expert Panel 3 determined the original 8th dimension of decision support and information systems, as well as telehealth practice, were technologies that support all dimensions.
3. Population health management became the new 8th dimension given the prominence it is assuming in outpatient care, even though there was little discussion of it in the literature reviewed.
4. Expert Panel 3 also determined methods to be used to enhance teamwork and interprofessional collaboration in outpatient settings.
5. Nationally recognized core competencies for interprofessional collaborative practice, QSEN competencies, and public health nursing competencies overlap with the dimensions and competencies needed for the CCTM RN (see Table 1-1 on p. 13).
E. Expert Panel 4 was convened in Summer 2013. This panel was charged with writing the *CCTM Core Curriculum*. Names of panelists are in the contributor list in the beginning of this text.

VIII. Logic Model

As we prepared to work with the expert panelists who were writing chapters for the *CCTM Core Curriculum*, we developed a Logic Model to guide the organization of the chapters to identify not only activities, but also processes and outcomes involved in each dimension. We knew from analyzing other care coordination and transition models that the main outcomes identified were emergency room visits and hospital readmission rates. When other quality-of-life outcomes were reported, there was a great variety of outcomes specified, but often, there was no distinction as to whether they were short-, medium-, or long-term outcomes. We decided to try to plot the CCTM Model within a logic model as illustrated in Appendix 1-1.

IX. **Mechanics**

A. This second edition of the CCTM text has been enhanced with the addition of content. When the first edition was published, AAACN was developing its *Scope and Standards of Practice for Registered Nurses in Care Coordination and Transition Management*. The relevant *Scope and Standards* (2016) are now integrated in each chapter of the second edition of the *CCTM Core Curriculum*. To prepare for the second edition of the *CCTM Core Curriculum* text, two surveys were developed and sent to purchasers of the first edition of the *CCTM Core Curriculum*. Based on survey responses and our review of health care issues and challenges over the past 4 years, multiple content areas were added or enhanced. First, pediatric and geriatric content were added to chapters where appropriate. Behavioral health, dementia care, opioid addiction, palliative and end-of-life care, health literacy, and social determinant content were also added to appropriate chapters. Case studies and care plans have been added and are designed to provide scenarios depicting the use of evidence within activities in each dimension and to assist in understanding how the dimensions and competencies pertain (relate) to practice. Chapter 11 includes examples using the Society of Hospital Medicine's Project BOOST tools. Additionally, content and a glossary listing "Apps" that can assist with practice in many of the dimensions have been added.

B. Throughout the text of the *Core*, you will see the Care Coordination Transition Management Registered Nurse (CCTM® RN) written as it refers to the RN practicing in the role of CCTM. It also indicates this role is one in which RNs in any setting have within their scope of practice. If the RN has the certification credential, they will use CCCTM® in their title. In addition, you will see the use of the terms *individual* and *person* rather than *patient*, changing the paradigm from caring for patients to caring for people.

C. Content in the *CCTM Core Curriculum* is presented in outline format for easy review and reference. Key terms defined in the text are captured in the Glossary. Resources and published references are identified throughout the text and at the end of chapters for further information. It is important to realize this content captured the best evidence and information available at a point in time, and the reader is encouraged to seek current sources of information as new research and evidence on CCTM are being published.

D. Organization of each chapter.
 1. Learning outcome statement: Broad outcome statement or goal that summarizes the specific topic and aim of the chapter.
 2. Learning objectives: Brief, clear statements that describe what the reader is expected to achieve as a result of reading the chapter.
 3. Competency definition for the chapter using evidence from literature reviewed and enhanced where necessary by expert opinion.
 4. A listing of the *Scope and Standards of Practice for Registered Nurses in Care Coordination and Transition Management* (2016) included in the text.
 5. Brief introduction to the competency.
 6. Content outline for the competency.
 7. Competencies: Sets of knowledge, skills, and attitudes that enable a nurse to perform in a specific role, such as the CCTM RN.
 8. Finalized list of knowledge, skills, and attitudes for each competency modeled after the QSEN (Cronenwett et al., 2007) entry/pre-licensure competencies.
 9. Nationally recognized core competencies for interprofessional collaborative practice (Interprofessional Education Collaborative, 2016), QSEN competencies (Cronenwett et al., 2007), and public health nursing competencies (Quad Council Coalition of the Public Health Nursing Organizations, 2018) overlap with the dimensions and competencies needed for the CCTM RN.
 10. Suggested process and outcome indicators for competencies where available.

X. **Contents**

A. The majority of the book is composed of nine chapters listed below, one for each evidence-based dimension, written by nurse experts. This

Chapter 1

compilation is the work of many nurse leaders representing practice, education, and research across all settings and the community. The authors would like to acknowledge the collaboration with the leadership from the Academy of Medical-Surgical Nurses (AMSN) on the four Expert Panels.
1. Advocacy.
2. Education and Engagement of Individuals and Families.
3. Coaching and Counseling of Individuals and Families.
4. Person-Centered Care Planning.
5. Support for Self-Management.
6. Nursing Process (Proxy for Monitoring and Evaluation).
7. Teamwork and Collaboration.
8. Cross Setting Communications and Care Transitions.
9. Population Health Management.

B. One chapter is dedicated to the transition from acute care to ambulatory care and the critical nature of hand-offs in ensuring safety and quality of care.

C. Two chapters are devoted to technologies that provide decision support and information systems for all dimensions of care coordination and transition management.
1. Informatics Competencies to Support Nursing Practice.
2. Telehealth Nursing Practice.

XI. Who Will Benefit from This Book?

This text is written for you, the RN – whether you are a nurse working in ambulatory care, in a hospital, an extended care facility, an individual's home, or a community setting; are a student nurse, a nurse educator, or a nurse who functions in any of the other diverse places where nurses are coordinating care and managing transitions. Whatever your role, you will find this groundbreaking new and now updated text a source for development of knowledge, skills, and attitudes to competently provide care coordination and transition management for individuals and families no matter what setting you work in or are preparing to work in. It will be useful to both RNs and students aspiring to become licensed as an RN. It is also a reference book and indispensable guide to the state of research evidence for CCTM. Finally, it is designed to be a source to enrich understanding of dimensions, activities, knowledge, skills, and attitudes requisite to sit for the CCCTM Certification Exam.

XII. How Can I Use This Book?

This core resource on CCTM is ideal for:
A. Orienting nurses transitioning into ambulatory care settings as well as acute, subacute, and home care across the continuum about CCTM.
B. Orienting existing nursing staff in any settings about CCTM.
C. Orienting nurses' transition into the RN care coordination and transition management role.
D. Developing competencies, standards, policies, and procedures.
E. Developing position descriptions for nurses in CCTM RN roles in any practice setting across the health care continuum and community.
F. Revising performance appraisal instruments for nurses in any practice setting along the health care continuum and community CCTM RN roles.
G. Enhancing educational materials/programs for nurses in CCTM RN roles.
H. Identifying CCTM RN structure and process activities that contribute to quality outcomes.
I. Enhancing outcomes of high-risk individuals in a pay-for-performance environment and complex care programs.
J. Delineating the value proposition of the CCTM RN in the context of interprofessional team-based care.
K. Expanding/enhancing the use of evidence-based longitudinal care planning by CCTM RNs for individuals across providers of care and settings of care.
L. Developing, implementing, and evaluating quality improvement projects in your organizations around the implementation of CCTM RN Model dimensions.
M. Developing and implementing evidence-based projects and research projects guided by the CCTM RN Model dimensions.
N. Planning and implementing action plans to meet the new Magnet® standards related to ambulatory care.

Chapter 1

Table 1-1.
Crosswalk of Dimensions for Care Coordination and Transition Management (CCTM®) with Core Competencies of Other Organizations

Dimension RN Care Coordinator and Transition Manager (CCTM RN)	Quality and Safety Education for Nurses (QSEN) Core Competencies	Interprofessional Education Collaborative Core Competencies (2016)	Public Health Nursing Competencies (2018)
Support Self-Management	Person-Centered Care		
Education and Engagement of Individual and Family	Person-Centered Care		
Cross Setting Communication and Transition	Person-Centered Care	Interprofessional Communication	Domain #3: Communication Skills
Coaching and Counseling of Individuals and Families	Person-Centered Care		Domain #4: Cultural Competency Skills
Nursing Process: Assessment, Plan, Intervention, Evaluation	Evidence-Based Practice Quality Improvement	Roles and Responsibilities	Domain #1: Assessment and Analytic Skills
Teamwork and Collaboration	Teamwork and Collaboration	Teams and Teamwork	Domain #8: Leadership and Systems Thinking Skills
Person-Centered Planning	Person-Centered Care	Values/Ethics for Interprofessional Practice	Domain #1: Assessment and Analytic Skills
Population Health Management	Quality Improvement Informatics		Domain #5: Community Dimensions of Practice Skills Domain #6: Public Health Sciences Skills
Advocacy	Person-Centered Care Safety	Values/Ethics for Interprofessional Practice	Domain #2: Policy Development/ Program Planning Skills

Source: Haas, Swan, & Haynes, 2013; Updated 2018.

Chapter 1

Appendix 1-1.
Program: The CCTM® RN Model Logic Model

Situation: The Care Coordination Transition Management – Registered (CCTM® RN) Nurse Model evolved to standardize work of all registered nurses using evidence from nursing and interprofessional literature on care coordination and transition management. The CCTM RN Model specifies dimensions of CCTM and associated competencies – knowledge, skills, and attitudes – essential for the CCTM RN to meet the needs of individuals and families across the continuum of care. The preparation and work as a CCTM RN is recognized with the CCCTM credential from the Medical-Surgical Nursing Certification Board (MSNCB).

Inputs/Competencies	Activities	Outputs – Participation	Outcomes – Short	Outcomes – Medium	Outcomes – Long
Support for Self-Management	Enhance health literacy	CCTM RN, MD, APRN, pharmacist, social worker	Baseline comprehensive needs assessment reflects individual values, preferences, goals	Solutions to most critical socioeconomic issues	Engaged, educated individual/family, increased ability to "cope" with care interventions
Advocacy	Negotiate and secure individual services; coach person in self advocacy	CCTM RN, MD, APRN, pharmacist, social worker	Individual/family concerns and goals heard, able to access providers, community services, medications	Individual/family compliance with treatment plan, medications	Keep primary care appointments, appointments in community agencies
Education and Engagement of Individual and Family	Assess readiness to learn/learning styles	CCTM RN, pharmacist, social worker, dietician, psychologist	Individual/family can "teach back" info on care interventions	Increased engagement in preventative care and use of telehealth learning modalities	Engaged, educated individual/family
Cross Setting Communication and Transition	Coordination/collaboration between specialty and primary providers who develop and share the Individual Care Plan across settings	CCTM RN, MD, APRN, pharmacist, social worker, dietician, psychologist, MD specialists, acute care, long-term care and home care RN	Care Plan transmitted between setting, changes and updates communicated	Use of electronic Individual Care Plan for handoffs	Decreased errors, duplication, decreased costs

continued on next page

Care Coordination *and* Transition Management *Core Curriculum* – 2nd Edition – 2019

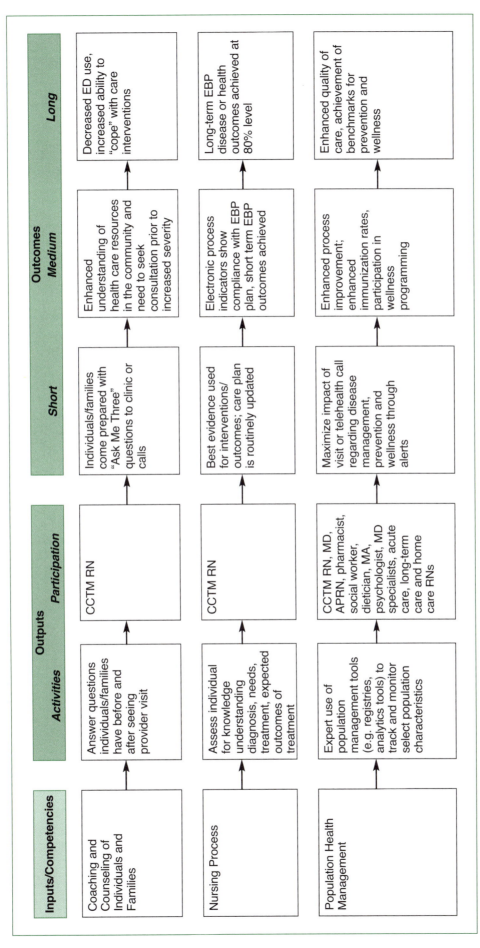

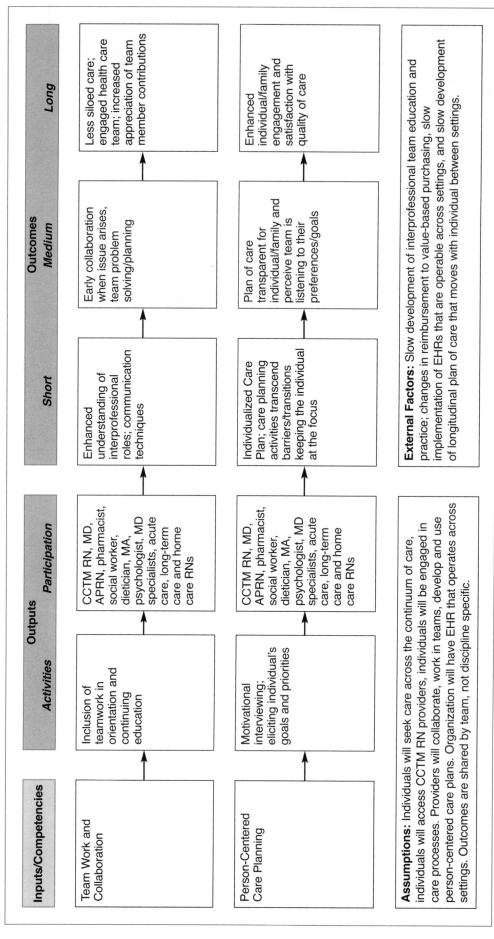

Appendix 1-1. (continued)
Program: The CCTM® RN Model Logic Model

Chapter 1

References

Agency for Healthcare Research and Quality (AHRQ). (2010). *Care coordination measures atlas* [AHRQ Publication No. 11-0023-EF]. Rockville, MD: Author. Retrieved from https://pcmh.ahrq.gov/sites/default/files/attachments/Care%20Coordination%20Measures%20Atlas.pdf

Altman, S.H., Butler, A.S., & Shern, L. (Eds.). (2015). *Assessing progress on the IOM report: The future of nursing.* Retrieved from http://www.nationalacademies.org/hmd/Reports/2015/Assessing-Progress-on-the-IOM-Report-The-Future-of-Nursing.aspx

American Academy of Nursing (AAN). (2012). *The imperative of patient, family, and population centered interprofessional approaches to care coordination and transitional care: Policy brief.* Washington, DC: Author.

American Association of Colleges of Nursing (AACN). (2018). *Vision for nursing education.* Washington, DC: Author.

American Nurses Association (ANA). (2008). *Position statement on competence and competency.* Silver Spring, MD: Author.

American Nurses Association (ANA). (2012). *Care coordination and registered nurses' essential role: Position statement.* Silver Spring, MD: Author.

Berwick, D.M., Nolan, T.W., & Whittington, J. (2008). The triple aim: Care, health, and cost. *Health Affairs, 27*(3), 759-769.

Bidassie, B. (2017). The Veterans Affairs Patient Aligned Care Team (VA PACT), a new benchmark for patient-centered medical home models: A review and discussion. In O. Sayligil (Ed.), *Patient-centered medicine* (pp. 139-160). doi:10.5772/66415

Boult, C., Karm, L., & Groves, C. (2008). Improving chronic care: The "guided care" model. *The Permanente Journal, 12*(1), 50-54.

Centers for Disease Control and Prevention (CDC). (2018). *Chronic disease prevention and health promotion.* Retrieved from https://www.cdc.gov/nccdphp/dch/pdfs/00-making-life-easier-nidcdp.pdf

Centers for Medicare & Medicaid Services (CMS). (2013). *Summary of 2015 physicians' value-based payment modifier policies.* Baltimore, MD: Author. Retrieved from https://www.cms.gov/Medicare/Medicare-Fee-for-Service-Payment/PhysicianFeedbackProgram/Downloads/CY2015ValueModifierPolicies.pdf

Coleman, E.A., & Boult, C. (2003). Improving the quality of transitional care for persons with complex care needs. *Journal of the American Geriatrics Society, 51*(4), 556-557.

Coleman, E.A., Parry, C., Chalmers, S.A., Chugh, A., & Mahoney, E. (2007). The central role of performance measurement in improving the quality of transitional care. *Home Health Care Services Quarterly, 26*(4), 93-104.

Commission for Case Manager Certification. (2018). *Definition and philosophy of case management.* Retrieved from https://ccmcertification.org/about-ccmc/about-case-management/definition-and-philosophy-case-management

Craig, C., Eby, D., & Whittington, J. (2011). *Care coordination model: Better care at lower costs for people with multiple health and social needs.* Cambridge, MA: Institute for Healthcare Improvement. Retrieved from http://www.ihi.org/resources/Pages/IHIWhitePapers/IHICareCoordinationModelWhitePaper.aspx

Cronenwett, L., Sherwood, G., Barnsteiner, J., Disch, J., Johnson, J., Mitchell, P., ... Warren, J. (2007). Quality and safety education for nurses. *Nursing Outlook, 55*(3), 122-131.

Haas, S., Swan, B.A., & Haynes, T.S. (2013). Developing ambulatory care registered nurse competencies for care coordination and transition management. *Nursing Economic$, 31*(1), 44-49, 43.

Haas, S., Swan, B.A., & Haynes, T.S. (Eds.) (2014). *Care coordination and transition management core curriculum.* Pitman, NJ: American Academy of Ambulatory Care Nursing.

Haas, S.A., & Swan, B.A. (2014a). Developing the value proposition for registered nurse care coordination and transition management role in ambulatory care settings. *Nursing Economic$, 32*(2), 70-79.

Haas, S., & Swan, B.A. (2014b). Emerging care coordination models for achieving quality and safety outcomes for patients and families. In G. Lamb (Ed.), *Care coordination: The game changer.* Washington, DC: American Nurses Association.

Haas, S.A., Vlasses, F., & Harvey, J. (2016). Developing staffing models to support population health management and quality outcomes in ambulatory care settings *Nursing Economic$, 34*(2), 126-133.

Harada, N.D., Traylor, L., Rugen, K.W., Bowen, J.L., Smith, C.S., Felker, B., ... Gilman, S.C. (2018). Interprofessional transformation of clinical education: The first six years of the Veterans Affairs Centers of Excellence in Primary Care Education. *Journal of Interprofessional Care.* doi:10.1080/13561820.2018.1433642

Humowiecki, M., Kuruna, T., Sax, R., Hawthorne, M., Hamblin, A., Turner, S., ... Cullen, K. (2018). *Blueprint for complex care: Advancing the field of care for individuals with complex health and social needs.* Chicago, IL: National Center for Complex Care and Social Needs.

Institute of Medicine. (IOM). (2010). *The future of nursing: Leading change, advancing health* (1st ed.). Washington, DC: National Academies Press.

Interprofessional Education Collaborative. (2016). *Core competencies for interprofessional collaborative practice.* Washington, DC: American Association of Colleges of Nursing.

Kangovi, S., Barg, F.K., Carter, T., Long, J.A., Shannon, R., & Grande, D. (2013). Understanding why patients of low socioeconomic status prefer hospitals over ambulatory care. *Health Affairs, 32*(7), 1196-1203.

Lobelo, F., Trotter, P., & Heather, A.J. (2016). *Chronic disease is healthcare's rising risk [white paper].* Retrieved from http://www.exerciseismedicine.org/assets/page_documents/Whitepaper%20Final%20for%20Publishing%20(002)%20Chronic%20diseases.pdf

McDonald, K.M., Schultz, E.S., Albin, L., Pineda, N., Lonhart, J., Sundaram, V., ... Malcolm, E. (2011). *Care coordination measures atlas* [AHRQ Publication No.11-0023-EF]. Rockville, MD: Agency for Healthcare Research and Quality. Retrieved from https://pcmh.ahrq.gov/sites/default/files/attachments/Care%20Coordination%20Measures%20Atlas.pdf

McDonald, K., Sundaram, V., Bravata, D., Lewis, R., Lin, N., Kraft, S.A. ... Owens, D.K. (2007). Care coordination. In K. Shojania, K. McDonald, R. Wachter, & D. Owens (Eds.), *Closing the quality gap: A critical analysis of quality improvement strategies* [AHRQ Publication No. 04(07)-0051-7]. Rockville, MD: Agency for Healthcare Research and Quality. Retrieved from https://www.ahrq.gov/downloads/pub/evidence/pdf/caregap/caregap.pdf

Morgan, S., Vogel, D.C., Hryznk Lind, P., Shear, J.M., Smith, A., Richardson, J., & Bethel, M. (2015). Expanding the primary care RN case manager and RN case manager roles in VA care program. In C. Rick & P. Beck Kritek (Ed.), *Realizing the future of nursing: VA nurses tell their story* (pp. 165-211). Washington, DC: United States Department of Veterans Affairs.

National Quality Forum (NQF). (2010). *Preferred practices and performance measures for measuring and reporting care coordination: A consensus report.* Washington, DC: Author.

National Quality Forum (NQF). (2016). *Looking back to plan ahead* [NQF Care Coordination Standing Committee Quarterly Off-Cycle Webinar]. Washington, DC: Author.

Naylor, M.D., Aiken, L.H., Kurtzman, E.T., Olds, D.M., & Hirschman, K.B. (2011). The importance of transitional care in achieving health reform. *Health Affairs, 30*(4), 746-754. Retrieved from https://www.healthaffairs.org/doi/10.1377/hlthaff.2011.0041

Naylor, M., & Sochalski, J. (2010). Scaling up: Bringing the transitional care model into the mainstream. *Issue Brief (Commonwealth Fund), 103,* 1-11.

Oncology Nursing Society (ONS). (2017). *2017 oncology nurse navigator core competencies.* Retrieved from https://www.ons.org/sites/default/files/2017-05/2017_Oncology_Nurse_Navigator_Competencies.pdf

Patient Protection and Affordable Care Act. (2010). Public Law 111-1148, §2702, 124 Stat. 119, 318-319.

Quad Council Coalition of the Public Health Nursing Organizations. (2018). *Community/public health nursing [C/PHN] competencies.* Retrieved from http://www.quadcouncilphn.org/documents-3/2018-qcc-competencies/

Sullivan, J.L., Eisenstein, R., Price, T., Solimeo, S., & Shay, K. (2018). Implementation of the geriatric patient-aligned care team model in the Veterans Health Administration (VA). *Journal of the American Board of Family Medicine. 31*(3), 456-465.

Swan, B.A. (2012). A nurse learns firsthand that you may fend for yourself after a hospital stay. *Health Affairs, 31*(11), 2579-2582.

Swan, B.A., & Haas, S. (2011). Health care reform: Current updates and future initiatives for ambulatory care nursing. *Nursing Economic$, 29*(6), 331-334.

Swan, B.A., Haas, S., & Chow, M. (2010). Ambulatory care registered nurse performance measurement. *Nursing Economic$, 28*(5), 337-339, 342.

Thorpe, K.E. (2013). Treated disease prevalence and spending per treated case drove most of the growth in health care spending in 1987-2009. *Health Affairs, 32*(5), 851-858.

True, G., Butler, A.E., Lamparska, B.G., Lempa, M.L., Shea, J.A., Asch, D.A., & Werner, R.M. (2012). Open access in the patient-centered medical home: Lessons learned from the Veterans Health Administration. *Journal of General Internal Medicine, 28*(4), 539-545.

Wagner, E.H. (1998). Chronic disease management: What will it take to improve care for chronic illness? *Effective Clinical Practice, 1*(1), 2-4.

Additional Reading

American Nurses Association (ANA). (2012b). *The value of nursing care coordination [White paper].* Silver Spring, MD: Author.

American Nurses Association (ANA). (2013). *Framework for measuring nurses' contributions to care coordination.* Silver Spring, MD: Author.

Cipriano, P.F., Bowles, K., Dailey, M., Dykes, P., Lamb, G., & Naylor, M. (2013). The importance of health information technology in care coordination and transitional care. *Nursing Outlook, 61*(6), 475-489.

Haas, S., & Swan, B.A. (2014). Care coordination models for achieving quality and safety outcomes for patients and families. In G. Lamb (Ed.), *Care coordination: The game changer – How nursing is revolutionizing quality care.* Silver Spring, MD: American Nurses Association.

Institute of Medicine (IOM). (2003). *Health professions education: A bridge to quality.* Washington, DC: National Academies Press.

Lamb, G. (Ed.). (2014). *Care coordination: The game changer – How nursing is revolutionizing quality care.* Silver Spring, MD: American Nurses Association.

Lamb, G., & Newhouse, R. (2018) *Care coordination: A blueprint for action for RNs.* Silver Spring, MD: American Nurses Association.

Lampman, L., Solimeo, S.L., Stewart, G., & Stockdale, S.E. (2017). Enhancing PACT implementation through qualitative research. *FORUM: Translating Research Into Quality Health Care for Veterans, Spring,* 5.

Naylor, M.D. (2000). A decade of transitional care research with vulnerable elders. *Journal of Cardiovascular Nursing, 14*(3), 1-14.

Stewart, K.R., Stewart, G.L., Lampman, M., Wakefield, B., Rosenthal, G., & Solimeo, S.L. (2015). Implications of the patient centered medical home for nursing practice. *Journal of Nursing Administration, 45*(11), 569-574.

United States Department of Veteran Affairs. (n.d.). *What is PACT?* Retrieved from https://www.visn4.va.gov/VISN4/CEPACT/pact.asp

Chapter 2

Instructions for Continuing Nursing Education Contact Hours
Continuing nursing education credit can be earned for completing the learning activity associated with this chapter. Instructions can be found at aaacn.org/CCTMCoreCNE

Advocacy

Mary Hines Vinson, DNP, RN-BC
William Duffy, RN, MJ, CNOR, FAAN

Learning Outcome Statement

After completing this learning activity, the learner will be able to define and describe the dimension of advocacy as an important element of the Care Coordination and Transition Management (CCTM®) model.

Learning Objectives

After reading this chapter, the CCTM registered nurse (RN) will be able to:
- Demonstrate person advocacy in all CCTM activities.
- Describe the application of professional practice standards to the CCTM role.
- Discuss the concept of person advocacy as it relates to ethical principles in nursing.
- Describe a plan of care developed in collaboration with the individual and family that reflects advocacy needs, interventions, and outcomes.
- Explain the importance of addressing behavioral and mental health needs of individuals, families, and populations.
- Discuss how social determinants of health impact the overall wellbeing of individuals, families, and communities.
- Describe the effects of health literacy on the health of individuals, families, communities, and populations.
- Discuss the importance of advocacy in the care of children.
- Discuss the importance of CCTM nurses' participation in organizational and public policy formation.
- Describe ways in which nurses can practice advocacy by working to influence policy development at the organizational, local, regional, state, or national level on behalf of individuals, families, and the profession of nursing.
- Describe leadership behaviors related to CCTM.
- Demonstrate the knowledge, skills, and attitudes required for the advocacy dimension (see Table 2-1 on page 43).

AAACN Care Coordination and Transition Management Standards

Standard 1. Assessment
Standard 3. Outcomes Identification
Standard 4. Planning
Standard 5. Implementation
Standard 5a. Care Coordination
Standard 5b. Health Teaching and Health Promotion
Standard 6. Evaluation
Standard 7. Ethics
Standard 8. Education
Standard 9. Research and Evidence-Based Practice
Standard 10. Performance Improvement
Standard 11. Communication
Standard 12. Leadership
Standard 13. Collaboration
Standard 15. Resource Utilization
Standard 16. Environment

Source: AAACN, 2016.

Competency Definition

Advocacy in nursing practice is a process that involves a series of strategies and actions for preserving, representing, and/or safeguarding the best interests and values of individuals, families, and populations within the health care system (Bu & Jezewski, 2007; Water, Ford, Spence, & Rasmussen, 2016).

Systems level advocacy in nursing refers to nurses' actions that promote health broadly at a systems level by remaining focused on the context of the health care delivery system and policymaking at the organizational, local, state, and national levels (Water et al., 2016).

Chapter 2

Medical science, technology, and the U.S. health care system have evolved rapidly over the past decade. This has brought continuous change in health care delivery systems and the policies that support them. Today's health care involves multiple disciplines and rapid turnover, which often leaves individuals and families moving between services, providers, specialties, departments, and locations, while having only brief contact with a number and range of health care professionals. Despite good intentions, health-related services may be fragmented and information difficult to access and understand, resulting in confusion and difficulty making decisions (Choi, 2015). These factors have led to the critical need for care coordination by registered nurses (RNs) working within interprofessional teams to assist individuals, families, and populations in negotiating and navigating health care systems. Although the importance of advocacy in nursing practice is widely recognized, the concept is not universally defined, nor are the processes, strategies, or activities that compose its framework (Bu & Jezewski, 2007). At the individual and family level, there is agreement that humanistic relationships between the nurse and the individual/family are the foundation for integrating advocacy into practice (Choi, 2015; Water et al., 2016). *The Code of Ethics for Nurses with Interpretive Statements* (American Nurses Association [ANA], 2015) delineates the role of advocacy at the individual, organizational, and system levels. To practice effectively, nurses in care coordination and transition management (CCTM®) require an understanding of the meaning and importance of advocacy in professional nursing practice. This chapter will focus on the dimension of advocacy as it relates to the CCTM RN model. In addition, the chapter includes an in-depth discussion of several areas of health care closely related to and affected by the practice of advocacy, including behavioral/mental health, social determinants of health, and health literacy.

I. Advocacy in Nursing Practice

Nursing theorists have continued to work toward a common description of advocacy in nursing practice. Bu and Jezewski (2007) summarized the evidence related to nursing advocacy published between 1974 and 2006 (Bu & Jezewski, 2007).

A. Three core attributes of the concept of advocacy were identified.
  1. Assuring individual autonomy and self-determination.
  2. Acting on behalf of individuals.
  3. Championing social justice in health care.

B. Antecedents of advocacy in health care are described by the context (level) of care in which they occur.
  1. Microsocial level. Refers to advocacy directed toward individuals, families, or groups. Antecedents of advocacy at this level include:
     a. Vulnerability. Refers to individuals or groups who are unable to protect their own needs and rights or to make decisions due to:
        (1) Language or literacy issues.
        (2) Learning disabilities.
        (3) Socioeconomic status.
        (4) Minority status.
        (5) Conditions.
           (a) Unconsciousness.
           (b) Mental illness.
           (c) Advanced disease processes.
     b. Lack of confidence in health-related decision-making, which creates a need for nursing intervention in support of the individual right of self-determination.
  2. Macrosocial level. Refers to advocacy directed toward a population, organization, or society in general. Antecedents of advocacy at the macro level include:
     a. Health disparities related to:
        (1) Minority populations.
        (2) Socioeconomic status.
     b. Complexity of health care system, including:
        (1) Advanced technology.
        (2) Health care costs.
        (3) Complexity of changing health care policies.
     c. Contributing societal factors, including:
        (1) Access to health care services.
        (2) Poverty.
        (3) Cultural barriers.
        (4) Racism.
        (5) Health literacy.
C. Outcomes evaluation of advocacy (Choi, 2015).
  1. At the microsocial level, positive outcomes of advocacy suggest the rights, values, well-being, and best interests of individuals and families have been upheld through the advocacy practices of the nurse.
     a. Individuals and families receive adequate information.
     b. Health care professionals with specific expertise are involved directly.
     c. Views of the individual/family are accurately relayed to the health care team.
     d. Individuals' rights to decision-making are respected.

Chapter 2

Figure 2-1.
Advocacy

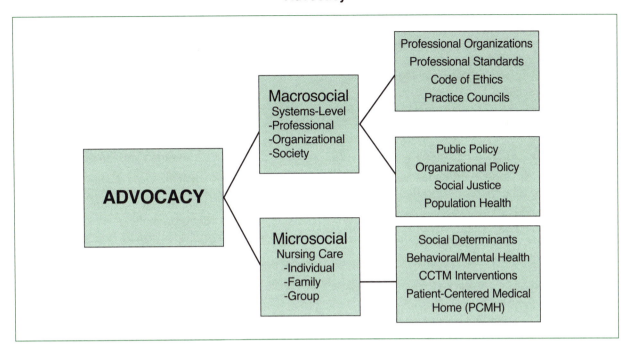

2. At the macrosocial level, positive outcomes suggest advocacy practices of nurses have resulted in desirable changes in health care policies and well-being of the organization, community, society, and the nursing profession.
   a. Improvement in access to services.
   b. Measureable improvements in population health.
   c. Enhanced public image of nurses.
   d. Increased satisfaction and autonomy of nurses (see Figure 2-1).

II. Ethics in CCTM Nursing

Because nursing exists to offer care and support to society at varying levels, ethical issues and questions are an inherent element of the profession. CCTM RNs are in a unique position of influence by virtue of their roles as caregivers and advocates. CCTM RNs often form close relationships with individuals, families, and communities, and therefore, observe and experience their life stories. Milliken and Grace (2017) describe ethical nursing care as those actions taken by nurses to address needs that are in accordance with the profession's goals and perspectives. CCTM RNs should be aware of those areas of their practice that are central to ethical standards (Milliken & Grace, 2017). The development of ethical sensitivity and decision-making skills is as important in day-to-day CCTM practice as it is in more obvious ethical situations (Grace & Milliken, 2016).

A. Ethical sensitivity.
   1. Begins with an awareness of the ethical implications of all actions in nursing practice.
   2. Ethical sensitivity is the first step in developing moral reasoning and moral agency.
B. Moral agency.
   1. Refers to ethical obligations inherent in nursing practice as established in professional codes of ethics.
   2. Involves the willingness and ability to take action on behalf of individuals and groups for the purpose of bringing about positive change.
   3. Is important in achieving individual and population health-related goals, as well as in preventing adverse outcomes.
C. Moral action.
   1. Achieved through the development of ethical awareness, moral agency, and ethical decision-making skills.
   2. Elements of moral action include:
      a. Problem analysis.
      b. Mediation.
      c. Effective communication.
D. Moral distress.
   1. Describes a temporary or repeated sense of uneasiness caused by one's inability to stop a perceived harm or carry out a beneficial action on behalf of another.
   2. Occurs when nurses recognize the actions to take but are constrained from taking

them.
3. Can lead to feelings of powerlessness, but importantly, can also lead to activism, a form of advocacy.
4. Can be mitigated by nurses working within their organizations to promote ethical sensitivity and decision-making in day-to-day practice.

> Ethical sensitivity begins with an awareness of the ethical implications of all actions in nursing practice.

E. ANA's (2015) *Code of Ethics for Nurses with Interpretive Statements* establishes ethical standards for professional nursing in the United States. An ethical code provides professional self-regulation and accountability, defines client-professional obligations and peer relationships, and serves as a resource for analysis, decision, and action. The Code is applicable in all settings in which nurses practice. This important document outlines the values, moral norms, and ideals that guide nurses and nursing organizations. CCTM RNs are expected to embrace these ethical standards in all nursing actions. The Code should also inform all aspects of life, both personal and professional (ANA, 2015). The following provisions of the Code of Ethics for Nurses are specifically and directly applicable to the advocacy dimension of the CCTM model:
1. The CCTM RN practices with compassion and respect for the inherent dignity, worth, and unique attributes of every person.
   a. Relationships with individuals.
      (1) CCTM RNs establish trusting relationships with individuals and families.
      (2) Individual factors are considered in establishing plans of care.
         (a) Culture.
         (b) Value systems.
         (c) Spiritual beliefs.
         (d) Social support systems.
         (e) Gender and sexual orientation considerations.
         (f) Communication and language.
   b. The right to self-determination refers to the individual's right to determine what will be done with and to their own person.
      (1) Individual rights are both moral and legal.
      (2) Information must be presented accurately, completely, and in a manner understandable to the individual and family.
         (a) CCTM RNs assess the individual's understanding of the information presented.
         (b) Self-determination is dependent on awareness of the decision and can be impacted by cognitive ability, literacy, language proficiency, educational level, visual or hearing impairment, anxiety, or fear.
      (3) Information must be provided in a manner that facilitates informed decision-making.
      (4) Individuals must be assisted with weighing available benefits and risks related to available options in treatment.
      (5) Individuals have the right to accept, terminate, or refuse treatment without coercion or deceit.
      (6) Individuals and families must be provided with support throughout the decision-making and treatment process.
         (a) CCTM RNs include family members and significant others in decision-making, as desired by the individual.
         (b) CCTM RNs include other expert and knowledgeable nurses and other health care providers in decision-making.
2. CCTM RNs maintain a primary commitment to the individual, family, group, community, or population. CCTM advocacy involves many levels of care and responsibility.
   a. CCTM RNs ensure that honest discussions regarding available resources and treatment options occur at all levels.
   b. CCTM RNs evaluate the capacity for self-care at individual, family, and population levels.
   c. CCTM RNs recognize and consider the individual's place within the family and other relationships.
   d. CCTM RNs value collaboration and shared decision-making, as well as participation of all appropriate health professions in coordinating care.
3. CCTM RNs promote, advocate for, and protect the rights, health, and safety of

individuals and families.
   a. CCTM RNs respect privacy and confidentiality.
      (1) Individuals have the right to control access to personal information, including disclosure and nondisclosure of personal information.
   b. CCTM RNs acquire and maintain appropriate practice competencies to support professional practice.
      (1) CCTM RNs demonstrate personal integrity, relational maturity, and professional commitment.
   c. CCTM RNs participate in the development, implementation, and review and adherence to organizational and professional policies that promote individual health and safety, reduce errors and waste, and sustain a culture of safety (see Section IX).
4. The CCTM RN owes the same duties to self as others.
   a. CCTM RNs have a duty to take the same care for their own health and safety as that of others.
      (1) CCTM RNs should be role models of health maintenance and health promotion.
      (2) CCTM RNs should seek appropriate health care services, as needed.
      (3) CCTM RNs avoid taking unnecessary risks to their own health and safety.
      (4) CCTM RNs mitigate fatigue and compassion fatigue.
         (a) Healthy diet.
         (b) Adequate rest.
         (c) Healthy relationships.
         (d) Adequate leisure.
         (e) Spiritual needs.
5. CCTM RNs contribute to nursing and health policy development (see Section X).
6. CCTM RNs collaborate with other health professionals and the public to protect human rights, promote health diplomacy, and reduce health disparities (see Section V).
7. CCTM RNs integrate social justice into nursing and health policy (see Section V).
   a. Justice refers to equal and fair distribution of resources.
   b. Justice implies an equal right to resources, regardless of what a person has contributed or who they are (ANA, 2015).

III. **Advocacy and the CCTM Standards of Practice**

RNs practice advocacy when they identify with and understand the professional standards that exist to guide their practice. For CCTM RNs, the *Scope and Standards of Practice for Registered Nurses in Care Coordination and Transition Management* (American Academy of Ambulatory Care Nursing [AAACN], 2016) provide this structure. These 16 standards are organized within the domains of Clinical Practice and Organizational and Professional Performance and serve as authoritative statements that describe the responsibilities for which CCTM RNs are accountable.

A. The first six standards describe responsibilities within the Clinical Practice domain. These standards reflect the nursing process, addressing each step as it applies to the practice of nursing within the CCTM model. The following elements of these standards in particular reflect the practice of advocacy in CCTM nursing practice.
   1. Standard 1: Assessment.
      a. CCTM RNs perform assessments which focus on health needs as well as the unique concerns of individuals, families, groups, and populations.
      b. CCTM RN executives advocate to ensure information technologies support input and retrieval of assessment data across the care continuum.
   2. Standard 2: Nursing Diagnoses.
      a. Prioritize nursing diagnoses based not only on an individual's physical condition, but also on personal and cultural preferences, age-specific needs, areas of risk, and psychosocial vulnerabilities.
   3. Standard 3: Outcomes Identification.
      a. Include input from individual, family, and/or caregiver in the process of identifying specific, concise, and measurable goals.
         (1) Prioritize goals based upon individual and family preferences and values.
         (2) Use a holistic, person-centered, evidence-based approach to achieve expected outcomes.
      b. CCTM RN executives advocate for administrative guidelines that ensure

continuity of care across the care continuum.
   c. CCTM RN executives serve as advocates at the systems level by developing collaborative relationships to ensure that integrated systems are available to support the delivery of person-centered care across the continuum.
   d. CCTM RN leaders and executives practice advocacy at the systems level when they initiate activities that improve nursing practice, organizational performance, and optimal person and population outcomes.
4. Planning.
   a. In defining a plan of care, CCTM RNs practice advocacy when they consider individual and population needs, including issues related to gender, race, cultural values and practices, ethical and legal considerations, and environmental factors, as well as anticipated risks and benefits of proposed interventions.
   b. CCTM RNs practice systems-level advocacy by assuring the plan of care complies with organizational policies, guidelines, and evidence-based practices.
   c. CCTM RNs advocate for the individual's desired outcomes in providing direction for members of the interprofessional team.
   d. At the systems level, CCTM RNs facilitate the development and maintenance of staff competency in planning and change processes.
5. Standard 5: Implementation.
   a. Prioritize interventions based on an individual's or population's condition, situation, and needs along the health care continuum.
   b. Assure that interventions are consistent with organizational policies and regulatory requirements.
   c. Collaborate with the interprofessional health team across health care settings to effectively implement population or individual care coordination plans.
   d. Provide population-specific and age-appropriate care in a compassionate, caring, and culturally and ethnically sensitive manner.
   e. CCTM leaders and executives practice systems-level advocacy by:
      (1) Establishing organizational systems that ensure implementation strategies are consistent with evidence-based practice guidelines, state and regulatory agency standards, and organizational policies and procedures.
      (2) Advocating for staff participation in decisions to improve population health interventions and interprofessional communication.
6. Standard 5a: Coordination of Care.
   a. Demonstrate advocacy across care settings by:
      (1) Recognizing and maximizing opportunities to improve the quality of care.
      (2) Continuously communicating relevant information to individuals, caregivers, and members of the interprofessional health care team.
   b. At the systems level, CCTM leaders and executives demonstrate advocacy by:
      (1) Building relationships with stakeholders across the care continuum.
      (2) Establishing practice standards that reflect evidence-based care delivery.
      (3) Developing and validating staff competencies consistent with standards of nursing practice and organizational policies for CCTM.
      (4) Ensuring regulatory compliance with external accrediting organizations.
7. Standard 5b: Health Teaching and Health Promotion.
   a. Provide health teaching that advocates for healthy lifestyles, risk-reducing behaviors, disease management strategies, psychosocial needs, and self-care.
      (1) Advocate for the development of self-efficacy skills as a strategy to effect positive health choices for individuals and groups across the lifespan.
      (2) Use health promotion and health teaching methods, which reflect individual, family, or group values, beliefs, health practices, developmental level, learning

needs, language preference, spirituality, culture, and socioeconomic status.
            b. Acting as an advocate, seek opportunities for individual and/or health care consumer feedback and evaluation of the effectiveness of teaching strategies.
            c. Advocate for and support self-care activities and stress management for all caregivers.
      8. Standard 6: Evaluation.
         a. Include individuals, their caregivers, interprofessional team members and community resources in the ongoing evaluation of the plan of care.
         b. CCTM leaders and executives practice advocacy at the systems level by:
            (1) Facilitating diverse groups of transition management professionals and other health care professionals to develop and evaluate processes, systems, and tools that will enhance the evaluation of outcomes.
            (2) Encouraging and empowering nursing staff and stakeholders to participate in the decision-making process related to outcome evaluation.
   B. The organizational and professional performance standards define competencies related to professional behavior in CCTM nursing practice.
      1. Standard 7: Ethics.
         a. In the role of advocate, CCTM RNs integrate principles of professional nursing codes of ethics to ensure individual's rights in all areas of practice.
            (1) Actively participate in the identification of ethical concerns within the organization.
            (2) Serve on organizational ethics and patient rights committees.
            (3) Maintain awareness of emerging ethical trends that affect the rights of individuals, groups, and populations.
            (4) Deliver nursing care that reflects and respects diversity.
               (a) Cultural.
               (b) Spiritual.
               (c) Intellectual.
               (d) Educational.
               (e) Psychosocial.
            (5) Practice nursing in a manner that preserves the individual's autonomy, dignity, and rights.
            (6) Individual informed decisions by the patient or legally designated representative.
            (7) Advocate for individuals who are unable to act in their own best interest or do not understand the consequences of their decisions.
            (8) Advocate to ensure that individuals, caregivers, and staff have a voice with regard to offering feedback related to care and services without recrimination.
            (9) Promote access to quality health services that encompass equality, confidentiality of information, and continuity of care.
         b. CCTM RNs practice systems-level advocacy by assuring that written policies exist in their organizations to:
            (1) Support individual's rights and responsibilities.
            (2) Assure confidentiality of information and personal privacy.
            (3) Encourage individual self-determination.
         c. CCTM leaders and executives practice advocacy at the systems level when they:
            (1) Create and sustain organizational environments that reflect the inherent self-worth and rights of individuals and groups.
            (2) Develop and update policies that define process and outcome indicators related to CCTM.
      2. Standard 8: Education.
         a. CCTM RNs practice professional advocacy by attaining knowledge and competence that reflects current evidence-based nursing practice.
      3. Standard 9: Research and Evidence-Based Practice.
         a. CCTM RNs practice professional advocacy by integrating relevant research and evidence into practice to optimize standards of care and best practice.
         b. CCTM RN leaders and executives practice advocacy at the systems level by:
            (1) Using research findings and/or evidence-based practices in the development of all applicable policies, procedures, and guidelines.
            (2) Ensure that research conducted in the clinical and/or organizational

environment undergoes review and approval by an Institutional Review Board (IRB) and adheres to ethical principles.
4. Standard 10: Performance Improvement.
   a. Serve as an advocate for continuous improvement in CCTM nursing practice within the organization.
      (1) Identify and eliminate barriers to care in CCTM practice.
      (2) Advocate for initiatives that identify and define nurse-sensitive indicators.
      (3) Foster communication, collaboration, and coordination of improvement efforts across the health care continuum.
   b. CCTM RN executives and leaders practice systems-level advocacy by implementing organizational policies and procedures specific to the practice of CCTM.
      (1) Ensuring policies are consistent with applicable federal and state statutes, rules, and regulations.
      (2) Ensuring policies reflect accepted standards and scope of nursing practice.
5. Standard 11: Communication.
   a. CCTM RNs practice advocacy when they:
      (1) Share best practices with peers, requesting feedback and evaluation.
      (2) Seek opportunities to create positive mentoring relationships.
   b. CCTM RN leaders and executives practice advocacy at the systems level by:
      (1) Creating and contributing to positive environments of collegiality and trust through shared professional communication and decision-making among new and experienced CCTM staff.
      (2) Acting as a resource and serving as an example of positive, professional communication.
      (3) Recognizing individual or group accomplishments.
6. Standard 12: Leadership.
   a. CCTM RNs demonstrate advocacy by:
      (1) Showing respect for human dignity and worth by valuing people as the central asset of the work setting, the profession, and the community.
      (2) Assuming an active role as a team player and team builder to create and maintain healthy, safe work environments.
      (3) Leading and actively participating in projects, community education, committees, and councils.
   b. CCTM RN executives and leaders practice advocacy at the systems level by:
      (1) Defining a clear vision for CCTM.
      (2) Advocating for organizational environments conducive to innovation, communication, and positive change.
      (3) Representing CCTM nursing on decision-making boards and committees.
7. Standard 13: Collaboration.
   a. CCTM RNs advocate for the promotion and restoration of health in populations through partnership with interprofessional team members in diverse settings.
      (1) Collaborate with local and community resources to improve the health of populations.
      (2) Partner with colleagues to promote changes that will improve outcomes for individuals, groups, and populations.
      (3) Serve as an advocate for nurses practicing in CCTM roles by identifying issues and celebrating successes.
8. Standard 14: Professional Practice Evaluation.
   a. CCTM RNs advocate for excellence in CCTM nursing practice through ongoing and systematic evaluation of work processes, personal performance, evidence-based practices, and quality measures.
9. Standard 15: Resource Utilization.
   a. CCTM RNs serve as advocates for appropriate resource allocation by partnering with individuals and their caregivers to identify unique needs and advocate for the resources needed to achieve desired outcomes.
   b. At the systems level, CCTM leaders advocate for resources, including technology, to enhance CCTM nursing practice and improve organizational performance.
10. Standard 16: Environment.
    a. CCTM RNs practice advocacy through:

(1) Ensuring the environment is accessible, safe, and functional for individuals, staff, and visitors.
(2) Mitigating occupational exposure and related risks by:
   (a) Utilizing preventive and screening programs.
   (b) Maintaining confidentiality of employee exposures.
   b. CCTM RN executives and leaders practice advocacy at the systems level by:
      (1) Utilizing applicable federal and state rules, regulations, organizational policies, and evidence-based practice to determine the level of resources needed for safe, quality individual care.
      (2) Implementing policies and procedures that address training in the use of personal protective equipment.
      (3) Implementing written policies and procedures regarding:
         (a) Confidentiality.
         (b) Infection control.
         (c) Fire and safety.
         (d) Security.
         (e) Harassment.
         (f) Equipment management.
         (g) Hazardous waste handling.
         (h) Emergency response.

IV. **Advocacy and Nursing Practice in the CCTM Model**

CCTM RNs must demonstrate an understanding of the dimension of advocacy in the following areas to optimize the CCTM needs of individuals and families.
A. Nursing assessment.
   1. Encompasses the total individual, including medical, psychosocial, behavioral, socioeconomic, cultural, and spiritual needs.
   2. Comprehensive assessment includes identification of actual or potential barriers.
      a. Financial.
      b. Transportation.
      c. Psychosocial.
      d. Health literacy.
   3. Document using standardized or electronic tools when available to ensure portability of care plan.
B. Plan of care: Development of the plan of care in the CCTM model is a collaborative process that prioritizes the goals and values of the individual and family.
   1. Acting as advocates, CCTM RNs facilitate and ensure effective communication between the individual/family and the health care team, provide information about treatment options and plans, assess the individual's skills and expectations, assist the individual/family in understanding health care benefits, and communicate with other health care providers (Camicia et al., 2014).
   2. The primary purpose of care planning in CCTM nursing is to provide continuity of care, ensuring the individual's needs are met on a long-term basis across the care continuum, and to serve as a communication tool for other providers and the individual/family. Care plans are valuable tools that can facilitate coordination between different clinicians' services, but also outline an expected course of care for individuals that provides a sense of security and a basis for shared decision-making (Haggerty, Roberge, Freeman, & Beaulieu, 2013).
   3. In developing a plan of care, CCTM RNs, acting as advocates, negotiate appropriate services with the individual and family; the goal of negotiating services is to maintain flexibility and engagement, moving toward optimal levels of health.
      a. Practice cultural competence with awareness and respect for diversity.
      b. Promote evidence-based care.
      c. Include preventive care measures.
      d. Provide optimal individual safety.
      e. Integrate behavioral change science through motivational interviewing.
C. Nursing Interventions.
   1. Provide support and assistance with accessing appropriate type and level of services.
      a. Educate regarding available resources and options.
      b. Link with community services.
         (1) Medical equipment.
         (2) Transportation.
         (3) Housing.
         (4) Supplemental food.
      c. Assist with navigating the health care system.
   2. Assist with medication management.
      a. Medication review and reconciliation at every encounter.
         (1) Review schedule.
         (2) Discuss actions and possible

reactions.
- (3) Alert to potential drug interactions.
- (4) Discuss pharmacy services and support.
3. Recognize, prevent, and eliminate disparities related to:
   a. Culture.
   b. Race.
   c. Ethnicity.
   d. National origin.
   e. Migration background.
   f. Gender.
      (1) Gender identity.
      (2) Gender expression.
      (3) Sexual orientation.
      (4) Marital status.
   g. Religious, political beliefs.
   h. Mental or cognitive disability.
4. Serve as the voice of the individual across settings and disciplines.
   a. Empower individuals and families to problem-solve by exploring options of care when available and alternative plans of care when necessary.
   b. Promote self-determination through:
      (1) Informed and shared decision-making.
      (2) Autonomy.
      (3) Growth.
      (4) Self-advocacy.
5. Educate other health care providers and disciplines in recognizing and respecting individual and family needs, strengths, preferences, and goals.
6. Provide frequent communication and education to facilitate timely and informed decisions regarding:
   a. Choices in treatment plan.
   b. Disease management.
   c. Community resources.
   d. Insurance benefits.
   e. Socio-emotional concerns.
7. Identify individual and family/caregiver goals.
8. Develop and maintain proactive, person-centered relationships with the individual, family, caregiver, and other necessary stakeholders to maximize outcomes.
   a. Use mediation and negotiation to improve communication and relationships.
   b. Use problem-solving skills and techniques to reconcile differing points of view between individual and family and/or individual, family, and provider, or between providers.

D. Evaluation. CCTM RNs, acting as advocates, understand the unique situation of the individual and family, which allows the nurse to evaluate the effectiveness of the plan of care in meeting the individual's needs over time. Acting as advocate, CCTM RNs:
1. Provide frequent review of goals and outcomes over time.
2. Understand that reassessment of the needs of the individual and family over time is essential.

V. **Social Determinants of Health and Advocacy**

In their role as advocates, CCTM RNs must understand the importance of attention to social factors in the coordination of care. The World Health Organization (2018) defines social determinants of health as "the conditions in which people are born, grow, work, live, and age," (para.1) and the wider set of forces and systems shaping the conditions of daily life. These forces and systems include poverty, educational level, housing, food insecurity, and the presence of toxins or violence in the environment, among others. There is a growing body of evidence that supports the link between social determinants of health and health status, health-related risks, and response to health interventions (Lathrop, 2013; Persaud, 2018). Over time, these "upstream factors" have influenced the growth of health disparities, or avoidable system-wide inequities, which may be directly attributed to social conditions. For these reasons, advocacy on the part of nurses and other members of the interprofessional team has become an increasingly important element of CCTM professional practice.

A. Individuals and families within high socioeconomic groups have access to resources, including higher-paying jobs, better food, higher levels of education, and better access to health care services. Such resources provide protective barriers against chronic illness, injuries, food insecurity, and emotional health issues (Lathrop, 2013).
1. Individuals and families living in poverty have a higher exposure to violence, environmental toxins, and poor nutrition, which directly influences health and well-being.
2. Individuals and families living in low socioeconomic environments experience higher levels of chronic stress, which can result in lower levels of immunity and higher levels of disease.
3. Low socioeconomic status (SES) early in life is a determinant of adult health behaviors, such as smoking, substance abuse, and mental illness.

Chapter 2

4. A growing body of knowledge has confirmed that adverse childhood experiences, which include traumatic experiences occurring during the childhood years, are associated with long-term health-related outcomes that may manifest later in life (Chung et al., 2016).
    a. Childhood adversity may lead to the presence of long-term toxic stress.
        (1) Toxic stress, left untreated, may continue from one generation to the next, negatively impacting health and SES.
B. There is evidence that models of care coordination that integrate health care, social services, and community outreach demonstrate improved health outcomes, as well as cost savings (Brewster, Brault, Tan, Curry, & Bradley, 2017). Recent studies demonstrate that attention to social needs consistently improves health outcomes.
    1. Care coordination and advocacy efforts related to community outreach resulted in improved health outcomes, including all-cause mortality in mothers and improved birth weight in infants, as well as lower overall costs (Taylor et al., 2016).
    2. Referrals for housing support were associated with lower health care costs and improved health outcomes (Taylor et al., 2016).
    3. Advocacy related to nutritional support was consistently associated with significantly improved health outcomes (Taylor et al., 2016).
    4. Studies reporting referrals to services related to income support, including Social Security income, demonstrated positive health outcomes (Taylor et al., 2016).
C. Impact of social determinants of health on children.
    1. Pediatric health care providers, including CCTM RNs caring for children, must be aware of the effects of poverty and social factors that directly impact the health of infants and children (Chung et al., 2016; Garg, Toy, Tripodis, Silverstein, & Freeman, 2015).
        a. A growing body of evidence indicates adverse childhood experiences are associated with developmental delays, chronic health issues, and behavioral consequences, which lead to toxic stress in children.
        b. Without attention, such issues often follow children throughout their growing years, impacting their ability to succeed in school, and ultimately, in life.
    2. Surveillance and screening for social determinants of health in children is an important element of advocacy related to care coordination, which should be addressed in the pediatric primary care medical home (PCMH). Few child health care providers address social and psychosocial issues regularly during routine well-child and primary care visits (Chung et al., 2016; Garg et al., 2015).
        a. Surveillance refers to a continuous process of skilled observation over time, which occurs during the provision of health care services. Examples include:
            (1) Child maltreatment.
            (2) Availability of childcare services.
            (3) Availability of early education programs.
            (4) Family financial status.
            (5) Physical environment/housing.
            (6) Family social support.
            (7) Intimate partner violence.
            (8) Maternal depression.
            (9) Family mental illness.
            (10) Household substance abuse.
            (11) Firearm exposure.
            (12) Parental health literacy.
        b. Screening refers to the use of standardized tools that provide specific measures.
            (1) Developmental milestones.
                (a) Physical.
                (b) Emotional development (expression, interacting, play, bonding).
                (c) Language development (communication, vocabulary).
            (2) Parental health literacy.
D. Barriers to including advocacy interventions among practicing nurses (Persaud, 2018).
    1. Nurses describe low levels of confidence in assessing social issues, including:
        a. Food insecurity.
        b. Job security.
        c. Unemployment.
        d. Social isolation.
        e. Education and literacy.
    2. Nurses describe perceived barriers to addressing social determinants of health:
        a. Discomfort with discussing social issues.
        b. Reliance on other disciplines.
        c. Lack of preparation, skill set.

d. Lack of support, including time.
e. Attitudes and beliefs regarding the relevance of social issues to nursing.
f. Attitudes and beliefs regarding the importance of social issues.
E. Implications for nursing leadership (Persaud, 2018).
1. CCTM RN leaders must commit to their role as advocates through the development of a nursing workforce with the knowledge, skills, and attitudes to address social issues directly impacting the health and well-being of individuals and families.
a. Trauma-informed care (TIC) provides a framework for providing care to traumatized individuals in a variety of service settings (Kenny, Vazquez, Long, & Thompson, 2017).
(1) The impact of traumatic stress may be long-lasting and can interfere with an individual's sense of safety, self-efficacy, self-control, and relationships.
(2) As advocates, CCTM RNs may benefit from an understanding of the effects of adversity and the basic tenets of TIC.
2. Nursing leaders should continue to support downstream interventions that may impact social issues.
a. Smoking cessation programs.
b. Coordination of services addressing transitional and supportive care.
c. Transportation and access services.
3. Nursing leaders should also begin to shift emphasis to include organizational efforts that influence upstream interventions at the systems level.
a. Advocate for interprofessional collaboration and education.
b. Become an advocate for decision-making at the health system, community, state, and national levels.

> Recent reports estimate that 77 million Americans, or 88% of the adult population, have limitations related to health literacy.

VI. Health Literacy

Although health literacy may be considered a social determinant of health based on its impact on health outcomes, it is presented separately here for purposes of addressing its importance as an element of advocacy in CCTM RN practice. General health literacy is reported to be the greatest individual factor affecting health status (Scotten, 2015). Recent reports estimate that 77 million Americans, or 88% of the adult population, have limitations related to health literacy, meaning they may struggle with the appropriate use of information for routine self-management tasks, such as discharge follow-up instructions and accurate medication management at home (Loan et al., 2018). Health literacy is not well understood, nor is there a single approach to addressing it across health care systems. Nurses must understand the dimensions and importance of health literacy to successfully practice in CCTM roles and settings.

A. Definition and context of health literacy.
1. At the individual and family level (microsocial level), health literacy refers to the personal and relational factors that affect a person's ability to acquire, understand, and use information related to health and health services (Batterham, Hawkins, Collins, Buchbinder, & Osborne, 2016).
a. Health literacy is a necessary precursor to the achievement of high levels of health and well-being (Barton et al., 2018).
b. The number and range of tasks required of consumers in today's health care system is complex.
2. At the systems (macrosocial) level, health literacy refers to characteristics of populations or communities and to public health efforts focused on health promotion and empowerment of people to access, understand, and use information to maintain good health (Loan et al., 2018).
a. A culture of health reflects a commitment on the part of individuals, families, organizations, communities, and governments to create a healthy society (Barton et al., 2018).
b. Evidence exists for a cost imperative related to improving the health literacy of individuals, organizations, and communities (Loan et al., 2018).
(1) It is estimated that health care costs for individuals with low health literacy are more than four times those of individuals with high health literacy.
(2) Boyle and colleagues (2017) reported that among hospitalized individuals, low health literacy is independently associated with increased risk for adverse transitional care outcomes, including readmission.
B. Health literacy and CCTM RN practice.
1. Nurses have direct and indirect influence

on health literacy at the individual and organizational levels (Loan et al., 2018).
  a. Nurses are often the first point of contact for individuals in health care settings, providing assessment and individualized care planning services.
     (1) The American Academy of Nursing (AAN) Health Literacy Task Force reinforced the need for nurses to assess and address health literacy for every individual in every health care encounter (Loan et al., 2018).
     (2) Nurses must encourage self-management of health by ensuring that individuals understand what they need to do after each health care encounter (Loan et al., 2018).
  b. Nurses are leaders in organizations and advocates for health care transformation at all levels.
     (1) CCTM RNs should engage in organizational policy development related to health literacy, as well as widespread promotion of the importance of health literacy.
     (2) Health literate organizations implement strategies that support system-wide navigation and use of health information to support and improve health (Loan et al., 2018).
C. Health Literacy Universal Precautions – Agency for Healthcare Research and Quality (AHRQ).
  1. A universal approach to health literacy, which assumes all individuals may potentially have some level of difficulty managing health information, is recommended (AHRQ, 2017; Barton et al., 2018; Loan et al., 2018). Elements of this approach include:
     a. Spoken communication.
     b. Written communication.
     c. Self-management and empowerment.
     d. Supportive systems.
  2. Health Literacy Universal Precautions have the following aims:
     a. Simplify communication and confirm comprehension for all individuals to minimize the risk of miscommunication.
     b. Address navigation issues within the office, health system, and community.
     c. Support individuals and families in efforts to improve their health.
  3. Elements of health literacy universal precautions include:
     a. Verbal communication.
        (1) Communicate clearly.
        (2) Use the teach-back method.
        (3) Follow up with individuals.
        (4) Improve telephone access.
        (5) Address language differences.
        (6) Consider culture, customs, and beliefs.
     b. Written communication.
        (1) Assess, select, and create easy-to-understand materials.
        (2) Use health education materials effectively.
     c. Self-management and empowerment.
        (1) Encourage questions.
        (2) Create action plans.
        (3) Provide assistance in managing medications.
        (4) Elicit feedback.
     d. Supportive systems.
        (1) Connect individuals and families to non-medical services.
        (2) Refer individuals and families to medical resources.
        (3) Provide links to resources for math and literacy skills.
D. Health literacy and care of children.
  1. In pediatric health care settings, practitioners have the responsibility of assessing and addressing the literacy of both parents and children.
     a. There is growing evidence that parental health literacy is associated with children's health status and access to care (Scotten, 2015).
     b. Studies reveal that children of parents with low literacy skills have worse health outcomes (Scotten, 2015). Studies have shown:
        (1) More emergency room visits and hospital admissions for children with asthma.
        (2) Lower parental comprehension of information regarding newborn screening and required vaccination schedules.
        (3) Parental difficulty understanding medication administration.
        (4) Decreased rates of breastfeeding.
        (5) Higher rates of parental smoking.
     c. Studies related to adolescent health literacy reveal a relationship between level of health literacy and health-related decisions. Adolescents with lower health literacy levels are more likely to:
        (1) Carry guns.
        (2) Smoke tobacco.
        (3) Engage in fighting.
  2. A survey of pediatricians revealed that

enhanced communication techniques are used with varying frequency to address parental literacy issues (Scotten, 2015). These communication strategies include:
a. Avoiding medical jargon.
b. Speaking slowly.
c. Repeating key points when giving instructions.
d. Presenting only two to three concepts at a time.
e. Providing detailed instructions regarding amounts of medication to be given for prescription drugs.
f. Providing written treatment plans for parents.
g. Reinforcing key elements of the visit.
h. Underlining or highlighting key information on written materials.

E. Nursing call to action for health literacy (Loan et al., 2018).
1. The AAN Health Literacy Task Force issued a white paper in 2017 that addresses the importance of health literacy to the nursing profession.
a. Nursing must collaborate with other professions and lead efforts to:
(1) Promote the use of existing resources to support and improve health literacy in the United States.
(2) Use health information technology, enhanced communication strategies, and individual self-management competencies to improve health literacy.
(3) Use evidence-based models and guidelines to improve health literacy in all health care settings.
(4) Recruit and retain a diverse workforce with health literacy expertise.
(5) Identify and engage with community partners to develop and evaluate health literacy initiatives.
(6) Integrate nursing models of care for health literacy into national quality health initiatives.
(7) Recommend that The Joint Commission require health literacy universal precautions as a component of accreditation.
(8) Advocate for funding to evaluate and support health literacy programs in nursing education and practice.
(9) Encourage the inclusion of health literacy initiatives and achievements as a component of Magnet® recognition.

VII. Advocacy and Behavioral/Mental Health

Mental health and behavioral disorders are common worldwide and continue to challenge the quality of overall health and well-being of individuals, families, and populations. In the United States, it is estimated that only one-third of those persons in need of mental health services actually receive appropriate care (Kilbourne et al., 2018). Significant gaps remain in access to mental and behavioral health services, and the rate of improvement has not kept pace with that of other general medical conditions. Despite a call for parity in coverage for physical and mental health conditions, insufficient attention has been given to the reporting of adequacy or intensity of behavioral health services (Kilbourne et al., 2018). The Centers for Disease Control and Prevention (CDC) reports that 8.1% of U.S. adults suffered from major depression between 2013-2016 (Brody, Pratt, & Hughes, 2018). An estimated 5.7 million Americans are living with dementia, most over age 65 years. In addition, the United States is in the midst of an overwhelming opioid crisis, which has escalated to more than 33,000 deaths annually as a result of the overuse of both prescription and illegally obtained opioids (Soelberg, Brown, Du Vivier, Meyer, & Ramachandran, 2017). Finally, an estimated 25% of children in primary care settings have a chronic mental health condition (Brown, Green, Desai, Weitzman, & Rosenthal, 2014). Recent efforts to embed mental health services within primary care medical home settings offer some promise for individuals and populations in need of these services. CCTM RNs in primary and specialty care settings with an understanding of their role as advocates are well-positioned to influence the quality of care and mental health outcomes at both the microsocial and macrosocial levels of care.

A. Improving access to effective treatment for individuals with mental health disorders is one of the great challenges facing the U.S. health care system (Olfson, 2016).
1. It is estimated that from onset of symptoms to receiving treatment is often more than a year for many mental health conditions.
a. Delays in seeking treatment may be due to:
(1) Attitudes and self-perceptions regarding need for treatment.
(2) Perceived stigma related to mental health conditions.
(3) Uncertainty regarding the effectiveness of treatment.

Chapter 2

                (4) Desire to handle problems independently.
         2. The current number of mental health specialists is insufficient to fill the growing demand for services.
         3. In an effort to mitigate delays in access, primary care physicians (PCPs) are providing behavioral and mental health services to an increasing volume of individuals within their practices.
            a. PCPs are managing a broad array of behavioral conditions and prescribing more psychotropic medications to support the needs of individuals.
            b. Depression, the most common psychiatric disorder, is managed by many PCPs.
                (1) Depressed individuals are more likely to receive antidepressant medications than counseling or psychotherapy.
            c. New models of collaboration between PCPs and mental health specialists are needed to optimize care and meet the needs of the growing number of individuals with behavioral and mental health conditions.
         4. Individuals with low incomes, those who lack health insurance, and those with disabilities are at even greater risk for experiencing delays in accessing needed mental health services.
         5. CCTM RNs in all settings should expand their skills to include assessment of behavioral and mental health needs of individuals and families.
    B. Health care providers and payers need defined and validated person and population-specific structures, processes, and outcomes to define quality measures for mental health services (Kilbourne et al., 2018).
         1. Many barriers exist to strengthening the infrastructure of measurement-based mental health services, including:
            a. Lack of provider training and support.
            b. Limited scientific evidence for mental health quality outcome measures.
            c. Cultural barriers to integration of mental health care within the primary care environment.
            d. Policy limitations.
            e. Limitations in technology.
         2. Post-acute transitional care models for mental health are needed.
            a. It is estimated that less than half of individuals with publically supported health insurance receive appropriate follow up after hospitalization for mental health diagnoses (Kilbourne et al., 2018).
            b. A study reporting interventions linking primary and specialty care services post-hospitalization for common mental disorders resulted in improved engagement during the immediate post-discharge period (Bonsack et al., 2016).
            c. Disparities in quality and outcomes of mental health services are greater for those of low SES.
                (1) Individuals with low incomes, those who lack health insurance, and those with disabilities are at even greater risk for experiencing delays in accessing needed mental health services.
                (2) Psychiatric/mental health nurse practitioners (NPs) are well prepared to provide coordinated specialty mental health care services for vulnerable populations (Baker, Travers, Buschman, & Merrill, 2018).
         3. Few studies have reported mental health care process measures that are directly associated with clinical outcomes. Additional research in this area is needed.
            a. CCTM RNs are in a position to track clinical outcomes by virtue of their relationships, communication, and care coordination activities over time. Quality measures may include:
                (1) Plans of care which are evidence-based.
                (2) Measurable clinical outcomes.
                (3) Use of information technology for documentation.
                (4) Policies and measurable standards of care.

> The United States is in the midst of an overwhelming opioid crisis, which has escalated to more than 33,000 deaths annually as a result of the overuse of both prescription and illegally obtained opioids.

    C. The opioid crisis.
         1. Opioid prescription drug use and resulting addiction has become a national crisis in America (Soelberg et al., 2017).
            a. Early in the 21st century, guided by The Joint Commission, the assessment of pain became the "5th Vital Sign," and health care providers turned attention to screening and assessment of pain in all sectors of health care.

b. This led to an increase in attention to the presence of pain and its management by health care providers.
   (1) Between 2000-2010, prescriptions for opioids increased dramatically, from 164 million to 234 million.
   (2) Between 2004 and 2011, emergency department encounters related to prescription opioids increased by 150% to 200%.
   (3) In the 4 years between 2010 and 2014, deaths due to overdose of prescription drugs increased by more than 2,000, from 16,651 to 18,893.
   (4) More than 63,000 deaths involving opioids were reported in 2016.
   (5) As a result of this epidemic, the life expectancy for Americans has experienced a decrease of 2 years, to 78.6 years (Dobbs & Fogger, 2018).
c. Policies and regulations at the state and federal level have been enacted to:
   (1) Reduce risks related to opioid overdose.
   (2) Increase resources for treatment.
d. Prescription drug monitoring programs (PDMPs) have been implemented in many states as a means of reducing the supply of opioids and modifying prescriber behavior (Soelberg et al., 2017).
   (1) A PDMP is an electronic database that tracks information related to prescription drugs, including:
      (a) Individual.
      (b) Drug and dose prescribed.
      (c) Prescriber.
      (d) Dispensing pharmacy.
   (2) Studies to date have not been conclusive regarding decreased use of schedule II or III drugs after implementation of PDMPs.
      (a) Dowell, Zhang, Noonan, and Hockenberry (2016) reported a reduction in prescribed opioids and opioid overdose death rates in a review of PDMP and pain clinics.
      (b) Efficacy of PDMPs is limited by minimal interstate sharing of data.
      (c) CCTM RNs should give particular attention to medication reconciliation for those individuals maintained on controlled medications for pain management.
2. Chronic pain. Individuals receiving treatment for chronic pain compose a significant subpopulation of this epidemic.
   a. It is estimated that more than 11% of the U.S. population present with complaints of chronic pain.
   b. 3% to 4% of the population are maintained on long-term opioid therapy (LTOT).
   c. Evidence suggests that between 11% to 25% of individuals on LTOT for chronic pain may become dependent or addicted.
3. In 2016, the CDC issued a guideline for managing chronic pain (Dobbs & Fogger, 2018).
   a. The guideline offers evidence-based strategies for managing chronic pain (not related to cancer, palliative care, or end-of-life care) in primary care settings.
      (1) Care providers should evaluate quality-of-life factors to determine if risks outweigh benefits of continued LTOT.
         (a) Current evidence related to the effect of LTOT on pain, functional health, and quality of life is weak.
         (b) Tapering and discontinuing the use of LTOT for chronic pain is an important first step in mitigating the flow of opiates that floods many communities.
         (c) CCTM RN advocates are well positioned to integrate risk assessment strategies into their roles.
            i. Use evidence-based screening tools or ask individuals about substance use at each encounter.
            ii. Counsel individuals and families regarding the risk of accidental overdose when combining prescribed opioids with other drugs or substances.
            iii. Support individuals in the use of non-pharmaco-

logical or non-opioid pain therapy.
4. The opioid epidemic is further magnified by the increasing supply of illegally obtained fentanyl and heroin (Dobbs & Fogger, 2018).
   a. Although efforts directed toward changing prescriber practices have been effective in decreasing the prescription opiate supply, illegally manufactured and distributed substances are readily available and present barriers to rapid mitigation of the addiction epidemic.
   b. It is important for CCTM RN advocates to build trusting relationships with individuals and families that support frequent assessment of issues related to pain management and substance use.

D. Dementia.
   1. Alzheimer's disease is the most common cause of dementia, accounting for 60% to 80% of dementia cases (Alzheimer's Association, 2018).
      a. An estimated 5.7 million Americans are living with Alzheimer's disease.
      b. This number is expected to reach nearly 14 million by 2050.
   2. Alzheimer's disease is currently the most expensive disease in the country.
      a. The 2018 cost of Alzheimer's disease is estimated at $277 billion.
      b. $186 billion of this expense is in Medicare and Medicaid costs.
   3. Morbidity and mortality of Alzheimer's disease.
      a. Deaths due to Alzheimer's disease increased 123% between 2000-2015. In comparison, deaths due to heart disease during the same period decreased by 11%.
      b. In 2017, more than 16 million family members and unpaid caregivers provided an estimated 18.4 billion hours of care to individuals with Alzheimer's disease.
         (1) This care is valued at more than $232 billion.
         (2) Caregivers are at increased risk for emotional distress and increased mental and physical health outcomes.
         (3) It is important for CCTM RN advocates to ensure that plans of care for this population include interventions for caregivers, as well as for individuals suffering from dementia.
   4. Transitions between acute care hospitals and skilled nursing facilities, community settings, or home occur frequently in this population (Hirschman & Hodgson, 2018).
      a. These frequent transitions increase the risk for poor health outcomes.
         (1) Hospital-acquired complications.
         (2) Increased morbidity and mortality.
         (3) Increased cost of care.
      b. CCTM RNs should advocate with their organizations for specific transitional care processes to facilitate care and mitigate adverse outcomes in this population.
      c. Hirschman and Hodgson (2018) conducted a review of available evidence-based transitional care interventions specific to this population.
         (1) Enhanced counseling and support for caregivers.
         (2) Dementia caregiver training program.
         (3) Structured care planning video and discussion for skilled nursing facility staff.
         (4) Augmented care using Naylor's Transitional Care Model.
         (5) Structured dementia care coordination at home (MIND at home).
         (6) Partners in dementia care.
         (7) Geriatrics team intervention for assisted living settings.
      d. There is a shift toward community-centered care for individuals suffering from dementia and their caregivers.
      e. CCTM RNs are in a position to advocate for evidence-based interventions to support enhanced care at the person, family, and community levels.

E. Behavioral and mental health services for children.
   1. An estimated 25% of children in primary care settings have a chronic mental health condition (Brown et al., 2014).
      a. Only 1 in 5 of these children receive mental health services.
      b. These children have co-morbidities and social conditions in need of care from multiple providers.
   2. Pediatric primary care practices are increasingly providing behavioral health services for children and adolescents (Kolko & Perrin, 2014).
      a. Positive features of this approach include:

(1) Local setting.
(2) Familiar provider.
(3) No stigma.
　　b. Common pediatric behavioral health problems seen in primary care settings include:
(1) Anxiety and depression.
(2) Autism spectrum disorders.
(3) Attention deficit and hyperactivity disorder (ADHD).
(4) Oppositional or aggressive behavior.
(5) Learning problems
(6) Substance use.
3. Care coordination needs of children with behavioral health conditions.
　　a. Brown and colleagues (2014) identified children with at least one of four chronic mental health conditions with a defined need for care coordination.
(1) ADHD.
(2) Anxiety disorder.
(3) Conduct (behavior) disorder.
(4) Depression.
　　b. The study concluded that care coordination for high-risk children and their families to address their medical, social, and behavioral health issues is needed.
　　c. More studies are needed to define the care coordination needs of this population.
4. Integrated pediatric primary care services for families experiencing traumatic stress (Dayton et al., 2016).
　　a. Care based on evidence of high prevalence of traumatic stress in childhood, often linked to social determinants, which impacts the behavioral and mental health needs of families.
(1) Children and families are exposed to trauma from multiple sources.
　　(a) Violence in communities.
　　(b) Substance abuse.
　　(c) Domestic violence.
　　(d) Parental mental health issues.
　　(e) Racism.
　　(f) Bullying.
　　(g) Family financial stressors.
　　　　i. Job insecurity.
　　　　ii. Decline in wages and benefits.
　　　　iii. Household debt.
　　　　iv. Food insecurity.
　　b. Children's response to trauma.

(1) Child traumatic stress occurs when a child is exposed to trauma and reacts in ways that affect well-being and day-to-day functioning.
　　(a) Achieving developmental milestones.
　　(b) Learning and school success.
　　(c) Interactions with adults and other children.
　　(d) Neurological and social development.
　　　　i. Behavior and emotional regulation.
　　　　ii. Ability to form trusting relationships.
　　　　iii. Attention deficits affecting learning.
　　(e) Disruptive physiological impact.
　　　　i. A growing body of evidence has demonstrated a link between childhood traumatic stress and a variety of chronic illnesses lasting through the adult years.
　　c. Trauma-informed integrated care (Brown, King, & Wissow, 2017).
(1) Refers to a collaborative service model which integrates primary care, mental health services, and community programs.
　　(a) Model has as its foundation an evidence-based approach, which integrates knowledge of the impact of trauma on all aspects of health and well-being.
　　(b) Primary care clinicians focus on the prevention, detection, and care that occurs as a consequence of trauma.

> There is a growing body of evidence which indicates that adverse childhood experiences are associated with developmental delays, chronic health issues and behavioral consequences which lead to toxic stress in children.

VIII. Advocacy in the Care of Children

A. CCTM RNs in all settings should be aware of advocacy issues specific to the pediatric population. Particularly in primary care settings, such issues should be discussed in the initial nursing assessment of children and updated over time. CCTM RNs should advocate at both the microsocial and macrosocial levels to assure that individual, family, community, and population-specific actions are endorsed. Nurses serving as activists for children's health-related issues are well received in legislative settings. The American Academy of Pediatrics (AAP) (2018) maintains an updated database of current advocacy and policy initiatives on its website. These initiatives include the following:

1. Poverty. At all levels of government, policies and programs that affect the health of children and families living in poverty should be supported.
    a. Nutrition assistance programs.
        (1) Women, Infants, and Children (WIC).
        (2) Supplemental Nutrition Assistance Program (SNAP).
        (3) School nutrition.
        (4) Summer meals.
    b. Early childhood education.
    c. Quality childcare standards.
    d. Low-income housing support.
    e. Access to quality health care.
        (1) Children's Health Insurance Program (CHIP).
        (2) Medicaid.
2. Childhood immunizations.
    a. Appropriate funding for public immunization programs should be supported to ensure all children have access to vaccines as outlined by CDC schedules.
    b. State laws permitting non-medical exemptions to school entry immunization requirements should be eliminated.
3. Child passenger safety.
    a. Motor vehicle accidents are the leading killer of children older than age 1 year.
    b. State laws must include provisions related to rear-facing safety seats until age 2 years.
    c. Children should ride in approved safety seats with a 5-point harness up to the highest weight and height allowed by the manufacturer.
    d. School-age children should ride in a belt-positioning booster seat until at least age 8 years or until the seatbelt fits correctly per AAP and National Highway Traffic Safety Administration standards.
    e. Children should ride in the rear seat until age 13 years.
4. School physical education.
    a. Physical activity is necessary to promote health and mitigate obesity in children.
        (1) All children should have at least 1 hour of physical activity per day.
        (2) Schools should provide quality physical education, which helps students develop motor skills, knowledge, positive attitudes, and confidence in physical activity.
5. Concussion management.
    a. Cognitive and physical rest following a head injury is imperative.
    b. Coaches and athletic trainers should be educated in identifying and reporting signs of concussion.
6. Gun safety.
    a. Firearm safety counseling should be provided to families.
        (1) Promote regulation of sale, purchase, ownership, safe storage, and use of firearms.
    b. Background checks for purchasers of firearms should be mandatory.
    c. Mental health restrictions for gun purchases should be enforced.
    d. Firearm regulation should include a ban on assault weapons and high-capacity magazine sales as a strategy to reduce firearm-related injuries.
7. Confidentiality for adolescents and young adults.
    a. Confidentiality is vital to the delivery of quality preventive health care services in this population due to fear of disclosure, which may lead to delay in seeking needed services.
        (1) Reproductive health.
        (2) Behavioral and mental health issues.
        (3) Substance abuse.
        (4) Tobacco cessation.
        (5) Abuse, neglect, and intimate partner violence.
    b. State laws and health system policies should provide for adolescent confidentiality in documentation within electronic health records.
8. Distracted driving.
    a. The National Transportation Safety Board recommends that states ban the use of all portable electronic devices (including hands-free) while driving.
    b. Evidence shows that distractions may present greater risks for inexperienced drivers.

c. The use of mobile phones while driving should be prohibited.
9. Electronic nicotine delivery systems (ENDS).
    a. ENDS are increasingly marketed to adolescents and young adults.
    b. Sale of ENDS to minors younger than age 21 years should be prohibited.
    c. Candy and fruit-flavored ENDS, which encourage youth smoking initiation, should be banned.
    d. Federal, state, and local governments should enforce laws ensuring smoke-free environments, including ENDS vapor, in public places (AAP, 2018).
10. Compassionate and appropriate care for refugee children (Linton, Griffin, & Shapiro, 2017).
    a. Immigrant and refugee children should be treated with dignity and respect, and provided appropriate care that supports their health and well-being.
    b. Children should be provided with appropriate medical care that is culturally and linguistically sensitive throughout all phases of the immigration processing pathway.
    c. Children should not be exposed to settings or conditions that may cause traumatic stress, such as detention centers.
    d. Children should not be separated from their parents or primary caregivers.
    e. The Department of Homeland Security should consider community-based alternatives for family detention.

IX. **The Role of Advocacy in Organizational Policy Development**

Nurses' close interaction with individuals and their scientific knowledge of the care continuum places them in a unique position to lead in the redesign of health care systems from local practice environments to achieving system-wide change (Institute of Medicine [IOM], 2011). Improving the local practice environment through policy development is an excellent avenue for nurses to begin to influence the design of our health care system. Policies and procedures provide blueprints for the behavior of an organization and a framework that guides organizational consistency. Nursing policies define the standards of care and outline the necessary conditions required for appropriate care to occur (Burke, 2016). Once established, these policies will guide the ongoing development of consistent and measurable outcomes for individuals and families.

A. Advocacy and involvement for the CCTM RN includes developing and updating organizational policies that define process and outcome indicators related to care coordination.
  1. Participation on clinical practice committees (CPCs). Membership on departmental, service line, hospital, or health system CPCs is an excellent opportunity for nurses to contribute to the shaping of the care environment. CCTM RNs can ensure proper CCTM is part of the nursing process throughout the care continuum.
  2. Nursing policies, procedures, and standards provide evidence-based rationales for the practice of nursing.
  3. Nursing process standards define nursing practice and provide consistency in the delivery of care
B. Nurses with diverse practice expertise can provide insight for evidence-based rationales to support policy acceptance and implementation across the continuum of care. The care continuum covers multiple nursing specialties, all of which influence individuals' transition from acute care to ambulatory care.
  1. Acute care RNs will benefit from the involvement of CCTM ambulatory care RNs on interprofessional committees.
      a. Share expertise on effective CCTM.
      b. Educate colleagues on the importance of ambulatory care in preventing readmissions.
  2. Organizations striving for Magnet designation will benefit from ambulatory RN involvement and expertise.
      a. Ambulatory care nursing perspective and demonstration of improvement in individual care are essential elements to an organization's story.
      b. RNs should measure their organization's performance on recognized ambulatory nurse-sensitive individual indicators, such as the Ambulatory Care Nurse Sensitive Indicator Report (Mastal, Matlock, & Start, 2016).
          (1) Care coordination: Medication review and education.
          (2) Care coordination: Diagnostic tests.
          (3) Safety: Wrong site, wrong side, wrong individual, wrong procedure, wrong implant.
          (4) Safety: Individual burns.
          (5) Safety: Falls.
          (6) Transfer or admissions to acute care.

C. Nurses should continue to advance the science and care effectiveness of ambulatory care nursing by participating in the development of new ambulatory care-focused nurse-sensitive indicators (Mastal et al., 2016).
1. Potential indicators include:
   a. Readmissions across lifespan.
   b. Pain assessment and follow up.
   c. Screening for high blood pressure.
   d. Screening for depression.
   e. Screening for future fall risk.
   f. Screening for body mass index.
   g. Ambulatory care nursing demographics.
   h. Satisfaction with ambulatory nurse care.

X. **Advocacy, Public Policy Development, and Health Care Reform**

As the national health care system evolves, trends in where and how care is provided are transitioning from acute care to the ambulatory environment. It is critical nurses take an active role in the development of our nation's evolving health care system to ensure improvements in CCTM are embedded in our country's health care policies at the local, regional, and national levels.

The call for nurses to engage in health policy leadership has been growing, not only within the ranks of the nursing profession, but from governmental and health care organizational leaders (Ellenbecker et al., 2017). The time has arrived to ensure the importance of CCTM RN activities by ambulatory care nurses, as well as nurses in CCTM roles in other settings across the continuum, is inherently reflected in public policy.

A. Nurses must respect and utilize their power to achieve change.
   1. Nursing is viewed as the most honest and ethical profession (Brenan, 2017).
   2. Nursing is the largest medical profession (Brokaw, 2016).
   3. Nurses' knowledge of health care systems, combined with their analytic and communication skills, supports their qualifications to participate in developing health policy (Ellenbecker et al., 2017).
   4. This combination of public respect, professional size, and expertise places nursing in the unique role to influence change.

B. The first strategy is to embrace a sense of activism towards policy development.
   1. Historically, nurses have been indifferent to policy making (Ellenbecker et al., 2017).
   2. "As nurses, we need to think of policy as something we can influence, not just something that happens to us" (Brokaw, 2016, p. 1).
      a. Policy decisions impact departmental, organizational, professional, and societal environments.
      b. Policy decisions will be made regardless of participation, thus nursing input is needed.
   3. Take action to make your voice heard.
      a. Assume a leadership position at any level.
      b. Vote.
      c. Advocate to your leaders (both professional and political).
         (1) Call or write elected officials.
         (2) Testify at public hearings.
         (3) Join your professional association.

C. To achieve change, embrace the power of coalitions.
   1. Developing partnerships with physicians, pharmacists, and other health care professionals can influence transformative improvements at the organizational, local, and national levels.
      a. Interprofessional coalitions are effective political strategies for influencing health policy.
      b. Interprofessional support eases decision-makers' concerns regarding potential conflicts and turf battles regarding policy changes.
      c. Participation within professional associations and organizations can provide nurses the opportunity to influence policy.
         (1) Gaining professional organizational support adds the weight of the membership and goodwill of the organization to the proposed changes.
         (2) Organizations and associations open access to regional and national networks of professional colleagues.
         (3) Many organizations have policy advocacy expertise that can support nursing efforts to achieve change.
         (4) Hone skills engaging professional colleagues in association policy discussions and governance debates.

D. Educate the public.
   1. Public support can be a powerful tool in achieving policy improvements.
   2. Reach out to media outlets.
   3. Perform community education.

Chapter 2

E. Policy initiatives for care coordination. Efforts by nursing organizations and stakeholders to advance the benefits of care coordination and improve the practice environment for CCTM RNs have been ongoing for several years. It is important that nurses not only stay informed about ongoing efforts to improve the practice environment, but take an active role whenever possible to support the adoption or implementation of these recommendations.
 1. In 2012, the AAN, representing various nursing stakeholders, put forth recommendations to the Centers for Medicare & Medicaid Services (CMS) and the payer community (Cipriano, 2012). Recommendations included:
    a. Adopt clear definitions of care coordination and transitional care that can be used by all stakeholders.
    b. Implement payment models for evidence-based care coordination and transitional care services delivered at the community level.
    c. Ensure that approved care coordination and transitional care models are sustainable and replicable.
    d. Expedite funding to develop performance measures and supportive analytics.
    e. Invest in workforce development directly related to care coordination and transitional services.
 2. In 2014, the Care Coordination Task Force (CCTF) of the AAN was convened to develop recommendations for federal policy priorities that would sustain nursing contributions to care coordination across health care delivery environments, while reducing barriers to nurses practicing to the full scope of their education and experience (Lamb et al., 2015). Two major areas of policy priorities evolved through the work of the CCTF.
    a. Recommended that reimbursement for care coordination services be consistent for all qualified health professionals delivering those services.
       (1) Approve provisions for payment to specified providers of care coordination based on defined tasks and supportive documentation.
       (2) Advocate for inclusion of team-based models of reimbursement.
       (3) Recognize full scope of practice for advanced practice registered nurses (APRNs).
       (4) Recognize BSN-prepared nurses as qualified providers of care coordination services.
    b. Recommended the design and implementation of evidence-based care coordination measures should be accelerated, including those activities central to the domain of nursing practice.
       (1) Include nurses in the process of defining care coordination measures.
       (2) Convene stakeholders at the national level to identify pathways toward increased funding sources for the development and testing of measures central to nursing practice.
       (3) Ensure nurses are included on national review panels that are charged with developing care coordination measures.
 3. Primary care in the United States is changing rapidly to meet the evolving needs of individuals and families for care coordination (Bauer & Bodenheimer, 2017).
    a. Expanded roles for nurses are needed to improve quality and add capacity in primary care environments, particularly in chronic disease management.
       (1) The U.S. population of individuals age 65 years and older grew from 25.5 million in 1980 to 46.2 million in 2014.
       (2) This population is expected to increase by nearly 2 million annually up to 82.3 million in 2040.
       (3) 86% of older adult Americans have at least one chronic condition, and 33% have three or more chronic conditions.
    b. To assume expanded roles, several barriers must be overcome.
       (1) Payment reform.
       (2) Nursing education reform to include preparation of nurses for roles in primary care settings.
       (3) Scope of practice clarification for RNs performing care coordination activities using standardized procedures.
    c. Policy initiatives to address these needs include:
       (1) Recognition that primary care will be increasingly provided by NPs

as the number of PCPs continues to decrease.
                (2) To meet the needs of the millions of individuals with chronic health care needs, the number of RNs must expand, along with their scope of practice in chronic care management and care coordination.
    4. Opportunities for nurses to support these efforts and recommendations include:
        a. RN participation in the development of new care delivery models in state and local practice environments.
        b. Support efforts to build a more robust primary care model that will mitigate the need for more expensive acute care services.
        c. Assume roles (and seek leadership opportunities) essential to meeting the rapidly expanding demand for these services.
        d. Advocate for nurses to practice at the fullest extent of their licensure.

XI. **Leadership in CCTM**

Nurse leaders, acting as advocates, are responsible for the quality of care and services in their organizations. These leaders are positioned to use their professional knowledge base to lead care coordination initiatives and oversee models of care that manage services longitudinally across the health care continuum, as well as vertically among a variety of complex care delivery systems. CCTM roles are needed at all levels of organizations providing services across the care continuum. Nurse executives representing acute care, ambulatory care, and academic practice came together in early 2015 to collaborate around best leadership practices to enhance care coordination in health care organizations (Shulman, 2015).

A. Principles for establishing informed and collaborative care coordination processes:
    1. Know how care is coordinated in your setting.
        a. Understand the needs, requirements, and resources of your population.
        b. Track individuals' common pathways through your health care system.
        c. Understand your organization's transitional care infrastructure and how interprofessional leaders communicate.
    2. Know who is providing care.
        a. Conduct an organization-wide assessment of nurses and others providing CCTM services.
        b. Define evidence-based roles, responsibilities, and expected job results for all disciplines.
    3. Identify stakeholders among multiple entities involved in CCTM systems.
        a. Establish collaborative relationships and create a shared vision among leaders across the organizational continuum.
        b. Convene an interprofessional stakeholder group, which includes both internal and external team members involved in CCTM services.
        c. Seek input from all stakeholders to align and enhance communication.
    4. Understand the value of technology, and its impact on workflow and on the roles of CCTM team members.
        a. Assess the current state of technology and its impact on CCTM.
        b. Implement strategies to optimize information technology workflow to support CCTM roles.
        c. Leverage staff and leaders in technology to develop and disseminate data analytics in support of CCTM.
    5. Engage individuals and families.
        a. Utilize individual engagement strategies to assess and activate patient and family involvement in care.
        b. Ensure staff competencies in person and family engagement.
        c. Implement strategies and processes to engage individuals and families in the plan of care at all levels and among all providers.
        d. Identify structures and processes for providing individuals and families with a single point of contact for information.
        e. Include individuals and families on advisory boards and focus groups to ensure shared decision-making regarding CCTM processes.
    6. Engage all team members in CCTM.
        a. Identify senior leaders to serve as CCTM champions and leaders.
        b. Select physician and nurse-led leadership teams for CCTM initiatives.
        c. Educate leaders and staff regarding the value of CCTM in achieving the goals of the organization.

B. Five important CCTM leadership activities (Bower, 2016).
    1. Clarify the meaning and goals of care coordination specific to your organization.
        a. Goals provide a platform for ongoing evaluation.

b. A continuous evaluation and improvement process supports change and revision when and where needed.
c. Create new resources to address emerging problems.
2. Identify priorities specific to the populations served and the organization.
a. Define elements of CCTM for specific populations.
b. Integrate organizational priorities into the plan for CCTM.
3. Define roles, processes, and tools to support CCTM.
a. Identify individuals' care coordination needs.
b. Align individual needs with available resources.
4. Design continuum-based care.
a. Identify individual needs at all points of the care continuum.
b. Create roles and processes that support each element on the continuum.
5. Establish accountability for each CCTM role:
a. Define competencies for each role.
b. Educate staff continuously as the health care environment changes.

XII. Future Considerations for CCTM RN Practice

As the population of the United States continues to age, the work of government, health care systems, and health system leaders will be focused on the national priority of seamless, accessible, and affordable health care. Dr. Berwick's "Triple Aim" (Berwick, Nolan, & Whittington, 2008) accurately describes the goals that continue to challenge our country. Care coordination and transitional care innovations will be a priority in the years ahead. Advocacy will continue to be a critical element of CCTM nursing practice as we focus on emerging evidence-based interventions with the promise of improving individual, family, and population-centered care (Vinson, Toth-Lewis, & Grant, 2014). Leaders at the federal level should be urged to consider the issues discussed in this chapter as important decisions are made that impact the health of our nation. Addressing best practices in care coordination and transitional care within a framework of organizational ethics will assist leaders at all levels to design systems based on meeting the needs of individuals, families, and communities in this generation and the next (Naylor & Berlinger, 2016).

Chapter 2

Table 2-1.
Advocacy: Knowledge, Skills, and Attitudes for Competency

Advocacy in nursing practice is a process which involves a series of strategies and actions for preserving, representing, and/or safeguarding the best interests and values of individuals, families, and populations within the health care system.

Knowledge	Skills	Attitudes	Sources
Summarize principles of effective personal and professional communication.	Communicate individual, family, and community values, preferences, and expressed needs to members of the health care team.	Value active partnership with individuals and designated caregivers in planning, implementation, and evaluation of care.	Cronenwett et al., 2007
Discuss common barriers to active involvement of individuals and families in their own health care processes.	Assess level of individual and family decisional conflict and provide access to resources.	Value the individual and family expertise in defining self-care needs.	Cronenwett et al., 2007
Describe the impact of traumatic stress on overall health and well-being.	Demonstrate an understanding of the basic tenets of trauma-informed care.	Cultivate an awareness of the effects of trauma on physical, emotional, developmental, learning and social elements of health in children and adults.	Kenny et al., 2017 Beidas et al., 2016 Garg et al., 2015
Identify resources available to support individual and family needs.	Provide access to resources, including appropriate services, across settings and providers.	Respect individual and family right to access to personal health records. Appreciate the value of referrals across settings.	Cronenwett et al., 2007
Describe the importance of integrating behavioral and mental health assessment at each health encounter.	Demonstrate nursing assessment competencies which include behavioral and mental health needs of individuals and families.	Value and respect the impact of behavioral health issues on overall health and well-being.	Kilbourne et al., 2018 Soelberg et al., 2017 Olfson, 2016 Dobbs & Fogger, 2018
Integrate understanding of multiple dimensions of an individual's care. • Individual/family/community preferences and values. • Coordination and integration of care. • Transition and continuity.	Elicit and communicate the values, needs, and preferences of individuals, families, communities, and populations.	Value individual, family, and community expression of needs and preferences. Value the ability to see and understand health care situations through the eyes of individuals, families, and communities.	Cronenwett et al., 2007
Describe how diverse cultural, ethnic, and social backgrounds function as sources of individual, family, and community values.	• Practice cultural competency. • Deliver care with sensitivity and respect for the diversity of human experience.	Recognize personally held attitudes about working with individuals from different ethnic, cultural, and social backgrounds. Willingly support the care of individuals and groups whose values differ from our own.	Cronenwett et al., 2007

continued on next page

Table 2-1. (continued)
Advocacy: Knowledge, Skills, and Attitudes for Competency

Advocacy in nursing practice is a process which involves a series of strategies and actions for preserving, representing, and/or safeguarding the best interests and values of individuals, families, and populations within the health care system.

Knowledge	Skills	Attitudes	Sources
Discuss how health literacy is a necessary precursor to the achievement of health and well-being.	Assess and address health literacy for every individual and family at every health encounter. Integrate Health Literacy Universal Precautions into nursing practice. Demonstrate competency in health teaching as essential in providing nursing care.	Embrace the value of self-management of health by ensuring that individuals understand what they need to do after each health encounter. Cultivate an awareness that health literacy is often unrelated to socioeconomic status.	Loan et al., 2018 Barton et al., 2018 AHRQ, 2017
Describe strategies to empower individuals, families, and communities in all aspects of the health care process. Compare and contrast the role of CCTM nurses as advocates at the micro-social and macrosocial levels of care.	Assure individual's autonomy and self determination. Represent individual and family needs and preferences. Champion social justice in health care.	Defend the importance of establishing relationships with individuals and families in order to represent their needs and preferences at all levels.	Cronenwett et al., 2007 ANA, 2015 Bu & Jezewski, 2007
Demonstrate comprehensive understanding of the concepts of pain and suffering, including physiologic models of pain and comfort. Describe the importance of risk assessment in the CCTM nursing role. List evidence-based strategies for managing chronic pain.	Assess physical and emotional expressions of discomfort. Elicit expectations for relief of pain. Practice evidence-based strategies for managing chronic pain. Use evidence-based screening tools or ask individuals about substance use at each encounter. Counsel individuals and families regarding the risk of accidental overdose. Maximized use of non-pharmacological or non-opioid pain therapy. Practice medication review and reconciliation at every health care encounter.	Recognize personally held values and beliefs about the management of pain and discomfort. Appreciate the role of the nurse in relief of all types of and sources of pain and suffering. Recognize that individual and family expectations influence outcomes in the management of pain or suffering. Appreciate quality of life factors and weigh risks versus benefits in the use of opioids for treatment of chronic pain.	Cronenwett et al., 2007 Soelberg et al, 2017 Dobbs & Fogger, 2018

Source: Cronenwett et al. (2007). *Nursing Outlook, 55*(3), 122-131. Reprinted with permission from Elsevier.

Chapter 2

Case Study 2-1.
Exemplar in Nursing Advocacy: Achieving Universal Practice Change through Professional Organization Advocacy
Written by William Duffy, RN, MJ, CNOR, FAAN

Introduction

After the seminal *To Err Is Human* report (IOM, 2000), The Joint Commission issued its Universal Protocols that emphasized actions organizations should take to eliminate incorrect surgical procedures. However, The Joint Commission did not mandate a standard practice, and organizations adopted a variety of methods in implementing protocols. Variations in practice created a new set of problems for patients because members of the perioperative team often traveled between facilities that had different practices in implementing the protocol.

Advocacy

As president of the Association of periOperative Registered Nurses (AORN), I felt something must be done to standardize practice. This question was put to the AORN Board of Directors and staff, which debated the risks and benefits of acting. We knew this would require extreme effort and significant financial resources without a guarantee of success. But we recognized this was a chance to advocate for our patients at a national level. The Board agreed and allocated a significant portion of our financial reserves to spearhead the implementation of a standardized protocol. We knew we were doing the right thing but hoped the country and our membership would agree.

To create the protocol, we established a task force of nurses. We also invited nationally known safety experts to join our team to give fresh perspective, improve the quality of our work, and help ensure acceptance from stakeholders. This team developed the AORN Correct Site Surgery toolkit, which set out a step-by-step process for implementing the Universal Protocol (AORN, 2018).

Our next step was to develop a strategy to ensure implementation.

Strategy 1: Gaining support from organizational stakeholders. We knew the toolkit's success would depend on the support of various stakeholders in the perioperative process. We decided to build a consensus of supporting organizations, beginning with The Joint Commission and then expanding to the American College of Surgeons, the American Society of Anesthesiologists, and other professional organizations involved in surgical care. Next was the American Hospital Association, whose members would be key to gaining organizational support. With these professional organizations on board, we began building support among grassroots practitioners and organizations.

Strategy 2: Getting the toolkit out to practitioners. As nurses, we were acutely aware that getting research into practice takes years. We could not afford to wait that long because our coalition was united on the promise of action. So we decided to send a free toolkit (over 55,000) to every member of our association and every facility that performed invasive procedures. We then marketed the purpose and value of the toolkit through a variety of messaging to local chapter leaders and members.

Strategy 3: Gaining public support for the process. Then we focused on building public support to block resistors who could hinder implementation in practice environments. We invested in a public relations campaign and designated June 23, 2004, as AORN National Timeout Day.

Our campaign involved nurses giving interviews to local and national media on what patients should expect when having a procedure. Time Out Day was a resounding success and the top news story for weeks.

Clinical Implications

The practice of perioperative care has changed. The time out process has been adopted around the globe. Over the years, it has evolved and now has been incorporated in the World Health Organization Surgical Checklist. AORN members learned that nurses can change the way things are done. Our reputation for caring, our storytelling, and our compassion are powerful tools that can change the world.

Chapter 2

Case Study 2-2.
Enhancing Behavioral Health Services for Veterans

Introduction

Brad is a 30-year-old white male honorably discharged 1 year ago from the U.S. Army after 8 years of service that included two deployments to combat zones in Afghanistan and Iraq. Brad is married with one child and a second child expected in the next 3 months. He resides in a small town in the state of Washington, approximately 100 miles from Seattle. Brad sustained a right below the knee amputation secondary to combat during his last deployment. He has managed well through physical therapy and ambulates independently, but continues to experience chronic pain. Brad has had difficulty maintaining employment since his return home, and his wife reports concern that he is having difficulty managing stress related to his military service. He does not sleep well, uses alcohol moderately, and continues to use prescription pain medication to manage pain. Access to health care services is an issue for Brad due to the need to travel to the nearest VA facility.

Clinical Interaction

Prior to his appointment, Brad is contacted by Michelle, a VA RN care manager. Michelle confirms Brad's upcoming appointment, verifies demographic information, and asks a few brief assessment questions regarding Brad's general health and well-being. The following week, Brad travels to the nearest VA facility for his primary care visit. He meets initially with the primary care RN, who completes an intake assessment that includes brief screening for depression (PHQ2) and alcohol use (AUDIT-C). Following a complete physical and assessment with a primary care physician, Brad is introduced to Susan, a nurse whose role is with the Primary Care Mental Health Integration (PCMHI) team. Susan completes more in-depth screening for depression (PHQ9), for post-traumatic stress disorder (PTSD) using the PCL-5, and for anxiety using the General Anxiety and Depression (GAD) tool. Brad and Susan meet again with the primary care provider to discuss the plan of care. Brad is offered the opportunity to connect via video conference to a PCMHI psychiatrist who is available immediately to support Brad in his journey to wellness.

Clinical Plan and Implications

The plan of care includes weekly therapy sessions delivered via teleconference to Brad in his home. These services are part of the VA Video Connect program serving Veterans through an extensive network of telehealth services. Using the mHealth app, Brad is able to arrange weekly sessions with his mental health provider using his iPad from home. By using standardized screening tools, the PCMHI team is able to measure Brad's continuous progress or determine the need for additional services.

Brad's PTSD and anxiety have shown measured improvement, as evidenced by regular assessment using standardized tools. He is currently employed, and through the integrated specialty teams at the VA, is managing his pain without the use of opioid pain medications. He meets with a local physical therapist monthly to monitor mobility issues with his prosthesis and has joined a local Veterans' advocacy group which connects him to other Veterans.

Telehealth services are widely used in the VA system, as evidenced by the 702,000 Veterans (12% of the country's Veteran population) who have used telehealth or telemedicine in FY 2016, accounting for 2.17 million telehealth encounters. Approximately 45% of these encounters were delivered to Veterans like Brad who reside in rural communities (https://mhealthintelligence.com).

References

Agency for Healthcare Research and Quality (AHRQ). (2017). *AHRQ health literacy universal precautions toolkit* (2nd ed.). Retrieved from https://www.ahrq.gov/professionals/quality-patient-safety/quality-resources/tools/literacy-toolkit/index.html

Alzheimer's Association. (2018). 2018 Alzheimer's disease facts and figures. *Alzheimer's & Dementia, 2018*(14), 367-429. doi:10.1016/j.jalz.2018.02.001

American Academy of Ambulatory Care Nursing (AAACN). (2016). *Scope and standards of practice for registered nurses in care coordination and transition management.* Pitman, NJ: Author.

American Academy of Pediatrics (AAP). (2018). *State advocacy.* Retrieved from https://www.aap.org/en-us/advocacy-and-policy/state-advocacy/Pages/State-Advocacy.aspx

American Nurses Association (ANA). (2015). *Code of ethics for nurses with interpretative statements.* Silver Spring. MD: Nursebooks.org.

Association of periOperative Registered Nurses (AORN). (2018). *Correct site surgery toolkit.* Retrieved from https://www.aorn.org/guidelines/clinical-resources/tool-kits/correct-site-surgery-tool-kit

Baker, J., Travers, J.L., Buschman, P., & Merrill, J.A. (2018). An efficient nurse practitioner-led community-based service model for delivering coordinated care to persons with serious mental illness at risk for homelessness. *Journal of the American Psychiatric Nurses Association, 24*(2), 101-108. doi:10.1177/1078390317704044

Barton, A.J., Allen, P.E., Boyle, D.K., Loan, L.A., Stichler, J.F., & Parnell, T.A. (2018). Health literacy: Essential for a culture of health. *Journal of Continuing Education in Nursing, 49*(2), 73-78. doi:10.3928/00220124-20180116-06

Batterham, R.W., Hawkins, M., Collins, P.A., Buchbinder, R., & Osborne, R.H. (2016). Health literacy: Applying current concepts to improve health services and reduce health inequalities. *Public Health, 132*, 3-12. doi:10.1016/j.puhe.2016.01.001

Bauer, L., & Bodenheimer, T. (2017). Expanded roles of registered nurses in primary care delivery of the future. *Nursing Outlook, 65*(5), 624-632. doi:10.1016/j.outlook.2017.03.011

Beidas, R.S., Adams, D.R., Kratz, H.E., Jackson, K., Berkowitz, S., Zinny, A., ... Evans, A. (2016). Lessons learned while building a trauma-informed public behavioral health system in the City of Philadelphia. *Evaluation and Program Planning, 59*, 21-32. doi:10.1016/j.evalprogplan.2016.07.004

Berwick, D.M., Nolan, T.W., & Whittington, J. (2008). The triple aim: Care, health, and cost. *Health Affairs, 27*(3), 759-769. doi:10.1377/hlthaff.27.3.759

Bonsack, C., Golay, P., Gibellini Manetti, S., Gebel, S., Ferrari, P., Besse, C., ... Morandi, S. (2016). Linking primary and secondary care after psychiatric hospitalization: Comparison between transitional case management setting and routine care for common mental disorders. *Front Psychiatry, 7*, 96. doi:10.3389/fpsyt.2016.00096

Bower, K.A. (2016). Nursing leadership and care coordination: Creating excellence in coordinating care across the continuum. *Nursing Administration Quarterly, 40*(2), 98-102. doi:10.1097/NAQ.0000000000000162

Boyle, J., Speroff, T., Worley, K., Cao, A., Goggins, K., Dittus, R.S., & Kripalani, S. (2017). Low health literacy is associated with increased transitional care needs in hospitalized patients. *Journal of Hospital Medicine, 12*(11), 918-924. doi:10.12788/jhm.2841

Brenan, M. (2017). *Nurses keep lead as most honest ethical profession.* Retrieved from http://news.gallup.com/poll/224639/nurses-keep-healthy-lead-honest-ethical-profession.aspx

Brewster, A.L., Brault, M.A., Tan, A.X., Curry, L.A., & Bradley, E.H. (2017). Patterns of collaboration among health care and social services providers in communities with lower health care utilization and costs. *Health Services Research, 53*(Suppl. 1), 2892-2909. doi:10.1111/1475-6773.12775

Brody, D.J., Pratt, L.A., & Hughes, J.P. (2018). Prevalence of depression among adults aged 20 and over: United States, 2013-2016 *National Center for Health Statistics Data Brief, 303*, 1-8.

Brokaw, J. (2016). *The nursing profession's potential impact on policy and politics.* Retrieved from https://www.americannursetoday.com/blog/nursing-professions-potential-impact-policy-politics/

Brown, N.M., Green, J.C., Desai, M.M., Weitzman, C.C., & Rosenthal, M.S. (2014). Need and unmet need for care coordination among children with mental health conditions. *Pediatrics, 133*(3), e530-e537. doi:10.1542/peds.2013-2590

Brown, J.D., King, M.A., & Wissow, L.S. (2017). The central role of relationships with trauma-informed integrated care for children and youth. *Academic Pediatrics, 17*(7S), S94-S101. doi:10.1016/j.acap.2017.01.013

Bu, X., & Jezewski, M.A. (2007). Developing a mid-range theory of patient advocacy through concept analysis. *Journal of Advanced Nursing, 57*(1), 101-110. doi:10.1111/j.1365-2648.2006.04096.x

Burke, S.A. (2016). *Influence through policy: Nurses have a unique role.* Retrieved from https://www.reflectionsonnursingleadership.org/commentary/more-commentary/Vol42_2_nurses-have-a-unique-role

Camicia, M., Black, T., Farrell, J., Waites, K., Wirt, S., & Lutz, B. (2014). The essential role of the rehabilitation nurse in facilitating care transitions: A white paper by the association of rehabilitation nurses. *Rehabilitation Nursing, 39*(1), 3-15. doi:10.1002/rnj.135

Choi, P.P. (2015). Patient advocacy: The role of the nurse. *Nursing Standard, 29*(41), 52-58. doi:10.7748/ns.29.41.52.e9772

Chung, E.K., Siegel, B.S., Garg, A., Conroy, K., Gross, R.S., Long, D.A., ... Fierman, A.H. (2016). Screening for social determinants of health among children and families living in poverty: A guide for clinicians. *Current Problems in Pediatric and Adolescent Health Care, 46*(5), 135-153. doi:10.1016/j.cppeds.2016.02.004

Cipriano, P. (2012). American Academy of Nursing on Policy. The imperative for patient-, family-, and population-centered interprofessional approaches to care coordination and transitional care: A policy brief by the American Academy of Nursing's Care Coordination Task Force. *Nursing Outlook, 60*(5), 330-333. doi:10.1016/j.outlook.2012.06.021

Cronenwett, L., Sherwood, G., Barnsteiner, J., Disch, J., Johnson, J., Mitchell, P. ... Warren, J. (2007). Quality and safety education for nurses. *Nursing Outlook, 55*(3), 122-131.

Dayton, L., Agosti, J., Bernard-Pearl, D., Earls, M., Farinholt, K., Groves, B.M., ... Wissow, L.S. (2016). Integrating mental and physical health services using a socio-emotional trauma lens. *Current Problems in Pediatric and Adolescent Health Care, 46*(12), 391-401. doi:10.1016/j.cppeds.2016.11.004

Dobbs, G.C., & Fogger, S.A. (2018). Opiate dependence or addiction?: A review of the centers for disease control and prevention guidelines for management of chronic pain. *Journal of Addictions Nursing, 29*(1), 57-61. doi:10.1097/jan.0000000000000212

Dowell, D., Zhang, K., Noonan, R.K., & Hockenberry, J.M. (2016). Mandatory provider review and pain clinic laws reduce the amounts of opioids prescribed and overdose death rates. *Health Affairs, 35*(10), 1876-1883. doi:10.1377/hlthaff.2016.0448

Ellenbecker, C.H., Fawcett, J., Jones, E.J., Mahoney, D., Rowlands, B., & Waddell, A. (2017). A staged approach to educating nurses in health policy. *Policy, Politics & Nursing Practice, 18*(1), 44-56. doi:10.1177/1527154417709254

Garg, A., Toy, S., Tripodis, Y., Silverstein, M., & Freeman, E.R. (2015). Addressing social determinants of health at well child care visits: A cluster RCT. *Pediatrics, 135*(2), e296-e304. doi:10.1542/peds.2014-2888

Grace, P., & Milliken, A. (2016). Educating nurses for ethical practice in contemporary health care environments. *Hastings Center Report, 46*(Suppl. 1), S13-S17. doi:10.1002/hast.625

Haggerty, J.L., Roberge, D., Freeman, G.K., & Beaulieu, C. (2013). Experienced continuity of care when patients see multiple clinicians: A qualitative metasummary. *Annals of Family Medicine, 11*(3), 262-271. doi:10.1370/afm.1499

Hirschman, K.B., & Hodgson, N.A. (2018). Evidence-based interventions for transitions in care for individuals living with dementia. *The Gerontologist, 58*(Suppl. 1), S129-S140. doi:10.1093/geront/gnx152

Institute of Medicine (IOM). (2009). *To err is human: Building a safer health system.* Washington, DC: National Academies Press.

Institute of Medicine (IOM). (2011). *The future of nursing: Leading change, advancing health.* Washington, DC: The National Academies Press.

Kenny, M.C., Vazquez, A., Long, H., & Thompson, D. (2017). Implementation and program evaluation of trauma-informed care training across state child advocacy centers: An exploratory study. *Children and Youth Services Review, 73*, 15-23. doi:10.1016/j.childyouth.2016.11.030

Kilbourne, A.M., Beck, K., Spaeth-Rublee, B., Ramanuj, P., O'Brien, R.W., Tomoyasu, N., & Pincus, H.A. (2018). Measuring and improving the quality of mental health care: A global perspective. *World Psychiatry, 17*(1), 30-38. doi:10.1002/wps.20482

Kolko, D.J., & Perrin, E. (2014). The integration of behavioral health interventions in children's health care: Services, science, and suggestions. *Journal of Clinical Child and Adolescent Psychology, 43*(2), 216-228. doi:10.1080/15374416.2013.862804

Lamb, G., Newhouse, R., Beverly, C., Toney, D.A., Cropley, S., Weaver, C.A., ... Peterson, C. (2015). Policy agenda for nurse-led care coordination. *Nursing Outlook, 63*(4), 521-530. doi:10.1016/j.outlook.2015.06.003

Lathrop, B. (2013). Nursing leadership in addressing the social determinants of health. *Policy, Politics & Nursing Practice, 14*(1), 41-47. doi:10.1177/1527154413489887

Linton, J.M., Griffin, M., & Shapiro, A.J. (2017). Detention of immigrant children. *Pediatrics, 139*(5). doi:10.1542/peds.2017-0483

Loan, L.A., Parnell, T.A., Stichler, J.F., Boyle, D.K., Allen, P., VanFosson, C.A., & Barton, A.J. (2018). Call for action: Nurses must play a critical role to enhance health literacy. *Nursing Outlook, 66*(1), 97-100. doi:10.1016/j.outlook.2017.11.003

Mastal, M., Matlock, A.M., & Start, R. (2016). Ambulatory care nurse-sensitive indicators series: Capturing the role of nursing in ambulatory care – The case for meaningful nurse-sensitive measurement. *Nursing Economic$, 34*(2), 92-97, 76.

Milliken, A., & Grace, P. (2017). Nurse ethical awareness: Understanding the nature of everyday practice. *Nursing Ethics, 24*(5), 517-524. doi:10.1177/0969733015615172

Naylor, M., & Berlinger, N. (2016). Transitional care: A priority for health care organizational ethics. *Hastings Center Report, 46*(Suppl. 1), S39-S42. doi:10.1002/hast.631

Olfson, M. (2016). The rise of primary care physicians in the provision of U.S. mental health care. *Journal of Health Politics, Policy and Law, 41*(4), 559-583. doi:10.1215/03616878-3620821

Persaud, S. (2018). Addressing social determinants of health through advocacy. *Nursing Administration Quarterly, 42*(2), 123-128. doi:10.1097/naq.0000000000000277

Scotten, M. (2015). Parental health literacy and its impact on patient care. *Primary Care: Clinics in Office Practice, 42*(1), 1-16. doi:10.1016/j.pop.2014.09.009

Shulman, K.M. (2015). Joint statement: The role of the nurse leader in care coordination and transition management across the health care continuum. *Nursing Economic$, 33*(5), 281-282.

Soelberg, C.D., Brown, R.E., Jr., Du Vivier, D., Meyer, J.E., & Ramachandran, B.K. (2017). The U.S. opioid crisis: Current federal and state legal issues. *Anesthesia and Analgesia, 125*(5), 1675-1681. doi:10.1213/ane.0000000000002403

Taylor, L.A., Tan, A.X., Coyle, C.E., Ndumele, C., Rogan, E., Canavan, M., ... Bradley, E.H. (2016). Leveraging the social determinants of health: What works? *PloS One, 11*(8), e0160217. doi:10.1371/journal.pone.0160217

Vinson, M.H., Toth-Lewis, J.M., & Grant, V. (2014). Advocacy. In S.A. Haas, B.A. Swan, & T.S. Haynes (Eds.), *Care coordination and transition management core curriculum* (1st ed., pp. 13-21). Pittman, NJ: American Academy of Ambulatory Care Nursing.

Water, T., Ford, K., Spence, D., & Rasmussen, S. (2016). Patient advocacy by nurses – Past, present and future. *Contemporary Nurse, 52*(6), 696-709. doi:10.1080/10376178.2016.1235981

World Health Organization. (2018). *About social determinants of health.* Retrieved from http://www.who.int/social_determinants/sdh_definition/en/

Chapter 3

Instructions for Continuing Nursing Education Contact Hours

Continuing nursing education credit can be earned for completing the learning activity associated with this chapter. Instructions can be found at aaacn.org/CCTMCoreCNE

Education and Engagement of Individuals and Families

Cheryl Lovlien, MS, RN-BC
Denise Rismeyer, MSN, RN, RN-BC
Jayme M. Speight, MSN, RN-BC

Learning Outcome Statement

After completing this learning activity, the learner will be able to identify methods to assess individual, family/caregiver learning needs, create learning opportunities, and promote an open learning environment in which the learner works toward self-management and optimal health.

Learning Objectives

After reading this chapter, the Care Coordination and Transition Management registered nurse (CCTM® RN) will be able to:
- Identify individual, family/caregiver education needs, goals, and expected behavioral outcomes.
- Discuss steps to assess learning needs, readiness to learn, and health literacy needed to plan education.
- Implement and evaluate education and learning across the lifespan for individual, family/caregiver members.
- Employ methods to actively engage individual, family/caregiver in health care.
- Review educational principles and theories of learning.
- Apply methods of teaching and learning that focus on special populations and how they best learn, assimilate information, and improve outcomes.
- Use methods, such as 'teach back' to assess learning and health literacy.
- Demonstrate the knowledge, skills, and attitudes required for the education and engagement of individual, family/caregiver dimension (see Table 3-1 on page 61).

AAACN Care Coordination and Transition Management Standard
Standard 5b. Health Teaching and Health Promotion

Source: AAACN, 2016.

Competency Definition
Competency: Engaging individuals, families/caregivers. Creating a partnership with the individual, family/caregiver through communication, collaboration, and developing a trusting relationship. This includes assisting the individual, family/caregiver to be involved and preparing him/herself for a provider visit, encouraging the use of notes and reminders, encouraging questions, and identifying health goals (Agency for Healthcare Research and Quality [AHRQ], 2018c).

Nurses in care coordination and transition management (CCTM) have a role in serving the individual, family/caregiver in creating an open environment to identify learning needs, capacity to learn, and honoring the individual and his or her cultural background. The nurse will identify the method to support the learner through identifying opportunities to share information, considering each person's values and beliefs. Prioritizing information, the nurse identifies important aspects for self-management, assisting the individual, family/caregiver in becoming actively engaged in their health care. Time is taken to evaluate the effectiveness of learning and the effect of learning on health outcomes (American Academy for Ambulatory Care Nursing [AAACN], 2016).

Individual and family education has been accepted as a standard of practice for nursing. Traditions of caring for others through the translation of health care into knowledge for individuals and families were foundational from

Florence Nightingale and continue today. Methods of education have changed over time, but the need exists today and is a key component of nursing action (Bastable, 2017).

Health care information flow has traditionally been a one-way communication between a member of the care team and the receiver, as individual, family/caregiver, with little time or effort taken to identify if the education was clear, meaningful, or able to be accomplished. Cognitive learning theory identifies the need for the learner to gain attention, receive the information, and identify how that information is used. Learners need to process information to demonstrate understanding (Bastable, 2017).

Education of individuals, families/caregivers is a major dimension of the role of the registered nurse in care coordination and transition management (CCTM RN), with the expectation individual, and families/caregivers will adapt and apply health practices to improve health outcomes. Once the provider and/or CCTM RN completes the provision of care and the individual, family/caregiver leaves the care facility, it is up to the individual, family/caregiver to implement the continuing care plans and activities to promote or improve health. The success of the educational efforts will hinge upon the ability of the individual, family/caregiver to understand the disease process and treatment plan, and to incorporate that knowledge into actionable behaviors that will promote lifestyle changes. To achieve this goal, the individual, family/caregiver needs to understand health, illness, and influencing factors through communication that meets their level of understanding in a manner that is respectful and engaging and encompasses their culture and diversity (Hibbard, 2016). The CCTM RN must be aware of the individual, family/caregiver's level of health literacy and find resources that best help them learn new concepts, integrate and internalize those concepts, and be able to change behaviors with reinforcement of those concepts from members of the health care team. This is a collaborative relationship between the CCTM RN and individual, family/caregiver, and a relationship that must be constantly nurtured.

Engaging individuals in their health care through activation improves outcomes (Do, Young, Barnason, & Tran, 2015). Individuals within the context of the Patient-Centered Medical Home (PCMH) should receive person-centered care focused on the needs of that person, and within the context of his or her culture, values, and preferences (AHRQ, 2015). Individuals should receive support for self-care efforts and involvement with the health care plan. Providing education and information to individuals, families/caregivers is a core dimension in the CCTM RN that assists individuals and families/caregivers to anticipate needs and use tools to improve or maintain health (Naylor et al., 2017).

I. **Assess Readiness for Learning**

A. Identify the audience.
  1. Identify who will participate in learning: individual, family/caregivers.
  2.. Establish relationships with individuals, families/caregivers that are open to conversation and discussion. Individuals, families/caregivers are the experts of their health experience and will identify what they perceive as a learning need (Bastable, 2017).
  3. Age differences for education: See Table 3-2. As individuals change and grow, so do their learning abilities.
  4. Considerations of ability that may interfere or inhibit learning.
      a. Hearing loss may affect one in eight people over the age of 12 years. Two percent of adults aged 45 to 54 years have disabling hearing loss, 25% of those ages 65 to 74 years and 50% for those who are 75 years and older (U.S. Department of Health and Human Services [DHHS], 2016).
      b. Learning disabilities (e.g., dyslexia): Learning disabilities are a group of varying disorders that have a negative impact on learning. They may affect one's ability to speak, listen, think, read, write, spell, or compute. The most prevalent learning disability is in the area of reading, known as dyslexia (National Center for Learning Disabilities, 2014).
      c. Intellectual disability is evident through observed limitations in behaviors, such as social and practical skills in daily living. This does not mean the person cannot learn; however, the approach is important:
          (1) Focus on ability.
          (2) Support a relationship of trust.
          (3) Speak directly to the person, keep eye contact, and use plain speech.
          (4) Ask permission prior to using another person to help with his or her care.
          (5) Use many different methods to convey the information.

Chapter 3

Table 3-2.
Age Differences in Learning

Age Range	Ability to Learn	Methods
0-1 years/ 1-2 years	Driven by environment Through sensation Curious	Teach to the parent/caregiver Use sensory adapted play and use of objects
3-5 years	Concerned about self and needs Directed by fear Associates pain with punishment Active, uses body to learn Curious Imagination & play	Use calm, build trust through play Repeat information Reassure Safe secure environment Play with objects Use dolls Ask parents for information on child's abilities
6-11 years	Ability to reason maturing Concrete learning Makes associations with objects and events Concentrates on the present	Honest information Explain and ask questions Tell them honestly what it will feel like Use play: dolls, drawings, audio and video
	Prefer learning from parents based on the diagnosis; however, this is dependent on the literacy level of the parent	Health care providers need to adjust the way they share information with children based on their learning preference. Use of the internet: the health care provider should assist to identify reliable resources Diabetes Mellitus diagnosed: prefer learning from other kids with the disease African Americans preferred health care providers as a source of information (Johnson, Javalkar, Tilburg, Habrman, Rak & Ferris, 2015)
10-19 years		Rapid Estimate of Adult Literacy in Medicine-Teen (REAL-Teen); identifies the ability of adolescents in this age range to use written materials (Cohen, et al., 2015)
12-19 years	Reasons by logic Thinks things through Thinks about the future Desires acceptance Peers are important	Build trust through honesty Seek to understand concerns Allay fears Use peer groups Negotiate as needed Use electronic tools: internet, gaming, role play, reading materials May choose not to have parents present
		Successful Transition to Adulthood with Therapeutics Rx (STARx) Questionnaire: Identifies through self-report readiness related to chronic illness and the ability to engage in medication management, communication with providers, assuming adult responsibilities in regard to health and knowledge of resources (Cohen, et al., 2015)
20-40 years	Self-directed Bases learning on past lived experience Self-motivated	Focus on the problem and solution Provide avenue to read more Engage person as active participant Ask open-ended questions to identify perceptions and need for further education

continued on next page

**Table 3-2. (continued)
Age Differences in Learning**

Age Range	Ability to Learn	Methods
41-64 years	Self-directed Changes noticed related to aging Self-motivated Re-examines life and goals for the near future	Focus on future goals and maintenance of activities Assess learning needs, previous methods of learning and preferences
65 + years	Information processing takes time Thinks concretely Decreased short-term memory	Use concrete examples Use life experiences Allow time to process Introduce one concept and determine learning, then move on Encourage self-management Use materials that provide contrast Allow extra time

Source: Bastable, 2017.

      (6) Demonstrate and then have the person demonstrate (Werner, Yalon-Chamovitz, Tenne Rinde, & Heymann, 2017).
   d. Social networks and support improve the ability to self-manage related to health behaviors (Koetsenruijter et al., 2016).
B. Create an environment of learning (Bastable, 2017).
   1. Identify the 'right' time for the discussion: Provide education when the individual, family/caregiver is ready.
   2. Decrease distractions, such as environmental noise (e.g., TV, radio, other conversations).
   3. Arrange furniture that allows discussion.
   4. Prepare individual learning materials: Reading materials at the appropriate reading level, note taking, graphics, pictures, videos, computers.
C. Alternate learning environments.
   1. Convene shared medical appointments.
   2. Initiate telephone calls to individual, family/caregiver to engage in self-care and lifestyle counseling.
   3. Initiate programs, such as grocery shopping with dietitian, cooking demonstrations, and providing appropriate recipes.
   4. Provide small group informational seminars.
   5. Prepare and provide simple exercises that can be done at home; no gym required (Cesta, 2011).
D. Electronic methods of learning.
   1. Facebook formats, connecting stories from those who have had experience (Frederick, Bober, Berwick, Tower, & Kenney, 2017).
   2. Patient portal or eHealth.
   3. Smartphone utilization for medication adherence.
   4. Virtual provider care (remote patient care) (Harding, Mersha, Vassalotti, Webb, & Nicholas, 2017).

II. **Assessment of Knowledge and Abilities**
A. Health literacy. See Chapter 1, "Introduction."
   1. Health literacy is the ability to comprehend the language of health, process and use information to make health decisions, and take actions to self-care (Osborne, 2018).
   2. Low health literacy is associated with less-than-adequate caregiver support, lower level of understanding of the use of medical devices, and a higher risk of physical decline (Boyle et al., 2017).
B. Literacy assessment.
   1. Language: Greater than one-third of all adults cannot read or understand the written word. Most written patient education is at the 8th grade level or higher (Hersh, Salzman, & Snyderman, 2017).
   2. More than one-third of individuals may lack essential skills to handle their health (Hersh et al., 2017).
      a. Identify and determine the best way for the learner to understand information provided and their role in managing the information.
      b. Choose the method or modality that individual, family/caregiver members identify as an effective method for learning in the past.
C. Culture.

Chapter 3

1. Culture affects how people communicate, understand, and respond to health information. The ability to work with people in other cultures related to their health literacy requires cultural competence. This means sensitivity to and valuing the individual's cultural beliefs, values, attitudes, traditions, language, and health practices to work toward positive health outcomes (Narayan, 2017).
2. Use of interpreters:
    a. Allow sufficient time for interactions, speak slowly and clearly.
    b. Use simple sentences.
    c. Look at the individual not the interpreter.
    d. Avoid medical jargon.
    e. Use language tools available.
    f. Communicate with drawings such as:
        (1) Anatomical models.
        (2) Rating scales.
    g. Appreciate differences in body language.
    h. Notice signs of difficulty.
    i. Verify understanding, asking the individual, family/caregiver to explain in their own words or describe through an interpreter.

D. Social groups.
   Generations are social groups bound by a shared life experience usually grouped into 20-year spans of time. Each generation has expectations from the health care system, including how to learn about their health care.
   1. The Silent Generation (born prior to 1946): Respect the formality of the doctor as leader of health care. They want to learn from the expert.
   2. Baby Boomers (born 1946-1962): Are team players and prefer team aspects of the health care team. They want to participate in their health care and dialogue about many aspects and questions they may have.
   3. Generation X (born 1963-1980): Would like to have their health care delivered through electronic means, such as telehealth and education via electronic means. Education needs to be short and direct. This group is okay with seeking answers to their questions.
   4. Millennials (born 1980-2000): Are even more engaged in technology and seeking health care education. They are prone to close social groups, and want to get to know others and learn in group environments (Heath, 2016).
   5. Generation Z (born 2000+): Value for convenience. They would like it easy, using digital methods, and love gaming. They text in short phrases and want information in short bytes; however, they also like the human touch and being talked to as a person (Busenbark, 2017).

E. Assess styles in which people learn.
   1. Visual: Seeing/watching.
   2. Auditory: Listening.
   3. Kinesthetic: Hands-on learning (using touch and manipulatives).
   4. One or more of the above.

F. Assess individual, family/caregiver knowledge of health/disease.
   1. What does the learner know or not know about the following relating to his or her health/disease:
      a. Risk factors for disease.
      b. Symptoms.
      c. Infection control practices.
      d. Communication of errors and omissions.
      e. Resources regarding care for disease, health, and wellness.

III. **Methods to Provide Education**

A. Teach to meet needs of health literacy: Over 30% of U.S. adults have challenges in understanding health care information (Hersh et al., 2017).
B. Teach using a 'universal precautions' approach, so all communications are clear, assuming all individuals have trouble understanding.
   1. Design written materials, format, and information delivery to match learning needs.
   2. Multimedia: For those unable to process written materials, other techniques and modalities must be used, including illustrations, DVDs or CDs, streaming media, and podcasts.
   3. Use plain language to make written and oral information easier to understand for all people.
      a. Provide the most important information first.
      b. Break content into smaller, understandable "chunks" of information.
      c. Use simple words and define technical terms.
      d. Use active voice (Batterham, Hawkins, Collins, Buchbinder, & Osborne, 2016), which is writing sentences where the action is done by the subject.
   4. Picture-based instructions/illustrations.

Pictorial representations show individual, family/caregivers illustrative diagrams or pictures of anatomical representations of organs (e.g., show normal heart and then heart with signs of valve issues).
5. Graphs to illustrate health risk: Utilize graphs on disease morbidity and quantitative health risks in specific age groups and ethnic populations (Bastable, 2017).
6. Utilization of health information technology (HIT). The availability of technology across generations and income levels have changed the method of education delivery for health care. Technology and e-health tools support individual engagement in their skill and knowledge of disease by use of technology. This allows collaboration with the provider and communication with the health care team, as well as connection to education materials and resources. Methods include:
    a. Electronic access to health records.
    b. Use of mobile technologies.
    c. Use of health monitoring devices that connect to the health care organization with oversight by a health care provider.
    d. Secure email/messaging through patient portals.
    e. Access to Internet-based learning modules and resources.
    f. Video chat and consultation.
    g. Social media and chat rooms (Rozenblum, Miller, Pearson, & Marelli, 2015).
    h. Adolescents and young adults may benefit from engagement in technology-based learning and socialized learning (Coyne, Prizeman, Sheehan, Malone, & While, 2016).
C. Provide individualized education that includes components of communication, including active listening (Casimir, Williams, Liang, Pitakmongkolkul, & Slyer, 2014).
    1. Recognize words used and body language, eye contact, voice intonation.
    2. Listen for what is *not* said.
    3. Reinforce with positive comments when individuals learn well.
    4. Reiterate content that is missed and supplement with written instructions and illustrations.
    5. Break teaching into short manageable sections.
    6. Reinforce previously learned content prior to moving on to other areas of information.
D. Utilize "teach-back:" A method of teaching individuals and assessing learning; providing clear information for individuals, families/caregivers (Always Use Teach-back!, 2018; Peter et al., 2015).
    1. Use a clear, caring tone of voice.
    2. Keep an open and comfortable body position and speak to the person.
    3. Use plain language, no acronyms or words that are medical jargon.
    4. Have the person repeat back what you said in their own words
    5. Use open questions that explore understanding. Sentences that start with "what," "why," or "how" will assist to keep answers from just "yes" or "no."
    6. Create an open environment of exploration where the responsibility is on the nurse to identify how to help the person understand.
    7. Be patient and re-teach with the person explaining again from their perspective.
    8. Use reading materials with pictures/images that assist to explain difficult concepts.
E. Share information on how the individual and family can engage in the process of learning more about their health and concerns. (See the AHRQ [2018b] clinician guideline "Helping Patients and Families Prepare for an Appointment.")
F. Individuals, families/caregivers are encouraged to discuss their health care concerns in their own words and to re-explain or reiterate information to the health care provider. This process can improve individual health outcomes and provider communication (National Institutes of Health [NIH], n.d.).
    1. Assist individuals to ask questions.
        a. Offer a notepad.
        b. Allow time to write answers.
        c. Provide a writing surface.
    2. Acknowledge what individuals have already heard or read.
    3. Confirm they heard what you said.
    4. Confirm you heard what they said.
    5. Provide ways for individuals to learn more, offering pamphlets, websites, videos, and reliable sources of medical information.
    6. Ask questions that require more than a "yes" or "no" answer: Ask open-ended questions and examples of what the individual is most concerned about (e.g., *What concerns you most about this diagnosis?* or *Tell me about how you see your life changing?*).
    7. Encourage the individual to:
        a. Take note of symptoms: Timing, intensity, characteristics.

b. Invite individuals to bring the family/caregiver/advocate to learning sessions.
c. Use devices such as hearing aids/eyeglasses.
d. Learn only as much as they want to know.
e. Create personal medical record (NIH, 2017) (see Appendix 3-1).
8. Simplify language for translation (avoid using multisyllabic words, such as hypertension, replace with high blood pressure).
9. Inform individuals about availability of translations into their native language.
10. Use culturally appropriate/age-appropriate examples.
11. Avoid jargon, abbreviations (write it out), acronyms, homonyms (gait, stool), idioms ("heads up" or "feeling blue") (PlainLanguage.gov, 2011).
12. Talk about topics one at a time, gain an understanding, and then move on.
13. Build on the familiar: Ask individuals what they are currently doing to manage their condition and offer suggestions of ways to optimize what they are doing or to support problem solving.
14. Explain in plain language (make it real: 5 lb. bag of flour).
15. Prioritize information based on needs for survival.
   a. Actions for survival.
   b. Actions easy to do.
   c. Resources needed to get to actions (Osborne, 2018; Wein & Hicklin, 2015).
16. Watch for cues the discussion is moving too fast or slow, such as wandering eyes, shifting positions, looking to family/caregivers for support, etc.
17. Use 'Ask Me 3' as a tool for individuals, families/caregivers to use when discussing their healthcare with their provider (Institute for Healthcare Improvement, 2018).
   a. What is my main problem?
   b. What do I need to do?
   c. Why is it important for me to do this?
F. Peer or group discussions:
   1. Use community setting.
   2. Social networks may improve learning (Batterham et al., 2016).
G. Pediatrics.
   1. Talk to the child based upon developmental level and perceived understanding. Start early and repeat information over time (Frederick et al., 2017).
   2. Prepare for the procedure using models, visuals, and objects.
   3. Encourage and use laughter.
   4. Avoid teaching when there are obvious signs of pain, anxiety, confusion, medications, sleep deprivation, and frequent changes in regimen.
   5. Encourage "active" learning using dolls, toys, models, or other items that can be manipulated.
   6. Encourage engagement in self-advocacy early.
   7. Adolescents: Based on developmental level, the adolescent to early adult years begin the transition to self-management beyond parental control for chronic illnesses.
      a. Assess developmental readiness.
      b. May need re-teaching as they grow into assuming self-management.
      c. Methods/resources:
         (1) Use a workbook.
         (2) Use a friend or relative.
         (3) Create an open relaxed environment.
         (4) Develop a relationship of trust (Bashore & Bender, 2016).
   8. Consider appropriate anticipatory guidance counseling to direct children and parents to future issues that may arise. Guidance should be developmentally appropriate and focus on the pediatric patient or caregiver's concerns in-depth (Hay, Levin, Deterding, & Abzug, 2018).
      (1) Use oral and written materials.
      (2) Consider literacy levels.
      (3) Consider cultural and linguistic barriers.
H. Use of acronyms: Acronyms help learning by allowing the learner to attach words or mnemonics in order of actions to identify steps of a process for easier recall and retention. For example:
   1. PREPARED (Cibulskis, Giardino, & Moyer, 2011)
      a. **P**resenting history.
      b. **R**eceived therapies.
      c. **E**xisting baseline.
      d. **P**ending test for follow up.
      e. **A**nticipated needs.
      f. **R**ecords to be sent.
      g. **E**nd-of-life preferences.
      h. **D**iscussion with family/caregiver and provider.

Chapter 3

IV. **Collaboration and Teamwork**
(Interprofessional Education Collaborative [IPEC], 2016)
A. The health care team works collaboratively with the individual, family/caregiver, and other professions to maintain a climate of mutual respect and shared values working together toward a common goal.
1. Embrace cultural diversity and differences that characterize individuals, populations, and the health care team.
2. Respect the roles/responsibilities and expertise of all health professions and the impact they have on health outcomes and behavior change.
3. Develop a trusting relationship with the individual, family/caregiver, and all team members.
4. Utilize tools to support the communication and collaboration: "Be Prepared" (AHRQ, 2018a) and "Write It Down – Join Your Team!" (AHRQ, 2018d).
B. The CCTM RN uses the collective knowledge of one's own role, the health care team, and other professions to assess, plan, implement, and evaluate health care needs of the individual and to promote and advance the health of populations. They alter plans as needs change along the continuum of care.
1. Coordinate with entire care team so all members are targeting the same health literacy level.
2. Communicate one's roles and responsibilities clearly to the individual, family/caregiver, and other professionals.
3. Use the full scope of practice, including knowledge, skills, and abilities of all professionals to provide care that is safe, timely, efficient, effective, and equitable.
C. The CCTM RN moves fluidly within the organization and outside of the health system to forge interdependent relationships with other professionals as a basis for collaboration.
D. The CCTM RN communicates with the individual, family/caregiver, community resources, and professionals in other fields in a manner that supports a team approach to the promotion and maintenance of health and the prevention and treatment of disease.
1. Choose effective communication tools and techniques, including information systems and technologies (e.g., mobile applications for learning).
2. Communicate in a form that is understandable and tailor the message to fit understanding.
3. Evaluate the understanding of information given. Reframe the message to fit individual, family/caregiver needs. Assess when enough information is given and continually reassess.
4. Listen actively and encourage sharing of ideas and opinions from all team members, including the individual, family/caregiver.
E. The CCTM RN applies values and principles of team dynamics to perform effectively in different team roles to plan, deliver, and evaluate person-centered care and population health programs/policies.
1. Constructively manage disagreements about values, roles, goals, and actions that arise among team members and with the individual, family/caregiver.
2. Share accountability with all team members for outcomes.
3. Use process improvement to evaluate and increase effectiveness of collaborative teamwork for team-based education services, programs, and policies.
F. Pediatric considerations. Include parents and caregivers in care discussions (e.g., daily provider rounds, offering families opportunities to provide direct care, review of medication lists, allowing families to remain at the child's side for procedures).

V. **Evaluation of Learning**
A. Confirm understanding by asking an application question (Peter et al., 2015).
1. What will you do when you get home?
2. What is your greatest concern?
3. How can I help you to better understand what to do?
4. What will you tell your family/friend about what you must do?
B. Consider why the individual, family/caregiver may not understand and seek to assist with resources. Look to support in area of:
1. Learning disabilities.
2. Hearing loss.
3. Cognitive impairment.
4. Depression.
5. Limited literacy (cognitive decline, developmental disabilities, autism).
6. Language skills.
7. Cultural considerations.
8. Readiness to learn and adapt to the change needed to optimize outcomes.
C. Utilize 'teach-back' to validate understanding with children as well as adults (Peter et al., 2015).
1. Confirm understanding by having the individual teach-back in his or her own words.

Chapter 3

  2. Tailor questions to progress from learning to behavior change.
      a. Knowledge: What is the name of your medication?
      b. Attitudes: Why is it important to take your medication every day?
      c. Behaviors: How will you remember to take your medication every day?
  D. Communicate teaching that has been done with individual and family/caregiver through documentation in the medical record so all team members can collaborate and subsequent interactions can start from information already known and move onward to new information that is needed (Peter et al., 2015).

VI. **Accessing and Evaluating Reliable Health Information**

  A. Improves the individual, family/caregivers level of knowledge, skills, and attitudes to effectively adopt/reinforce healthy behaviors.
  B. Evaluate effectiveness of mediums of learning.
      1. Electronic media (CD, DVD, online, or Web-based).
      2. Mobile applications and social media websites (e.g., YouTube, Facebook, podcasts, webcasts, news, blogs, and Twitter).
      3. Printed: books, leaflets, magazines, newspapers.
  C. How to evaluate health information (National Cancer Institute, 2018).
      1. Look for authorship/sponsorship of material (NIH, 2017).
          a. Government: Identified as a part of federal or state-based organization (e.g., AHRQ, Centers for Disease Control and Prevention [CDC], NIH). For a list of government health sites, visit https://www.nia.nih.gov/health/online-health-information-it-reliable
          b. A website ending in .gov means it is a government agency.
          c. A website ending in .mil means it is a military agency.
          d. Education: Institutions of higher education may provide educational resources for individuals and families (e.g., created and sustained by the work of the educational institution, such as http://goaskalice.columbia.edu).
              (1) A website ending in .edu means it is an educational institution.
          e. Nonprofit organization: Health care, professional organization, or volunteer institutions (e.g., companies that serve the public to provide health services or to support disease-specific research and education).
              (1) A website ending in .org means it is a nonprofit organization.
          f. For-profit organization: Commercial or enterprise or business. Examples may be any company creating health-related products and services, such as drugs, medical equipment, insurance, health equipment, and supplies.
              (1) A website ending in .com or .net means it is a for-profit organization or business.
      2. Current: Look for updates and the date of posted information.
          a. Look at the back of a brochure or at the bottom of a website for the date published or reviewed. Is it within the past 5 years?
          b. If links to research articles are included, ensure links are intact. If links are broken, information may not be current.
      3. Fact-based information: Determine if the author(s) is (are) a subject matter expert in the field. Caution if only one author is listed; is the information fact or opinion-based?
          a. Look for clues that information is based on evidence or research; look for an authoritative source, such as a professional organization or government agency. There should be references citing the source of the information.
          b. Follow social media sites linked to reputable sources (e.g., the National Cancer Institute's Facebook or Twitter accounts) to ensure information is reliable and not personal accounts of experiences.
      4. Intent: Provided for the learner to receive accurate nonbiased information. The intention should be clear to provide health information to the learner. Information should be provided without bias to a particular service or product. Review the "About Us" section of a website.
      5. Website reliability.
          a. Most health information gets reviewed by someone with medical or research credentials (e.g., MD, PhD) prior to posting to ensure its accuracy.
          b. If information was originally published in a research journal or a book, this should be referenced to easily locate it for additional information.

Chapter 3

VII. **Engagement**
A. Identify the roles of care team and the individual, family/caregiver.
 1. Information and communication. The CCTM RN:
  a. Identifies how the medical system works and offers written and/or visual directions on how to navigate the system.
  b. Describes roles of team members and offers examples of how different members can address different needs.
  c. Assist the individual, family/caregiver to organize individual information. Identify decision-making role of CCTM RN and role of individual, family/caregiver (Smith, Swallow, & Coyne, 2015). The CCTM RN:
 2. CCTM RN values the knowledge and experiences of all.
 3. Provides support for each identified role.
 4. Forms trusting relationships based on a mutual dependency and shared responsibility for the care of the individual.
 5. Facilitates individual, family/caregiver participation in delivery of care, through process of negotiation, empowerment and shared goal setting.
B. Telehealth (Young & Nesbitt, 2016) provides:
 1. Health care to the individual both in the home and/or bringing specialty care to the primary care setting.
 2. E-consults, including live interactive conversations between health care professionals and the individual, family/caregiver.
 3. Coordination of care by reducing geographic disparities and allowing access to specialty care not located near the individual, family/caregiver.
C. Information technology provides new avenues of learning for the individual, family/caregiver.
 1. Access to electronic health record (McAlearney et al., 2016).
  a. Patient portals: Individual, family/caregiver controls access and has ability to manage, track, and participate in own care.
  b. Clinical notes: Provider progress notes, plan of care, and identified goals.
  c. Personalized health information: Individual education materials, including videos and/or brochures.
  d. Reminders with person-centered functionality.
 2. Mobile applications (Mohammadi, Ayatolahi Tafti, Hoveidamanesh, Ghanavati, & Pournik, 2018).
  a. Measurement: Digital blood pressure, camera for taking photos, transfer of information to a health care provider/organization.
  b. Adherence: Medications, reminders, schedule.
  c. Data tracking: Blood glucose levels, daily weight, activity/exercise, food intake, urine output.
  d. Consultation: diet recommendations, salt intake, nutrition, reading food labels.
 3. Wearable technology (Hilbert & Yaggi, 2018).
  a. Sensors: Tracking vital signs such as heart rate and breathing, activity, sleep, temperature.
  b. Disease management: Insulin pumps, pacemakers, seizure monitors.

VIII. **Self-Management Skills**
(Lorig, 2017)

The CCTM RN promotes self-management skills through actions in these areas.
A. Symptoms/management of symptoms
 1. May include pain, fatigue, stress, depression, etc.
 2. For chronic pain management and opioid use, engage the individual, family/caregiver in the plan of care to manage pain symptoms and appropriate goal setting (Quinn, Rubinsky, Fernandez, Hahm, & Sarnet, 2017).
B. Appropriate exercise.
 1. Focus on maintaining and improving strength, flexibility, and endurance.
C. Appropriate use of medications.
 1. Taking exactly as prescribed on a schedule or as needed, side effects, when to contact a provider, safe storage, and possible adverse effects.
 2. Opioids: Signs of misuse/abuse, proper disposal, tapering of medication, and antidote medication (Costello, 2015).
D. Communication with family/caregiver and friends (Pollack et al., 2016).
 1. Personal support systems contribute to emotional and informational needs of the individual.
 2. Peer support groups of individuals with similar conditions provide personal insight from previous experiences.
E. Communication with health care professionals.
 1. Gain knowledge and access to resources.

2. Assists with coordination across health care systems and population health resources.
3. Identifies individual cultural differences and how this impacts decision-making (Hawley & Morris, 2017).

F. Healthful eating.
 1. Reading food labels accurately to make good food choices.

G. Decision-making.
 1. Making daily decisions based on what the individual, family/caregiver know about the disease/wellness; how they will react based on their role, knowledge, and psychological involvement in the decision.

H. Problem solving.
 1. Defining problems, generating solutions, and gaining support and knowledge from health care professionals and friends.
 2. Goal setting, including development of action plans accounting for knowledge and access to resources.

IX. **Individual Education for Opioid Medications** (Costello, 2015)

A. Many individuals are given prescriptions for opioid analgesics and often lack the knowledge of how to appropriately take them. There are several risks associated with misuse of this type of medication. Nonmedical use of opioid medications is a rising public health concern. Individual, families/caregivers need to have adequate education, and the CCTM RN plays a key role in providing this.
 1. Misuse and abuse.
  a. Taking the medication exactly as prescribed by the health care professional. Not taking too large of a dose or dosing more frequently.
  b. Intent of opioid use is to increase functional status of the individual. Use of opioid for medical condition only, not as a sleep aid or to produce a euphoric effect to mask the pain.
 2. Risks.
  a. Use of opioid medication may result in several adverse effects, including respiratory depression, somnolence, increased risk of accidents, work and driving restrictions, addiction, and overdose.
  b. Educate family/caregivers to wake the individual if he or she is sleeping heavily or snoring. Contact emergency services if unable to wake the individual.
 3. Addiction.
  a. Inability of the individual to abstain from or control impulse to use the medication even with negative consequences.
  b. Monitor for signs/symptoms indicating addiction disease process. Often affects interpersonal relationships, produces a dysfunctional emotional response, and impairs behavioral control.
 4. Tolerance and withdrawal.
  a. Individual, family/caregiver knowledge about development of a tolerance to the medication over time, especially with misuse/abuse.
  b. Long-term opioid use often results in withdrawal symptoms during the taper schedule. CCTM RN discusses appropriate expectations of the individual, family/caregiver during this time.
 5. Storage and disposal.
  a. Safe storage of opioids while taking the medication includes proper labeling for dose and clear naming of the medication to help reduce errors.
  b. Disposal of opioids not used ensures no future misuse/abuse. Review local resources for take-back programs and other disposal options.
 6. For more information on opioids, refer to Chapter 2, "Advocacy."

X. **Patient Education Apps**

A. Applications for mobile devices serve to engage the individual and/or family/caregiver through active involvement in managing health parameters, such as diet, exercise, and some blood monitoring. Applications should be used with caution and with the discretion of the health care team so the person is informed of the benefits and risks (Groshek, Oldenburg, Sarasohn-Kahn, & Sitler, 2015).

B. Mobile apps for individual use:
 1. Simply Sayin' – Medical Jargon for Families.
  a. IOS devices.
  b. Uses pictures, sounds, and terms to assist with understanding medical jargon for a child or caregiver.
 2. Up-to-date for Patients and Caregivers.
  a. Access information for patients, including pictures, graphs, and charts.
 3. HeartMapp.

a. Android-based application intended to assist patients with heart failure in managing symptoms and medications.
4. mySugr Diabetes Training.
   a. Makes type 2 diabetes learning fun and easy to comprehend.
5. Mango Health.
   a. IOS.
   b. Medicine reminder app.
   c. Medication manager that assists to remind to take pills, tracks refills, identifies food and drug interactions.
6. MyRA.
   a. Rheumatoid arthritis tracker, picks, communications.
7. Fooducate.
   a. Diabetes nutrition and diet tracker.
   b. Identifies food content of groceries purchased and alternatives for people with diabetes.
8. iBGstar Diabetes Manager.
   a. Record, track, and manage diabetes data.
   b. Integrates with iBG start blood glucose monitors.
9. HealthTap.
   a. Gives tips and answers related to health concerns and other topics.
10. Diabetes App.
    a. Blood sugar, glucose, and carb counter.
11. Pillboxie.
    a. Helps to remember your medications.
12. goMeals.
    a. Identifies nutrition from meals and restaurants.
13. WebMD for iPad.
    a. Health information and tools to check symptoms.
    b. First aid information.
14. AAP Asthma Tracker for Adolescents.
    a. Education section is pre-populated with pediatric relevant educational content, instructions, and videos.
15. The Amazings.
    a. Gameplay to help kids recognize and avoid asthma triggers, such as pollen, cigarette smoke, and pollution, and stay vigilant about their health.
    b. Target audience is children with asthma aged 7 to 12 years.
16. Wizdy Pets.
    a. Health-oriented gaming start-up promoting self-management through engaging mobile games.
17. KidsDoc.
    a. AAP app to help parents know when to have their child seen by a doctor.
C. The following are mobile apps that may be of interest for nurses seeking information to share with individuals, families/caregivers. This list is not all inclusive but noted from the article by Aditi Pai (2013).
   1. Nursing Central.
      a. Knowledge app for nurses to find answers to questions about diseases, labs and procedures.
   2. NurseTabs.
      a. Fundamentals: step by step procedures for 120+ skills.
   3. NurseTabs – MedSurg.
      a. Offers the ability to search across diseases and disorders to have medical information easily available.
   4. Shots by STFM.
      a. A digital reference on immunizations.
   5. Lab Notes.
      a. A nurses' guide to lab and diagnostic tests with individual education.
      b. Provides information related to laboratory values and radiology imaging, with individual education and imaging.

Chapter 3

Table 3-1.
Education and Engagement of Individuals and Families: Knowledge, Skills, and Attitudes for Competency

Knowledge	Skills	Attitudes	Sources
Person-Centered Planning			
Identify care centered on the individual.	Elicit individual's values, preferences, and expressed needs as part of clinical interview, implementation of care plan, and evaluation of care.	Value seeing health care situations through individuals' eyes. Respect and encourage individual expression of patient values, preferences, and expressed needs.	Cronenwett et al., 2007, p.123
Seek to understand individual/family/community preferences and values regarding health and illness.			Scholl, Zill., Härter, & Dirmaier, 2014
Define assessment of physical, psychological, emotional, social, and cultural barriers to learning.		Support person-centered care for individuals and groups whose values differ from own. Believe individuals/families can follow a plan of care.	Del Monte & Mell, 2018
		Be flexible and seek to solve problems with a commitment to individual and family.	Del Monte & Mell, 2018
Identify components of a coordinated, integrated plan of care.			AAACN, 2018
Create an evidence-based plan of care, including promotion of individual engagement, self-management and monitoring of health condition, coaching on healthy behaviors, and recognition of emergent signs and symptoms.			AAACN, 2018
	Use evidence-based clinical care plan and evaluate effectiveness.		Casimir, Williams, Liang, Ptakmongkolkul, & Slyer, 2014
		Value individual/family involvement in planning health care changes and activities.	Del Monte & Mell, 2018
		Seek learning opportunities with individuals who represent all aspects of human diversity.	AAACN, 2018.
		Recognize personally held attitudes about working with individuals from different ethnic, cultural, and social backgrounds.	Cronenwett et al., 2007, p. 123

continued on next page

Table 3-1. (continued)
Education and Engagement of Individuals and Families: Knowledge, Skills, and Attitudes for Competency

Knowledge	Skills	Attitudes	Sources
Patient-Centered Planning			
Identify individual/family/caregiver need for physical comfort and emotional support.	Provide person-centered care with sensitivity and respect for the diversity of human experience.	Willingly support person-centered care for individuals and groups whose values differ from own. Value the person's expertise with own health and symptoms.	Cronenwett et al., 2007
Identify the support found through involvement of family and friends.			Hawley & Morris, 2017
Identify transition and continuity.			Darnell & Hickson, 2015
Integrate multiple dimensions of the individual/family to provide information, communication, and transition care.	Use motivational interviewing.	Interpersonal mutual respect and trust that supports individual learning. Accept changes in the plan and maintain flexibility in planning educational activities.	Bastable, 2017
		Respect and encourage expression of values. Create relationships where evaluation of progress is open and nonthreatening.	AAACN, 2018
Collaborative Teamwork			
Discuss principles of effective communication. Describe basic principles of consensus building and conflict resolution.	Assess own level of communication skill in encounters with individuals and families. Participate in building consensus or resolving conflict in the context of individual care.	Appreciate shared decision-making with empowered individuals and families, even when conflicts occur.	Cronenwett et al., 2007, p. 124
	Communicate care provided and needed at each transition in care.	Value continuous improvement of own communication and conflict resolution skills.	Cronenwett et al., 2007, p. 124 Smith, Swallow, & Coyne, 2015
		Act with honesty and integrity in relationships with individual, family, and caregivers.	Interprofessional Education Collaborative (IPEC), 2016

continued on next page

Table 3-1. (continued)
Education and Engagement of Individuals and Families: Knowledge, Skills, and Attitudes for Competency

Knowledge	Skills	Attitudes	Sources
Collaborative Teamwork (continued)			
Understand scope of practice to effectively highlight members of the team who are best prepared to handle the issue and delegate to appropriate team member.	Establish collaborative relationships with individual/family by explanations of care coordination collaborative care to meet individual's needs.	Identify one's own attitude concerning support of family members and expectations.	AAACN, 2016
	Use active listening and encourage ideas and opinions from members of the team.		IPEC, 2016
	Communicate individual values, preferences, and expressed needs to other members of health care team.	Value active partnership with individuals or designated surrogates in planning, implementing, and evaluating care.	Cronenwett et al., 2007, p.125
		Respect individual preferences for degree of active engagement in care process.	Connor et al., 2018
		Allow family members to determine their ability to provide support.	Smith, Swallow, & Coyne, 2015
Reach out to each provider to inform him or her of your role to assist in meeting health care needs of individuals with specific interventions.			AAACN, 2016
Explain the role and responsibilities of care providers and how members of the team work together to provide care.			IPEC, 2016
	Facilitate individual support groups for shared learning and coping.		Bastable, 2017
Knowledge of individual education, coaching process to support self-management.	Demonstrate coaching methods to engage and motivate individuals.	Belief that individuals and families can manage their chronic conditions.	Phillips et al., 2015
	Use motivational interviewing or other techniques.		Bastable, 2017
	Teach self-care actions, how to manage symptoms, how to manage care, and how to adapt to changes brought on by changing health.		Do, Young, Barnason, & Tran, 2015
		Accept individual self-management as important component of care management.	Phillips et al., 2015

continued on next page

Table 3-1. (continued)
Education and Engagement of Individuals and Families: Knowledge, Skills, and Attitudes for Competency

Knowledge	Skills	Attitudes	Sources
Education and Engagement of Individuals and Families			
Define information, communication, and education.		Creatively plan experiences for individual and family learning.	Aboumatar et al., 2017
Coordinate the provision of individual education and learning reinforcement across the team, and inform and update the care team as the plan evolves to meet the needs of the individuals.	Assess individual and family readiness, which is dependent on psychological readiness (aware of condition and implications, level of anxiety and/or depression), physiological readiness (level of pain, sedation), and social readiness (able to share with family and/or caregivers).	Value creativity in adapting learning to meet the need of the individual/family. Respect individual/family values, allowing space for discussion and common understanding.	Aboumatar et al., 2017
		Create an environment of communication and questioning that empowers individual/family to engage in planning care.	Bastable, 2017
	Identify primary support person/persons at first encounter.		Hawley & Morris, 2017
		Organize and communicate with individuals, families, and health care team in a way that is understandable, avoiding discipline-specific terminology when possible.	IPEC, 2016
Identify appropriate approach to convey teaching after evaluation of health literacy.	Assess cognition and aptitude and readiness to learn. Develop individual/family/caregiver ability to engage in decision-making.	Value active partnerships with individuals or designated surrogates in planning, implementing, and evaluating care.	Bastable, 2017
Examine common barriers to active involvement of individuals in their own health care processes.		Respect individual preferences for degree of active engagement in care process.	Asiedu, Ridgeway, Carroll, Jatoi, & Radecki Breitkopf, 2018
Demonstrate knowledge of engaging individuals and families in health care.	Assess and teach to meet the learner's need.	Belief that knowledge and education make a difference in health care outcomes.	Hilbert & Yaggi, 2018

continued on next page

Table 3-1. (continued)
Education and Engagement of Individuals and Families: Knowledge, Skills, and Attitudes for Competency

Knowledge	Skills	Attitudes	Sources
Education and Engagement of Individuals and Families (continued)			
Identify questions to ask and cues for physical, psychological, and social readiness. Identify ways to ask open-ended questions and seek to understand individual/family needs.	Address need for self-care. Engage and invite individual and others in learning. Create trusting relationships.		Lovell et al., 2014
	Enable individuals and families from multiple generations to cope and adapt to individual health stages, encouraging and engaging them in self-management.		Busenbark, 2017
Implement teaching.	Use teach back. Able to impart skills to individual/family.		Cronenwett et al., 2007
	Develop and use content that is appropriate to the age of the learner.	Acknowledge differences in learning abilities.	Peter et al., 2015
	Teach and coach self-management skills.	Flexible and creative in understanding that all individuals learn differently. Adapt a creative and engaging atmosphere for education.	Lorig, 2017
	Engage individuals or designated surrogates in active partnerships that promote health, safety and well-being, and self-care management. List resources available to meet individual/family needs.		Peter et al., 2015
	Identify priorities in education: • Provide critical information. • Provide printed documents and communicate during transitions in care. Identify when information exceeds ability of individual to absorb.		Archer et al., 2015

continued on next page

**Table 3-1. (continued)
Education and Engagement of Individuals and Families: Knowledge, Skills, and Attitudes for Competency**

Knowledge	Skills	Attitudes	Sources
Education and Engagement of Individuals and Families (continued)			
	Identify individual/family level of knowledge related to medication management.	Belief that individuals can manage their medications.	Acher et al., 2015
	Recognize the boundaries of therapeutic relationships.		Cronenwett et al., 2007, p. 124
Identify reliable resources. Describe reliable sources for locating evidence reports and clinical practice guidelines.	Read original research and evidence reports related to area of practice. Locate evidence reports related to clinical practice topics and guidelines.	Appreciate the importance of reading relevant professional journals regularly.	Cronenwett et al., 2007, p. 126
	Question rationale for routine approaches to care that result in less than desired outcomes or adverse events.		Cronenwett et al., 2007, p. 126
	Participate in structuring the work environment to facilitate integration of new evidence into standards of practice.	Value the need for continuous improvement in clinical practice based on new knowledge.	Cronenwett et al., 2007, p. 126
Evaluate understanding.	Identify the ability of the family member to comprehend the level of information given.		Peter et al., 2015
	Assess learning and retention through evaluation of key topics and how to implement self-care measures.		Acher et al., 2015
Advocacy			
Explore ethical and legal implications of person-centered care.	Recognize the boundaries of therapeutic relationships.	Acknowledge the tension that may exist between individual rights and the organizational responsibility for professional, ethical care.	Cronenwett et al., 2007, p. 124
Describe the limits and boundaries of therapeutic person-centered care.		Appreciate shared decision making with empowered individuals and families, even when conflicts occur.	Hawley & Morris, 2017
		Examine nursing roles in assuring coordination, integration, and continuity of care.	Cronenwett et al., 2007, p. 124

continued on next page

Table 3-1. (continued)
Education and Engagement of Individuals and Families: Knowledge, Skills, and Attitudes for Competency

Knowledge	Skills	Attitudes	Sources
Advocacy (continued)			
Identify the informed, motivated, and prepared individual and family.	Coach individuals and caregivers in resolving problems, writing down resources, and providing support during transitions.		Acher et al., 2015
		Value active partnership in individual/family/caregiver in health care process.	Smith, Swallow, & Coyne, 2015
	Assess the role of the family members in care and support.		Hawley & Morris, 2017
	Encourage individual and family communication of concerns and reinforce independent decision-making in their care.		Hawley & Morris, 2017

Source: Cronenwett et al. (2007). *Nursing Outlook,* 55(3), 122-131. Reprinted with permission from Elsevier.

Appendix 3-1.
National Institute on Aging U.S. Department of Health and Human Services

Your Health		
Topic	Date	Notes
Bone/joint pain or stiffness		
Bowel problems		
Chest pain		
Feeling dizzy or lightheaded		
Headaches		
Hearing changes		
Losing urine or feeling wet		
Recent hospitalizations or emergencies		
Shortness of breath		
Skin Changes		
Vision changes		

Your Diet, Medication, and Lifestyle		
Topic	Date	Notes
Alcohol use		
Appetite changes		
Diet/Nutrition		
Medicine		
Tobacco Use		
Weight changes		

Your thoughts and feelings		
Topic	Date	Notes
Feeling lonely or isolated		
Feeling sad, down, or blue		
Intimacy or sexual activity		
Problems with memory or thinking		
Problems with sleep or changes in sleep patterns		

Everyday living		
Topic	Date	Notes
Accidents, injuries, or falls		
Advance directives		
Daily activities		
Driving/transportation/mobility		
Exercise		
Living situation		

Source: National Institute on Aging, 2017.

Chapter 3

Case Study 3-1.
CCTM® Role in Diabetes Education

Introduction

Diabetes is a chronic disease that may have an early onset with individuals who are young and need to learn quickly how to change their lifestyle management to mitigate health outcomes of blood glucose levels that are not in control and may cause life-threatening illnesses as they age. Many individuals have complex situations such as this one where social, cultural and age-related issues intertwine.

- Nora is a 14-year-old Somali child whose parents immigrated to the United States 6 years ago. Nora is a student at one of the schools integrated through the English as a Second Language program. Nora was diagnosed over a year ago with diabetes mellitus type 1. She speaks English well and does some translation for her parents. They have three other children ranging from ages 5 to 16 years. Nora has not been successful in achieving goal range with her HbA1c. Nora's parents do not speak English well and a translator is used for the visit. The family has access to the electronic environment through school and a home computer.

The CCTM® RN prepares for her visit with Nora and her family by researching the Somali culture literature. She reviews common dietary menus for this culture, as well as beliefs about health and healing. The CCTM RN reviews websites and games that Nora may like that would support her own self-learning and management.

On the first visit with Nora and her family, the CCTM RN assesses the learning needs by getting to know Nora and her likes and dislikes. What are favorite foods, and what traditions do the family and Nora observe? Does Nora prepare food?

The CCTM RN then will explore with Nora and family what her biggest concerns are with diabetes.
- The CCTM RN will state the medical goal and reason why.
- Discuss with Nora and family, creating a mutual goal. One way to say this is:
  - "We've talked about your family and diabetes. My role is to help you manage your diabetes so you have a healthy life. I want to know what your goal(s) are."
  - "I can see now that we can work on how you manage food and insulin. What goals do you think we can work on?"
  - "Tell me what you normally eat in a week."
- The CCTM RN will work with Nora on an eating plan that meets her nutrition and insulin goals.
- At the end of the first session, the CCTM RN would use concepts of teach-back, having Nora and her family state back three things they will be able to do and how.
- The CCTM RN shares websites and diabetes games that might interest Nora, as well as a school-based support group for people with diabetes.
- Follow-up interactions for the CCTM RN would be related to:
  - Nursing considerations: The CCTM RN needs to review carefully the culture and family traditions. Using open-ended questions and understanding cultural differences are important.
  - Lifestyle: For adolescents who attempt to move toward independence, the CCTM RN will need to simplify expectations and look for alternatives that fit their peer group's eating style. It may be of interest to connect this person with someone in her age group who has the same disease, especially someone who is successful in managing his or her disease.
  - Cultural issues: Having an interpreter present if the family is not fluent in English is necessary because the adolescent should not feel the need to interpret, but should be free to express him/herself as the individual.
  - Family involvement is important for the adolescent. However, the stage of development for the adolescent is seeking independence, so asking if he or she wants to talk alone with the nurse or provider is important.
  - Environment: This should be in an open learning environment, not necessarily the clinic office. However, this depends on the person and family.

Resources

American Diabetes Association. (n.d.). *Teens*. Retrieved from http://www.diabetes.org/living-with-diabetes/parents-and-kids/teens/

Health Information Translations. (2016). *Diabetes*. Retrieved from https://www.healthinfotranslations.org/pdfDocs/Diabetes_Som.pdf

Minnesota Department of Health. (2008). *Somalia*. Retrieved from http://www.health.state.mn.us/divs/idepc/refugee/globalbbsom.pdf

Case Study 3-2.
CCTM® Role in Opioid Management and Chronic Pain Education

Introduction

Chronic pain impairs the physical, psychological, and social functioning of an individual and his or her family. The use of prescription opioids for chronic, non-cancer pain has dramatically increased in the last decade, leading to misuse/abuse and dependence as a current public health crisis. A collaborative care approach for chronic pain management focuses on individual and family engagement, care coordination, education, and shared decision-making with goal setting.

Larry is a 47-year-old construction worker who injured his back at work five months ago while lifting heavy equipment. He lives with his wife, Kelly, and three children ages 9, 13, and 15 years. Larry has high blood pressure controlled with metoprolol and is slightly overweight. He has a family history of depression, including his mother and sister. Larry was initially diagnosed with a herniated disk and was treated by an orthopedic spine specialist. His injury has medically healed, but he is still experiencing chronic pain, rating it a 6/7 out of 10 on an average day. He had been taking oxycodone 10 mg by mouth every 6 hours as needed since his initial injury. His current care plan includes a scheduled taper off the opioid medication and alternative pain management strategies.

The CCTM® RN reviews literature about chronic pain management, long-term opioid use, and goal setting prior to the visit with Larry. Engagement of family members is highlighted for individuals with chronic pain. The CCTM RN creates a suitable learning environment for Larry and his family prior to the visit.

Clinical Interaction (as Indicated by Dimension)

- Learning needs assessment.
  - The CCTM RN works with the individual and family to determine what learning needs exist overall and in relation to the current plan of care.
- Larry (Individual).
  - Literacy level – High school diploma.
  - No language barriers.
  - Preferred learning style – Listening and doing. Likes tactile learning with his hands to improve memory.
  - Denies any cultural or lifestyle barriers.
- Kelly (Family/Caregiver)
  - Literacy level – Associate's college degree. Works as a medical secretary.
  - Prefers plain language even though she's familiar with some medical terminology.
  - Preferred learning style – Reading. Likes pamphlets to take home to refer to in the future.
  - Denies any cultural or lifestyle barriers.
- Non-verbal cues.
  - The CCTM RN notes both Larry and Kelly are making good eye contact, and their body language toward each other indicates a good support system.
- Prioritize immediate learning need.
  - The CCTM RN works collaboratively with Larry and Kelly to determine the immediate learning need is the opioid tapering schedule. Larry identifies historically he has not been good about following a medication schedule but recognizes the importance of it.
  - CCTM RN explores tools/resources to assist.
  - Larry has a smart phone and enjoys using technology; the CCTM RN researches and recommends a mobile application for medication management with audible reminders and a chart/graph format for a visual aid.
- Address barriers.
  - Larry verbalizes a fear of an increase in pain and inability to manage it without the opioid medication. The CCTM RN reviews pain management strategies outlined by the care team.
- Goal setting.
  - The CCTM RN uses negotiation, empowerment and shared decision making to work together with Larry and Kelly to create short-term goals.
- Engagement.
  - Kelly plans to download the mobile application to her smart phone so she is aware of what the daily medication schedule is.
  - CCTM RN suggests Larry keep a daily journal to record his medication intake, pain levels, track his pain management strategies, and record questions or concerns as they arise.
- Evaluation of learning.
  - CCTM RN utilizes teach back strategies to evaluate learning. Asks questions, such as:
    - What will you do when you go home?
    - How will you explain to your children what you have to do?
    - What is your biggest concern about the learning we did today?

Clinical Implications (as indicated by dimension)

- Follow-up interactions for the CCTM RN would be related to:
  - Continued engagement of the individual and family/caregiver working towards a mutually agreed upon goal.
- Nursing considerations.
  - Evaluate learning and understanding as the medication schedule changes over time with the opioid taper. Evaluate the effectiveness of the mobile application as a useful tool. Identify alternatives as needed.
  - Ongoing discussion of barriers and fears.
- Environmental issues.
  - Ongoing ability to involve family/caregiver in each visit and expand support system as needed per individual's request.
- Lifestyle.
  - Assess for signs of misuse of the opioid medication. Assess for inappropriate symptoms indicating a relapse and overuse based on current dose per taper schedule.
- Significant other involvement.
  - Continue to engage family and expand caregiver support based on individual's needs. Future involvement of children may be indicated/preferred.

continued on next page

Case Study 3-2. (continued)
CCTM® Role in Opioid Management and Chronic Pain Education

Resources
Paice, J., Battista, V., Drick, C., & Schreiner, E. (2018). Nursing's role in providing pain and symptom management. *Journal of Hospice and Palliative Nursing, 20*(1), 30-35.
Pharmacy Times (2017). *The top medication reminder apps for patients*. Retrieved from http://www.pharmacytimes.com/contributor/christina-tarantola/2017/12/the-top-medication-reminder-apps-for-patients

References

Aboumatar, H., Naqibuddin, M., Chung, S., Adebowale, H., Bone, L., Brown, T., … Pronovost, P. (2017). Better respiratory Education and Treatment Help Empower (BREATHE) study: Methodology and baseline characteristics off a randomized controlled trial testing a transitional care program to improve patient-centered care delivery among chronic obstructive pulmonary disease patients. *Contemporary Clinical Trials, 62*,159-167.

Agency for Healthcare Research and Quality (AHRQ). (2015). *Creating patient-centered team-based primary care*. Rockville, MD. Retrieved from https://pcmh.ahrq.gov/page/creating-patient-centered-team-based-primary-care

Agency for Healthcare Research and Quality. (AHRQ). (2018a). *Be prepared*. Retrieved from https://www.ahrq.gov/sites/default/files/wysiwyg/professionals/quality-patient-safety/patient-family-engagement/pfeprimarycare/patient-prep-card.pdf

Agency for Healthcare Research and Quality (AHRQ). (2018b). *Helping patients and families prepare for an appointment: A guide for clinicians*. Retrieved from https://www.ahrq.gov/sites/default/files/wysiwyg/professionals/quality-patient-safety/patient-family-engagement/pfeprimarycare/clinician-info-poster.pdf

Agency for Healthcare Research and Quality (AHRQ). (2018c). *The guide to improving patient safety in primary care settings by engaging patients and families*. Rockville, MD.

Agency for Healthcare Research and Quality (AHRQ). (2018d). *Write it down – Join your team!* Retrieved from https://www.ahrq.gov/sites/default/files/wysiwyg/professionals/quality-patient-safety/patient-family-engagement/pfeprimarycare/bepreparedptnotesheet.pdf

Always Use Teach-back! (2018). *Using the Teach-back toolkit*. Retrieved from http://www.teachbacktraining.com/using-the-teach-back-toolkit

American Academy of Ambulatory Care Nursing (AAACN). (2016). *Scope and standards of practice for registered nurses in care coordination and transition management*. Pitman, NJ.

American Academy of Ambulatory Care Nursing (AAACN). (2018). *Ambulatory care nursing orientation and competency assessment guide* (3rd ed.), L. Brixey & C. Newman (Eds.). Pitman, NJ: Author.

Archer, A.W., LeCaire, T.J., Hundt, A.S., Greenberg, C.C., Carayon, P., Kind, A.J., & Weber, S.M. (2015). Using human factors and systems engineering to evaluate readmission after complex surgery. *Journal of the American College of Surgeons, 221*(4), 810-820.

Asiedu, G.B., Ridgeway, J.L., Carroll, K. Jatoi, A., Radecki Breitkopf, C. (2018). "Ultimately, mom has the call": Viewing clinical trial decision making among patients with ovarian cancer through the lens of relational autonomy. *Health Expectations,* 1-9. doi:10.1111/hex.12691

Bashore, L., & Bender, J. (2016). Evaluation of the utility of a transition workbook in preparing adolescent and young adult cancer survivors for transition to adult services: A pilot study. *Journal of Pediatric Oncology Nursing, 33*(2), 111-118.

Bastable, S. (2017). *Essentials of patient education*. Jones & Bartlett Learning. Burlington: MA.

Batterham, R.W., Hawkins, M., Collins, P.A., Buchbinder, R., & Osborne, R.H. (2016). Health literacy: Applying current concepts to improve health services and reduce health inequalities. *Public Health, 132*, 3-12.

Boyle, J., Speroff, T., Worley, K., Cao, A., Goggins, K., Dittus, R., & Kripalani, S. (2017). Low health literacy is associated with increased transitional care needs in hospitalized patients. *Journal of Hospital Medicine, 12*(11), 918-924.

Busenbark, M.M. (2017). *What different generations want from a health care experience*. Retrieved from https://www.childrenshospitals.org/Newsroom/Childrens-Hospitals-Today/Issue-Archive/Issues/Fall-2017/Articles/What-Different-Generations-Want-From-a-Health-Care-Experience

Casimir, Y.E., Williams, M.M., Liang, M.Y., Pitakmongkolkul, S., & Slyer, J.T. (2014). The effectiveness of patient-centered self-care education for adults with heart failure on knowledge, self-care behaviors, quality of life, and readmissions: A systematic review. *JBI Database of Systematic Reviews and Implementation Reports, 12*(2), 188-262.

Cesta, T. (2011). Reducing readmissions: Case management's critical role. *Hospital Case Management, 19*(3), 39-42.

Cibulskis, C.C., Giardino, A.P., & Moyer, V.A. (2011). Care transitions from inpatient to outpatient settings: Ongoing challenges and emerging best practices. *Hospital Practice, 39*(3), 128-139.

Connor, J.A., Antonelli, R.C., & O'Connell, C.A., Bishop Kuzdeba, H., Porter, C., & Hickey, P.A. (2018). Measuring care coordination in the pediatric cardiology ambulatory setting. *The Journal of Nursing Administration, 48*(2), 107-113.

Costello, M. (2015). Prescription opioid analgesics: Promoting patient safety with better patient education. *American Journal of Nursing, 115*(11), 50-56.

Coyne, I., Prizeman, G., Sheehan, A., Malone, H., & While, A.E. (2016). An e-health intervention to support the transition of young people with long-term illnesses to adult healthcare services: Design and early use. *Patient Education and Counseling, 99*(9), 1496-1504.

Cronenwett, L., Sherwood, G., Barnsteiner, J., Disch, J., Johnson, J., Mitchell, P., … Warren, J. (2007). Quality and safety education for nurses. *Nursing Outlook, 55*(3), 122-131.

Darnell, L.K., & Hickson, S.V. (2015). Cultural competent patient-centered care. *Nursing Clinics of North America, 50*(1),99-108.

Del Monte, P.S., & Mell, S. (2018). Organizational/systems role of the ambulatory care nurse competencies In L. Brixey, & C.A. Newman (Eds.), *Ambulatory care nursing orientation and competency assessment guide* (3rd ed.). Pitman, NJ: American Academy of Ambulatory Care Nursing.

Do, V., Young, L., Barnason, S., & Tran, H. (2015). Relationships between activation level, knowledge, self-efficacy, and self-management behavior in heart failure patients discharged from rural hospitals. *F1000Research, 4*, 150. Retrieved from https://f1000research.com/articles/4-150/v1

Frederick, N.N., Bober, S.L., Berwick, L., Tower, M., & Kenney, L.B. (2017). Preparing childhood cancer survivors for transition to adult care: The young adult perspective. *Pediatric Blood & Cancer, 64*(10), 1-9.

Groshek, M.R., Oldenburg, J., Sarasohn-Kahn, J., & Sitler, B. (2015). *mHealth App essentials: Patient engagement, considerations, and implementation.* Retrieved from http://www.himss.org/mhealth-app-essentials-patient-engagement-considerations-and-implementation

Harding, K., Mersha, T.B., Vassalotti, J.A., Webb, F.A., & Nicholas, S.B. (2017). Current state and future trends to optimize the care of chronic kidney disease in African Americans. *American Journal of Nephrology, 46*(2),176-186.

Hawley, S.T., & Morris, A.M. (2017). Cultural challenges to engaging patients in shared decision making. *Patient Education and Counseling, 100*(1),18-24.

Hay, W.W., Levin, M.J., Deterding, R.R., & Abzug, M.J. (2018). Ambulatory and office pediatrics. In *Current diagnosis & treatment* (24th ed.). New York, NY: McGraw-Hill Education.

Heath, S. (2016). *Understanding generational differences in patient engagement.* Retrieved from https://patientengagement hit.com/news/understanding-generational-differences-in-patient-engagement

Hersh, L., Salzman, B., & Snyderman,D. (2017). Health literacy in primary care practice. *American Family Physician, 92*(2), 118-124.

Hibbard, J.H. (2016). Patient activation and the use of information to support informed health decisions. *Patient Education and Counseling, 100*(1), 5-7.

Hilbert, J., & Yaggi, H.K. (2018). Patient-centered care in obstructive sleep apnea: A vision for the future. *Sleep Medicine Reviews, 37,*138-147.

Interprofessional Education Collaborative (IPEC). (2016). *Core competencies for interprofessional collaborative practice.* Washington, DC: Author.

Institute for Healthcare Improvement (IHI). (2018). *Ask me 3: Good questions for your good health.* Retrieved from http://www.ihi.org/resources/Pages/Tools/Ask-Me-3-Good-Questions-for-Your-Good-Health.aspx

Koetsenruijter, J., van Eikelenboom, N., van Lieshout, J., Vassilev, I., Lionis, C., Todorova, E., ... Wensing, M. (2016). Social support and self-management capabilities in diabetes patients: An international observational study. *Patient Education and Counseling, 99*(4), 638-643.

Lorig, K. (2017). Commentary on "evidence-based self-management programs for seniors and other with chronic diseases": Patient experience-patient health-return on investment. *Journal of Ambulatory Care Management, 40*(3),185-188.

Lovell, M., Luckett, T., Boyle, F., Phillips, J., Agar, M., & Davidson, P.M. (2014). Patient education, coaching, and self-management for cancer pain. *Journal of Clinical Oncology, 32*(16), 1712-1720.

McAlearney, A.S., Sieck, C.J., Hefner, J.L., Aldrich, A.M., Walker, D.M., Rizer, M.K., ... Huerta, T.R. (2016). High Touch and High Tech (HT2) proposal: Transforming patient engagement throughout the continuum of care by engaging patients with portal technology at the bedside. *JMIR Research Protocols, 5*(4), e221-e236.

Mohammadi, R., Ayatolahi Tafti, M., Hoveidamanesh, S., Ghanavati, R., & Pournik, O. (2018). Reflection on mobile applications for blood pressure measurement: A systematic review on potential effects and initiatives. *European Federation for Medical Informatics, 247,* 306-310.

Narayan, M.C. (2017). Strategies for implementing the national standards for culturally and linguistically appropriate services in home health care. *Home Health Care Management and Practice, 29*(3),168-175.

National Cancer Institute (NCI). (2018). *Using trusted resources.* Retrieved from https://www.cancer.gov/about-cancer/managing-care/using-trusted-resources

National Center for Learning Disabilities. (2014). *2014 state of LD.* Retrieved from https://www.ncld.org/archives/reports-and-studies/2014-state-of-ld

National Institute on Aging. (2017). *Discussing changes in your health: Worksheet.* Retrieved from https://www.nia.nih.gov/health/discussing-changes-your-health-worksheet

National Institutes of Health (NIH). (2017). *Online health information: Is it reliable?* Retrieved from https://www.nia.nih.gov/health/online-health-information-it-reliable

National Institutes of Health (NIH). (n.d.) *Quick guide to health literacy.* Retrieved from https://health.gov/communication/literacy/quickguide/factsbasic.htm

Naylor, M.D, Schaid, E.C., Carpenter, D., Gass, B., Levine, C., Li, J., ... Williams, M.V. (2017). Components of comprehensive and effective transitional care. *Journal of American Geriatric Society, 65*(6), 1119-1125.

Osborne, H. (2018). *Health literacy from A to Z: Practical ways to communicate your health message* (2nd ed.). Lake Placid, NY: Aviva Publishing.

Pai, A. (2013). *Apple's top 118 apps for doctors, nurses, patients.* Retrieved from http://www.mobihealthnews.com/23740/apples-top-118-apps-for-doctors-nurses-and-patients/page/0/9

Peter, D., Robinson, P., Jordan, M., Lawrence, S., Casey, K., & Salas-Lopez, D. (2015). Reducing readmissions using teach-back: Enhancing patient and family education. *The Journal of Nursing Administration, 45*(1), 35-42.

Phillips, R.L., Short, A., Kenning, A., Dugdale, P., Nugus, P., McGowan, R. & Greenfield, D. (2015). Achieving patient-centered care: The potential and challenge of the patient-as-professional role. *Health Expectations, 18*(6), 2616-28.

Plainlanguage.gov. (2011). *Federal plain language guidelines.* Retrieved from https://www.doi.gov/sites/doi.gov/files/migrated/open/upload/Plain_Language_PDF.pdf

Pollack, A.H., Backonja, U., Miller, A.D., Mishra, S.R., Khelifi, M., Kendall, L., & Pratt, W. (2016). Closing the gap: Supporting patients' transition to self-management after hospitalization. *Proc SIGCHI Conference on Human Factors in Computer Systems, 2016,* 5324-5336.

Quinn, A.E., Rubinsky, A.D., Fernandez, A.C., Hahm, H.C., & Sarnet, J.H. (2017). A research agenda to advance the coordination of care for general medical and substance use disorders. *Psychiatric Services, 68*(4), 400-404.

Rozenblum, R., Miller, P., Pearson, D., & Marelli, A. (2015). Patient-centered healthcare, patient engagement and health information technology: The perfect storm. In M.A. Grando, R. Rozenblum, & D. Bates (Eds.), *Information technology for patient empowerment in healthcare.* Boston, MA: DeGruyter.

Scholl, I., Zill, J.M., Härter, M., & Dirmaier,J. (2014). An integrative model of patient-centeredness: A systematic review and concept analysis. *PLoS ONE 9*(9), e107828. doi:10.1371/journal.pone.0107828

Smith, J., Swallow, V., & Coyne, I. (2015). Involving parents in managing their child's long-term condition: A concept synthesis of family-centered care and partnership-in-care. *Journal of Pediatric Nursing, 30*(1), 143-159.

U.S. Department of Health and Human Services. (2016). *Quick statistics about hearing.* Retrieved from https://www.nidcd.nih.gov/health/statistics/quick-statistics-hearing

Wein, H., & Hicklin, T. (2015). *Talking with your doctor: Make the most of your appointment.* Retrieved from https://newsinhealth.nih.gov/2015/06/talking-your-doctor

Werner, S., Yalon-Chamovitz, S., Tenne Rinde, M., & Heymann, A.D. (2017). Principles of effective communication with patients who have intellectual disability among primary care physicians. *Patient Education and Counseling, 100*(7), 1314-1321.

Young, H.M., & Nesbitt, T.S. (2016). Increasing the capacity of primary care through enabling technology. *Journal of General Internal Medicine, 32*(4), 398-403.

Additional Readings

Cohen, S.E., Hooper, S.R., Javalkar, K., Haberman, C., Fenton, N., Lair, ... Ferris, M. (2015). Self-Management and transition readiness assessment: Concurrent, predictive and discriminant validation of the STARx questionnaire. *Journal of Pediatric Nursing, 30*(5), 668-676.

Family Caregiver Alliance® National Center on Caregiving. (n.d.). *Resources by health issue or condition.* Retrieved from https://www.caregiver.org/resources-health-issue-or-condition

Horowitz, S.H., Rawe, J., & Whittaker, M.C. (2017). *The state of learning disabilities: Understanding the 1 in 5.* New York, NY: National Center for Learning Disabilities.

Johnson, M.A., Javalkar, K., van Tilburg, M., Haberman, C., Rak, E., & Ferris, M.E. (2015). The relationship of transition readiness, self-efficacy, and adherence to preferred health learning method by youths with chronic conditions. *Journal of Pediatric Nursing, 30*(5), e83-e90.

National Institute on Aging. (2017). *Talking with your doctor: Discussing changes in your health worksheet.* Retrieved from https://www.nia.nih.gov/health/discussing-changes-your-health-worksheet

NurseBuff Blog. (2016). *8 free apps you can use for patient education.* Retrieved from https://www.nursebuff.com/patient-education-apps/

Office of Disease Prevention and Health Promotion. (2018). *Health literacy.* Retrieved from https://health.gov/communication/

Scholle, S., Torda, P., Peikes, D., Han, E., & Genevro, H. (2010). *Engaging individuals and families in the medical home* [AHRQ Publication No. 10-0083-EF]. Rockville, MD: Agency for Healthcare Research and Quality.

U.S. Department of Health and Human Services (n.d.). *Quick guide to health literacy.* Retrieved from http://www.health.gov/communication/literacy/quickguide/Quickguide.pdf

Chapter 4

Instructions for Continuing Nursing Education Contact Hours
Continuing nursing education credit can be earned for completing the learning activity associated with this chapter. Instructions can be found at aaacn.org/CCTMCoreCNE

Coaching and Counseling of Individuals and Families

Karen Alexander, PhD, MSN, RN
Constance Dahlin, MSN, ANP-BC, ACHPN, FPCN, FAAN
Judy Dawson-Jones, MPH, BSN, RN
Mary Clare Houlihan, MS, RN, CCRN

Learning Outcome Statement

After completing this learning activity, the learner will be able to utilize the existing strengths of the care team to create innovative ways to engage individuals and families in the care plan.

Learning Objectives

After reading this chapter, the Care Coordination and Transition Management registered nurse (CCTM® RN) will be able to:
- Discuss methods of developing a relationship with individuals and families to capitalize on their strengths and identify the barriers to fulfilling care plan goals.
- Demonstrate respect and valuing of individuals and families' preferences, interaction styles, and goals.
- Describe strategies to empower individuals and families in all aspects of the health care process (Cronenwett et al., 2007).
- Discuss definitions and key aspects of health coaching in the literature.
- Explain how to equip individuals and families with the tools needed to fulfill their responsibilities.
- Discuss ways to maintain a relationship with individuals and families to guide and reinforce the care plan.
- Demonstrate competence by positive individual outcomes as evidenced by increased care team communication, decreased emergency department visits, and reduced hospital re-admissions.
- Demonstrate the knowledge, skills, and attitudes required for the coaching and counseling of individuals and families dimension (see Table 4-1 on page 86).
- Facilitate advance care planning conversations with individuals and families to determine care preferences and surrogate decision-makers.
- Demonstrate understanding of palliative care as it pertains to advance care planning.
- Discuss role as primary palliative care provider and access to quality palliative care for individuals, as appropriate.

AAACN Care Coordination and Transition Management Standards

Standard 1.	Assessment
Standard 5.	Implementation
Standard 5a.	Coordination of Care
Standard 5b.	Health Teaching and Health Promotion
Standard 7.	Ethics

CCTM Scope and Standards of Practice for the CCTM® RN

To achieve effective implementation of the Care Coordination and Transition Management (CCTM®) Model by the registered nurse, the CCTM RN will coach and counsel individuals and families as they work to understand and cope with chronic disease and address social factors that influence their health. Individuals accessing health care should be empowered in all aspects of their care so they can actively participate with the care team and positively influence their care plan goals. In this dimension, the CCTM RN will develop the knowledge, skills, and attitudes necessary to prepare individuals and families to confidently carry out their responsibilities within the care plan (see Table 4-1).

Source: AAACN, 2016.

Chapter 4

> **Competency Definition**
> Coaching and counseling of individuals and their families involves developing a relationship that emphasizes communication, personalized goals, teamwork, and skill development (Guglielmi et al., 2014). In some instances, individuals' caregivers may not be family members. For the remainder of this chapter these caregivers will be termed *families*. The registered nurse coaches by guiding individuals to set goals, providing them with health information, and supporting them in meeting their goals (Esposito, Rhodes, Besthoff, & Bonuel, 2016). The registered nurse gives feedback on successes and constructive counseling to empower individuals in all aspects of their care so they can actively participate and positively influence their health outcomes.

I. **Develop a Relationship with the Individuals and Families**

A. Acknowledge and utilize the strengths of patients' existing support structure at home.
   1. Identification and inclusion of family members and community partners in the care team is key to success (Guglielmi et al., 2014), but this cannot occur until shared goals, resources, and limitations are known.
      a. "Value seeing health care situations through the patient's eyes" (Cronenwett et al., 2007, p. 123).
      b. Communicate regarding limitations of each team member and have defined responsibilities for the family members or community partners.
      c. Acknowledge the limitations of the CCTM RN and set availability boundaries.
   2. Families bring familiarity with local, culturally competent resources in their neighborhood.
      a. Recognize personally held attitudes about working with individuals from different ethnic, cultural, and social backgrounds (Cronenwett et al., 2007).
      b. Willingly support person-centered care for individuals and groups whose values differ from own (Cronenwett et al., 2007).
B. Barriers to coping and participating in the care plan include individual readiness to change, limited resources, and physical, mental, and educational limitations to include low health literacy (Ridosh, Roux, Meehan, & Penckofer, 2017).
   1. Readiness to change may not be immediately present in individuals or families.
      a. Nurses allow an individual to identify his or her readiness to change, as well as his or her own health goals to create autonomous control over goals (Mallishamv & Sherrod, 2017).
      b. Assess level of individual's ambivalence or decisional conflict while providing access to resources when requested (Mallisham & Sherrod, 2017).
   2. DiClemente and Prochaska (1998) created and tested the Transtheoretical Model of Change to describe behavioral change, which takes into account the patient's desire to change.
      a. Pre-contemplation: The time when the individual is not aware of a need to change behavior.
      b. Contemplation: The intention to take action in the next 6 months.
      c. Preparation: The intention to take action in the next month, with some new behaviors tried in the last 12 months.
      d. Action: Initiation of behavioral modification.
      e. Maintenance: Continuation of the behavior for more than 6 months.
   3. Identify what stage of readiness the individual is in before initiating interventions as a nurse coach (Mallisham & Sherrod, 2017).
      a. Understanding that not all patients will be prepared for action, allow a relationship to build that has a foundation in trust.
      b. Health outcomes desired by the patient may not mesh with the outcomes the medical team desires; however, reflecting on best care may help the team come to a shared goal (Guglielmi et al., 2014).
   4. Educational level of the patient and family needs to be determined before a care plan can be best carried out.
      a. Medical jargon and low health literacy contribute to individuals not hearing the messages being delivered (Esposito et al., 2016).
      b. Education will be personalized to the individual's disease management needs and reading and health literacy levels.
C. Activities and skills that will develop a relationship with the individual and family.
   1. Motivational interviewing is a proven technique to encourage behavior change,

which was first established within addiction therapy and has translated well into all types of health coaching.
- a. Motivational interviewing is an effective behavior change tool where individuals are guided towards addressing ambivalence to change and setting personal goals (Mallisham & Sherrod, 2017).
- b. The CCTM RN can guide individuals through the stages of change as they identify their own health goals and create autonomous control over their choices (Mallisham & Sherrod, 2017).
2. Empathy and listening must be at the heart of the interview process (VanBuskirk & Wetherell, 2014). Communication, whether face to face, via telephone, or email, is at the core of a coaching relationship.
- a. "Respect the dignity and privacy of patients while maintaining confidentiality in the delivery of team-based care" (Interprofessional Education Collaborative [IPEC], 2016, p. 19).
- b. Participate in building consensus or resolving conflict in the context of individual care (VanBuskirk & Wetherell, 2014).

II. **Encourage Individuals and Families to Be Active Members of the Team**

A. The CCTM RN is the day-to-day communicator via telephone or email in many settings, and therefore, can strive to include individuals and families in the team (Fritz, 2017).
B. Place interprofessional team collaboration in high importance with the individual as a valued member.
1. Individual is a co-laborer in the health goals, not an observer or a recipient.
2. Person-centered practice means care will look different for different individuals.
C. Activities that demonstrate the value of a individual on the team.
1. If person-centered goals and participation are valued as team outcomes, then nurses will be able to communicate these goals with all members of the interprofessional team (Guglielmi et al., 2014).
    - a. Communicate individual values, preferences, and expressed needs to other members of the health care team (Cronenwett et al., 2007).
    - b. Promote individualized self-management goals.
2. Frequently incorporate reflective practice after initiating goals.
    - a. Benner (1985) initially identified coaching as a nursing skill, emphasizing relational support and the art of caring.
    - b. "Recognize one's limitations in skills, knowledge, and abilities" (IPEC, 2016, p. 21).
3. In-person nurse-only visits, as well as telephone and email communication, can facilitate this interaction effectively (Swoboda, Miller, & Wills, 2017).

III. **Strategies in Identifying the Best Family Members to Support the Patient in the Health Care Plan**

A. It is important for the care team to identify which family member can most effectively provide the necessary level of support required by the individual.
1. Value active partnership with individuals or designated surrogates in planning, implementation, and evaluation of care (Guglielmi et al., 2014).
2. Respect individual preferences for degree of active engagement in care process (Cronenwett et al., 2007).
B. Motivational interviewing promotes trust between the care team, individual, and family, promoting an atmosphere of safety and acceptance for individuals to explore and modify health-related behaviors (Östlund, Wadensten, Kristofferzon, & Häggström, 2015).
1. Developing trust builds a collaborative team between the nurse, individual, and family.
2. Motivational interviewing relies on individuals' self-efficacy and families' understanding and desire to improve patients' health outcomes.
C. Refined listening skills are essential for clinicians to identify the family member who is best suited to support the patient's recovery plan.
D. The Fundamental Guidelines for Motivational Interviewing include (Miller, 2010):
1. Encourage and promote confidence in the individuals' and families' ability to achieve positive health outcomes.
2. Resist the reflex to direct rather than guide the recovery plan. Encourage individual input and respect the individual's perspective.
3. Understand a individual's motivation and desired health outcome.

4. Listen to individuals and family members to understand their interpersonal dynamics as they relate to the practical support and care during the individual's recovery process.
5. Empower individuals to control their own personal health outcomes.
6. Encourage and celebrate participation and contributions to wellness by individuals and families.
7. Initiate and promote collaborative conversation with individuals and families.
8. Identify and discuss all available resources with individuals and families.
9. Respect a person's autonomy and privacy.

E. When utilizing motivational interviewing, consider four general principles in your approach to collaborating with the family.
 1. Use honesty regarding matters of health and be empathetic to the individual's challenges relative to recovery (Mallisham & Sherrod, 2017).
    a. Engaging in honest discussions regarding individuals' medical conditions, along with a structured path to recovery, fosters realistic expectations by individuals and their families.
    b. Managing expectations and expanding individuals' understanding regarding their condition is essential to positive behavioral change.
    c. Consistent feedback and recognition of individual progress is indispensable to patient stability and positive outcomes.
    d. Acknowledging the role of family caregivers in progress discussions is invaluable to continued support and progress.
    e. Recognizing that ambivalence is normal and often inherent in longer recoveries.
    f. Discuss potential discrepancies in desired outcomes and behaviors that are inconsistent with the recovery plan (Mallisham & Sherrod, 2017). The relationship between the clinician, individual, families, and caregivers should address the benefits of changing behaviors that will facilitate desired outcomes.
    g. It is important to help individuals recognize contradictions between what they want and what they are doing.
    h. Acknowledge resistance and frustration by the individual and caregivers, which should signal a need to return to individual's goals (Mallisham & Sherrod, 2017).
    i. Care and recovery plans must include alternative care options that will accomplish the same goals and outcomes. Resistance often stems from fear of change and fear of failure.
    j. Encouragement and recognition of the individual's efforts and family contributions by clinicians is critical to maintaining the individual's progress, recovery, and positive outcomes.
 2. Support self-efficacy (Mallisham & Sherrod, 2017).
    a. Individuals and families must understand the value of changed behavior and have a solid belief in their ability to accomplish the desired change.
    b. Appreciate shared decision-making with empowered individuals and families, even when conflicts occur (Guglielmi et al., 2014).

IV. Equip the Individual and Family

A. Health coaching is an interprofessional concept that has been defined by a variety of experts. The nursing literature defines the practice as a goal-oriented, person-centered partnership, with individual enlightenment and empowerment as the desired outcome (Olsen, 2014). Health coaching is ultimately a method that educates patients while promoting self-management of individualized health.
 1. A self-management model can engage individuals in activities that promote health.
 2. The use of a self-management model is critical in equipping individuals and families with tools needed to fulfill their responsibilities.
 3. A self-management model is a set of tools used collaboratively by both individuals and their health care providers.
    a. It is a systematic approach to assessing the individual's self-management beliefs, behavior, and knowledge.
    b. Use of a self-management model improves partnerships with the individual's health care team, aids in sustaining behavior changes, collaboratively identifies goals, and targets interventions to reduce barriers.

B. The 5 A's Behavior Change Model Adapted for Self-Management Support Improvement (Glasgow et al., 2002) is an interactive, closed-loop model for implementing self-management strategies (see Figure 4-1).

Chapter 4

Figure 4-1.
5 A's Behavior Change Model
Adapted for Self-Management Support Improvement

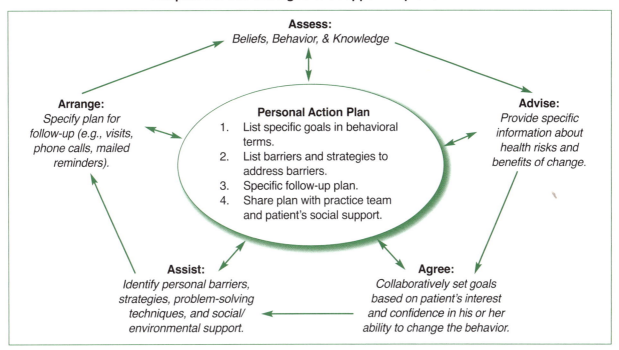

Source: Reprinted from Glasgow et al. (2002) with permission from Springer Science and Business Media.

Five A's Change Concept	Patient Level (Patient-Provider Interaction)	Office Environment (Standard Operating Procedure)	Community/Policy (Community Organization and Both Internal System and External Community Policy)
Assess CCM element: Have patient periodically complete valid health behavior surveys and provide him or her with feedback.	- Try brief behavior survey in (a) waiting room, (b) on computer. - Assess patient knowledge about his or her chronic condition. - Ask patient, "What about Self-Management (SM) is most important to talk about today?" - Ask patient, "What are your most challenging barriers?," recognizing physical, social, and economic barriers. - Provide patient with personalized feedback and results. - Assess conviction and confidence regarding target behaviors.	- Select or develop HRA survey. - Employ conviction and confidence rulers. - Revise self-care surveys to make appropriate. - Add fields to the medical record to record behavior status for smoking, weight, exercise. - Add behaviors to the problem list for patient. - Prompt staff to collect or update key behaviors status at each visit. - Have computer in waiting room for HRA assessment with printouts for providers and/or patients. - Employ outreach and population-based approach to assess all patients across multiple chronic illnesses. - Pilot approaches to providing feedback to patients; check for understanding.	*Community:* - Conduct needs assessment in partnership with community groups (e.g., include formative eval with potential users and non-users, small-scale recruitment studies to enhance methods). - Work on state health dept or other coalition to develop community health behavior survey or assess barriers to change. - Share data on BRFSS (Behavioral Risk Factor Surveillance System) items or other behaviors with other organizations. *Internal system policy:* - Employ longitudinal patient assessment system (e.g., using interactive computer technology). - Make screening on all four health behaviors a vital sign; and require reporting on all patients at some frequency.

continued on next page

Figure 4-1. (continued)
5 A's Behavior Change Model
Adapted for Self-Management Support Improvement

Five A's Change Concept	Patient Level (Patient-Provider interaction)	Office Environment (Standard Operating Procedure)	Community/Policy (Community Organization and Both Internal System and External Community Policy)
Advise *CCM element:* Provide personally relevant, specific recommendations for behavior change.	- Relate patient symptoms or lab results to patient behavior, recognizing patient's culture or personal illness model. - Inform patient that behavioral issues are as important as taking medications. - Provide specific, documented behavior change advice in the form of a prescription. - Share evidence-based guidelines with patients to encourage their participation.	- Develop list of benefits of behavior change/risk reduction. - Develop list of common symptoms that exercise, losing weight, or stopping smoking can improve. - Arrange prompt system to remind physicians to advise behavior change. - Provide prompt to have physician advise on importance of calling if any trouble taking medication as prescribed.	*Internal system policy:* - Reinforce/Recognize/Reward staff for documented advice to change behavior. *External policy:* - Recommend or lobby purchasers, health plan, and government to reimburse five A's/SM Action Planning.
Agree *CCM element:* Use shared decision-making strategies that include collaborative goal setting.	- Have patient develop specific, measurable, feasible SM goal for behavior change. - Provide options and choices among possible SM goals. - Do above with input from family or spouse, and with support/assistance from caregiver. - Share perspectives with patient on what is most important short-term goal; agree on a specific target. - Present evidence on benefits and harms to patient and let him or her decide on course.	- Make sure patient SM goals are in chart and all team members refer to them. - Provide staff with training in patient-centered counseling or empowerment training, which may include videos on motivational interviewing or goal setting. - Have in-service from expert on shared decision making. - Incorporate videos on patient role or choice into practice, and have patients see prior to consultation. - Develop multi-modal intervention to promote practice change rather than one utilizing single strategy.	*Community:* - Meet with organizations to identify agreed upon self-management support (patient education) priorities for coming year. *Internal system policy:* - Create field or permanent space in medical record for behavioral goals. - Develop assessment method to determine that goals were set in a collaborative fashion. - Require peer observation and feedback on real or simulated patients at a minimum of every 4 months. *External policy:* - Require or reimburse documentation of collaboratively set goals in medical records. - Recognize providers who have completed training in motivational interviewing; Bayer course on collaboration; etc.

continued on next page

Figure 4-1. (continued)
5 A's Behavior Change Model
Adapted for Self-Management Support Improvement

Five A's Change Concept	Patient Level (Patient-Provider Interaction)	Office Environment (Standard Operating Procedure)	Community/Policy (Community Organization and Both Internal System and External Community Policy)
Assist *CCM element:* Use effective self-management support strategies that include action planning and problem solving. Help patients create specific strategies to address issues of concern to them.	- Help patient develop strategies to address barriers to change (write on Action Plan form). - Implement patient discussion of SM Action Plan (a) during PCP visit, (b) immediately before or after with nurse. - Refer patient to evidence-based education or behavioral counseling (individual or group). - Elicit patient's views and plans regarding potential resources and support within family and community. - Use planned interactions to support evidence-based care. - Give care that patient understands and that fits with his or her cultural background. - During follow-up visits, review progress, experience, concerns; renegotiate goals and revise action plan.	- Select/develop SM Action Plan form. - Adapt SM Action. - Plan for your setting, specifically focusing on the four S's (size, scope, scalability, and sustainability) in planning any office restructuring. - Develop specific plan to enhance SM resources, by addressing the REAIM dimensions, to make sure you are addressing all key issues for panel wide or community impact. - Make sure blank Action Plan forms are in each exam room.	*Community:* - Work with community groups and referrals to develop Action Plans and communication avenues. - Get list of your patients who have used resources; get their feedback. *Internal system policy:* - Compile list of recommended quality resources that can be shared with staff and patients. - Evaluate adverse outcomes and quality of life for program revision and cost-benefit analysis. - Recognize/reward teams that have higher levels of documented action plans. *External policy:* - Add behavior change counseling to HEDIS criteria for each behavior for adult patients who receive such counseling. - Also, make problem solving, shared decision making, or approved SM support programs a HEDIS criterion.
Arrange *CCM elements:* Follow-up on action plans. Follow-up on referrals. Establish two-way communication and partner with community groups to improve services and linkages.	- Give patient copy of SM Action Plan. - Follow-up call to patient within a week after visit as "booster shot" for SM Action Plan. - E-mail follow-up or brief letter restating plan and inviting questions. - Arrange for patient to contact specific community resources that could support his or her goals. - Follow-up with goals set in action plan at each nonacute visit.	- Develop collaborative process that can facilitate communications and support with other practices. - Develop follow-up checklist/prompt to make sure follow-up is provided. - Include blank on Action Plan form for follow-up date.	*Community:* - Invite community program representatives to present at patient group visit, diabetes class, or health fair. - Follow-up with community programs to see how many patients attended and to get information on their progress. *Internal system policy:* - Employ longitudinal patient monitoring and feedback systems related to SM goals. - Provide time or incentives for follow-up contacts. *External policy:* - Recognize/reward social and economic environment in which these health systems interventions occur. - Reimburse follow-up phone calls, email contacts, etc., outside of face-to-face visit.

Source: Table developed by the authors from content in Glasgow et al. (2002).

C. The 5 A's are Assess, Advise, Agree, Assist, and Arrange. Each of the 5 A's feed into the individual's personal action plan (Glasgow et al., 2002).
1. Assess: Beliefs, behavior, and knowledge (Glasgow et al., 2002).
a. Assess individual's knowledge about his or her health status.
b. Elicit person's values, preferences, and expressed needs (Bednash, Cronenwett, & Dolansky, 2013; Cronenwett et al., 2007).
c. Assess levels of physical and emotional comfort (Bednash et al., 2013; Cronenwett et al., 2017).
d. Assess individual's confidence in dealing with his or her health goals and barriers.
e. Assess individual's knowledge, skills, and beliefs related to perceived health status.
2. Advise: Provide specific information about health risks and benefits of change (Glasgow et al., 2002).
a. Provide peron-centric recommendations to promote health.
b. Relate all health information to healthy behaviors.
c. Stress the importance of behavior changes.
3. Agree: Collaboratively set goals based on individual's interests and confidence in their ability to change behaviors (Glasgow et al., 2002).
a. Set collaborative goals.
b. Make SMART goals: Specific, Measurable, Attainable, Realistic, and Timely.
c. Incorporate family into plan to support and accomplish goals.
d. Communicate goals to all team members.
e. Consider both short- and long-term goals.
f. Discuss risks and benefits of proposed behavior changes.
4. Assist: Identify personal barriers, strategies, problem-solving techniques, and social/environmental support (Glasgow et al., 2002).
a. Promote creative strategies to lead to planned change.
b. Collaboratively design person-centric plans to address patient concerns.
c. Provide evidence-based care strategies.
d. Develop strategies and self-monitoring skills to address barriers to change.
5. Arrange: Specify plan for follow up (Glasgow et al., 2002).
a. Continually monitor and follow up on action plans that facilitate open communication.
b. Utilize strategies to monitor progress (email, phone calls, visits) as outlined in plan.
6. Personal action plan (Glasgow et al., 2002).
a. Identify specific goals.
b. List anticipated barriers.
c. Create strategies to minimize barriers.
d. Develop follow-up plan.
e. Communicate plan to patient/family and entire health care team.
D. Benefits to use of Self-Management Model.
1. Shared decision making.
2. Prompts behavior changes.
3. Relevant strategies and interventions.
4. Knowledge of treatment.
5. Individuals partner with health care team.
E. Awareness of person support structure within the health care team.
1. Telephone (and texting) contact.
2. Nurse-only visits.
3. Home visits.
4. Technology (Internet-based interventions).

V. **Maintain a Relationship with Individuals and Families**

A. Building a trusting relationship between clinicians, individuals, and families is a key component of successful coaching.
1. Establishing strong nurse-person relationships can determine the quality of individual outcomes, as well as the length of recovery (Guglielmi et al., 2014).
2. Development of a nurse-person relationship theory delineates conditions under which essential connections can be nurtured to attain desired health outcomes (Guglielmi et al., 2014).
3. The prerequisite for individual trust is the sense that the nurse is genuinely caring, compassionate, competent, and a knowledgeable expert regarding the individual's health care needs.
B. Halldorsdottir's (2008) theory was derived from an analysis of person/family perceptions of the nurse-person relationship. Building a relationship of trust between the nurse and patient can be categorized in six phases.
1. "Reaching out" (Halldorsdottir, 2008, p. 647).
a. Either the nurse or the individual reaching out to the other can

accomplish a connection; however, the other party needs to respond positively.
   b. If the individual reaches out to the nurse, the nurse needs to take the time to employ good listening skills to demonstrate a sense of genuine care.
   c. This initial communication can lay the foundation for building an effective bridge between nurse and individual/family members (Halldorsdottir, 2008).
2. "Removing the mask of anonymity" (Halldorsdottir, 2008, p. 647).
   a. Begin the development of removing the stereotypes of the individual and nurse.
   b. Nurse and individual acknowledge that each is essential to the individual's recovery program.
   c. Open discussion is an opportunity for the nurse to express interest and understanding of the broader dimension of the person's life (Halldorsdottir, 2008).
3. "Acknowledgment of connection" (Halldorsdottir, 2008, p. 647).
   a. At this juncture, the individual recognizes the connection because the nurse is responding to him or her as a whole person.
   b. Verbal, nonverbal, and body language are strong indicators of genuine caring.
   c. The nurse provides consistent eye-to-eye contact with the individual using dialogue, assuring the individual the nurse is listening and focused on his or her care and concerns (Halldorsdottir, 2008).
4. "Reaching a level of truthfulness" (Halldorsdottir, 2008, p. 647).
   a. In this progressive phase of connection, the individual has developed the feeling of being safe in the nurse's care.
   b. Individual will honestly share inner feelings, concerns, and level of knowledge and skill.
   c. Nurse acknowledges the patient's concerns, vulnerabilities, and feelings of uncertainty (Halldorsdottir, 2008).
5. "Reaching a level of solidarity" (Halldorsdottir, 2008, p. 647).
   a. Individual becomes more confident the nurse is on his or her side, and they are equal in the partnership.
   b. Feelings of mistrust disappear because the nurse demonstrates genuine care about the individual and understands the individual's personal life situation, goals, and expectations for recovery.
6. "True negotiation of care" (Halldorsdottir, 2008, p. 647).
   a. Nurse and individual work equally to develop the plan of care and goals.
   b. Nurse is able to be supportive while not creating a dependency. The nurse better understands the individual's world, and the individual has an increased sense of well-being (Halldorsdottir, 2008).
C. Careful, thoughtful navigation through these phases can influence an atmosphere that promotes a sense of support and well-being for individuals.

VI. **Advance Care Planning as Proactive Patient-Centered Care**
A. Defining advance care planning (ACP).
   1. A process of planning for an individual's future through discussion of goals, values, beliefs, and how they influence end-of-life care preferences and completion of appropriate documents (Izumi, 2017).
   2. ACP promotes the control of an individual's health care plan to guide care whether that person has decision-making capacity.
   3. Conversations are not a single or isolated instance, but rather, a process or series of conversations.
      a. Conversations should be initiated early and revisited.
      b. Conversations may change across the trajectory of illness.
      c. Conversations and context in which conversations occurred should be documented in the electronic health record.
   4. ACP is recommended for all children and adults regardless of age or health status because sudden events can occur that prevent individual decision-making (Izumi, 2017).
   5. ACP discussion includes three components:
      a. Identification of a surrogate decision-maker for health care, sometimes deemed a power of attorney for health care or a health proxy, to make medical decisions for an individual that is unable to make decisions.
      b. Description of medical and health care that the individual does or does not

want under certain conditions – depending on state where individual resides, usually referred to as advance directive and/or living will depending on state laws.
- c. Determination of resuscitation status (Do Not Resuscitate [DNR] and Do Not Intubate [DNI]) for the hospital and out of the hospital orders for life-sustaining treatment (a common form for this includes either Medical Orders for Life-Sustaining Treatment "MOLST" or Provider Orders for Life-Sustaining Treatment "POLST" forms).

B. Nurse's role in ACP conversation.
1. For the CCTM RN, ACP conversations are within the scope of practice of an RN, case manager, or care coordinator.
2. For the advanced practice registered nurse, case manager, or care coordinator, ACP may include prognostication and discussions about treatment decision-making in advanced illness.

C. Initiating ACP conversations.
1. Focus should be on open-ended questions to ascertain the values, beliefs, and care preferences of individuals and families.
2. Individual definitions of quality of life, religious/spiritual preferences, previous family/friend experiences with end-of-life care, and self-reflection should be considered during conversations.
3. Statements to normalize the conversation include (Dahlin & Wittenberg, 2015):
   - a. "I'd like to talk with you about possible health care decisions in the future."
   - b. "I would like to discuss something I discuss with those admitted to the hospital."
   - c. "I want to be sure I understand your wishes and preferences for aggressive care when there may be changes in your condition."
4. Questions to open the conversation include (Dahlin & Wittenberg, 2015):
   - a. "What is important to you?"
   - b. "What matters most to you?"
   - c. "How do you define quality of life?"
   - d. "If your health affects the things that matter or your quality of life, how would that change your health decisions?"
5. Resources for nurses to learn about how to initiate include:
   - a. End of Life Nursing Education Consortium (ELNEC): A collaborative education initiative between the City of Hope and the American Association of Colleges of Nursing (AACN) to improve palliative care (AACN, 2018).
   - b. The Conversation Project: Launched in collaboration with the Institute for Healthcare Improvement (IHI), The Conversation Project is a public engagement campaign with a simple goal to make sure that every person's wishes for end-of-life care are expressed and respected (The Conversation Project, 2018).
   - c. IMPACT ICU – Integrating Multi-disciplinary Palliative Care into the intensive care unit is a communication skills training program to provide education to bedside nurses (The Regents of the University of California, 2017).

D. Additional free ACP resources.
1. Five Wishes (Aging with Dignity, 2018).
   - a. A document that designates the health care power of attorney whom the individual wants to make decisions, what medical treatments the person wants, and other values and preferences about end-of-life care.
2. Choices for Care (Empath Health, 2018).
   - a. An affiliate of Suncoast Hospice. This site offers FAQs regarding advance directives and offers forms that list the individual's values and preferences for care of terminal illness and designation of a health care power of attorney.
3. Advance directive forms are available through the "Caring Info" page of the National Hospice and Palliative Care Organization; offers the forms from each state (National Hospice and Palliative Care Organization, 2018).
4. National Healthcare Decisions Day offers a plethora of resources from different organizations (National Healthcare Decisions Day, 2018).

VII. ACP and the Connection to Palliative Care

A. Definition of palliative care from the World Health Organization (2017).
1. Palliative care improves quality of life for individuals and families facing a life-threatening illness by providing adequate information; satisfying the physical, psychological, emotional, and spiritual needs of individuals; and facilitating prevention or alleviation of suffering.
2. Primary palliative care is defined as the basic palliative skills and competencies

required of all clinicians (Dahlin, 2015; Quill & Abernethy, 2013).
B. Specialized palliative care is defined by specialty consultation and care for complex cases (Weissman & Meier, 2011). Palliative care and ACP:
1. Palliative care begins at diagnosis of illness and involves an interprofessional and interdisciplinary team (Weissman & Meier, 2011).
    a. Early introduction promotes symptom management, decreases suffering, and improves overall quality of life (Temel et al., 2010; Vermylen, Szmuilowicz, & Kalhan, 2015).
    b. Appropriate interventions should consider disease process, symptom presentation, and goals of care (National Consensus Project for Quality Palliative Care, 2013).
    c. Care is based on ACP and goals of care, values, and preferences in health care.
2. Specific nursing considerations.
    a. Offer information to promote autonomy and decision-making.
    b. Assess and manage psychological, emotional, social, spiritual, and physical symptoms.
    c. Educate individuals on symptom management and clarify goals of care.
    d. The 4 C's of primary palliative care nursing interventions (Horton et al., 2013; Krimshtein et al., 2011).
        (1) Convening: Nurse ensures clinicians, individuals, and families come together to discuss care in a timely manner.
        (2) Checking: Nurse helps identify family needs, ensures families can voice concerns, and clarifies topics discussed.
        (3) Caring: Nurse supports family, responds appropriately to feelings, and assists interprofessional team with challenges.
        (4) Continuing: Nurse reinforces information and ensures decisions discussed are implemented.

C. Individuals demonstrate ability to seek help prior to escalation of symptoms.
D. Individuals demonstrate increased self-efficacy and ability to cope.

VIII. Evaluation and Outcomes

A. Individuals utilize the accessibility of the CCTM RN with increased phone, email, home, and office visits.
B. Individuals demonstrate increased understanding of resources available to meeting their self-management goals.

Table 4-1.
Coaching and Counseling of Individuals and Families: Knowledge, Skills, and Attitudes for Competency

Knowledge	Skills	Attitudes	Sources
Describe the benefit of the coaching relationship to the individual. Describe the benefit of the coaching relationship to the health care team.	Teach skills for self-management and supports individuals and families. Elicit individual values, preferences, and expressed needs as part of clinical interview.	Respect and encourage individual expression of values and preferences. Value the individual's expertise with own health and symptoms. Belief that individuals' and families' perspectives and participation are important in developing effective care plan.	Guglielmi et al., 2014 Ridosh et al., 2017
Describe motivational techniques. Understand SMART goals. Integrate understanding of multiple dimensions of person-centered care.	Assessment of life stressors motivating individuals towards self-care. Provide person-centered care with sensitivity and respect of health care team. Motivational interviewing may illicit shared, individual-centered goals.	Value involvement of individuals and families in shared decision-making. Individual as partner. Empathy and listening. Implement reflective practice and awareness of one's own limitations.	Östlund et al., 2015 Mallisham & Sherrod, 2017
Community resources and how to access services. Examine common barriers to active involvement of individuals in their own health care processes.	Assessment of family's strengths. Assessment of needs and barriers to health care goals.	Open and accepting attitude toward individuals and families. Person-centered care.	Mallisham & Sherrod, 2017
Demonstrate comprehension of self-management model.	Initiate 5 A's of Behavior Change.	Value involvement of individuals and families in self-management to prevent rehospitalization.	Glasgow et al., 2002
Understand role in ACP discussion.	Ability to discuss surrogate decision-maker, care options, and resuscitation orders within scope of practice.	Value individual and family involvement in conversations and participates in active listening during conversation.	Izumi, 2017; Dahlin & Wittenberg, 2015
Understand and describe palliative care.	Ability to discuss palliative care with individuals and describe palliative care as management of psychological, emotional, social, spiritual, and physical symptoms for individuals and families facing a life-threatening illness.	Encourage individual and family involvement in care plan and acknowledge individual concerns.	Quill and Abernethy 2012; Dahlin, 2015
Identify nurse role as primary palliative care provider.	Ensure clinicians, individuals, and families come together in a timely manner helps to identify family needs, and clarify topics of concern.	Support individual and family and respond appropriately to feelings.	Krimshtein et al., 2011; Horton et al., 2013

Chapter 4

Case Study 4-1.
Advanced Care Planning (ACP)

Introduction

Mr. Smith is a 65-year-old male who was recently hospitalized for a COPD exacerbation and is visiting the outpatient clinic for a follow-up appointment. After reviewing his chart and talking to him and his wife, you discover that he has been hospitalized five times in the last several years. You also discover that when Mr. Smith was initially admitted to the ICU, the clinical team discussed intubation and code status with him. Mr. Smith and his wife are [concerned] about his frequent hospitalizations and have several questions about prognosis and code status.

Clinical Interaction

Based on your assessment as the clinic nurse, you realize that Mr. Smith and his wife want to talk about advanced care planning (ACP). Together with Mr. and Mrs. Smith, you come up with a list of questions to discuss with the physician about prognostication and life-sustaining treatments he might need to consider in the future. While discussing this with Mr. Smith, you consider any spiritual or cultural issues that might affect any future decision-making, and provide him and his wife with resources about completing ACP paperwork. You also educate Mr. and Mrs. Smith on the importance of bringing any ACP paperwork with them whenever they visit the hospital to ensure that Mr. Smith's care wishes are met.

Clinical Implications

The CCTM® RN should ask open-ended questions and normalize the situation. Ask questions like, "You seemed to have a few concerns. Could you tell me more about them?" or "Many people have questions about ACP and planning for the future. Could you tell me more?"

First, does Mr. Smith want his wife involved in the conversation? Would another family member be a better surrogate decision-maker? Maybe this is the first time anyone has sat down with him to discuss these things. In this situation, the CCTM RN should stress that he does not have to make the decision at this exact moment, and that he can go home and discuss with his family.

Physicians and advanced practice registered nurses will discuss prognostication and end-of-life treatment decision-making; however, CCTM RNs can assess and manage physical symptoms, educate patients on symptom management, and clarify goals of care.

Often, nurses are unable to sign as a witness for power of attorney forms based on their clinical role. Nurses should discuss this with their employers.

Case Study 4-2.
Advanced Care Planning (ACP)

Introduction

Rayst Mohammed is an Arabic 10-year-old boy with asthma that is poorly managed. Over the last 7 months, he has had three hospitalizations and 10 emergency department visits, all driven by uncontrolled asthma. His last hospital discharge was 4 days ago, and he is now presenting to the primary care doctor with his mother because the discharging case manager made the appointment. The CCTM® RN meets with his mother to inquire about the reason for today's visit. What is the CCTM RN's primary objective?

Developing a trusting relationship with Rayst and his mother is essential. The CCTM RN must communicate in a manner that reassures both the mother and her child that the CCTM RN is there to help them develop a prescribed care plan to treat and control Rayst's asthma. Encouraging patients to embrace the CCTM RN as a partner in their care frequently improves outcomes (Hallidorsdottir, 2008, p. 647). In pediatrics, it is important to allow patients and their families to share their thoughts on the health situation because the care plan must include both the child and parents. Allowing the parents to own and drive decisions will not only support the child, but lead to more successful outcomes. The CCTM RN also explores the level of understanding for this patient and his mother. While the mother speaks English well, she quickly learns that her reading level of English is poor.

Clinical Interaction

The mother's concern is that Rayst keeps having asthma attacks and does not seem to be getting any better. She currently works at a restaurant and is having trouble at work because she is missing work too often as a result of Rayst's asthma. Rayst is outgoing, but overweight, and feels he is missing too many school days due to his asthma attacks. It has been determined that his mother uses the emergency department because it is available during her non-working hours. The CCTM RN needs to work with the family to set up appointments that are convenient and can be kept. In speaking with his mother, the CCTM RN realizes that she leaves for work before Rayst leaves for school, so the ability to monitor Rayst's compliance in using his inhaler is problematic.

Per the hospital discharge notes, Rayst is on a daily long-acting inhaler and also has his rescue inhaler and medications. An asthma action plan was given to his mother. The medical notes confirm the frequent visits to the emergency department and inpatient admissions, along with indications that Rayst and his family are non-compliant relative to his asthma care. The patient assessment was completed, and his respirations were 24, heart rate was normal, and his oxygen saturation was 98%. His breath sounds were clear with no audible wheezing upon auscultation. The CCTM RN asked his mother if she had his medications with her and to share

continued on next page

Case Study 4-2. (continued)
Advanced Care Planning (ACP)

any paperwork the hospital provided upon discharge. His mother shared his list of medications and his asthma action plan, and they were all written in English.

Clinical Implications

How does the CCTM RN begin developing a family care plan?

Rayst and his mother need to articulate their understanding of the treatment plan, their goals, and what works or does not work for them in a treatment plan. If there are any impediments they foresee, these need to be discussed as well. Ask Rayst what he wants to set as his health goals, making certain he understands his compliance is essential to a successful outcome. As the new/revised plan is developed, ask Rayst and his mother to describe their understanding of the step-by-step asthma action plan in detail. The plan should be translated into Arabic to meet his mother's comfort level with understanding. This assures the mother the CCTM RN recognizes the importance of their culture and language. The CCTM RN also offers to have an Arabic interpreter/family supporter in the appointments, for which his mother is very pleased. The CCTM RN must explain the details of the plan based on identifying symptoms and how exactly to respond to symptoms. Developing a plan with concise steps makes it more manageable. Ask if there are other family members who are involved in his care.

Check for resources that are available in the community to assist. A school nurse can assist in maintaining his compliance around medications and reinforce the need for compliance. Obtain a permit from his mother so you can contact the school nurse. Develop a family contract with all steps of the treatment plan detailed for the family. Encourage Rayst to be proactive in his care. Set weekly check-in phone calls or visits. Set attainable weekly goals for both Rayst and his mom.

The CCTM RN provides an asthma action treatment plan in Arabic and English for Rayst. Weekly appointments are set up with the goal of decreasing emergency department visits. The appointments are set during an evening clinic time with an Arabic translator. A process is created through the translator where they can rate each visit's experience and they both can share their thoughts on Rayst's progress; this begins the creation of a team, which includes the CCTM RN, family, and a support person.

Resource

Izumi, S., Barfield, P.A., Basin, B., Mood, L., Neunzert, C., Tadesse, R., ... Tanner, C.A. (2018). Care coordination: Identifying and connecting the most appropriate care to the patients. *Research in Nursing and Health, 41*(1), 49-56.

Chapter 4

References

American Academy of Ambulatory Care Nursing (AAACN). (2016). *Scope and standards of practice for registered nurses in care coordination and transition management.* Pitman, NJ: Author.

American Association of Colleges of Nursing (AACN). (2018). *About ELNEC.* Retrieved from www.aacnnursing.org/ELNEC/About

Aging with Dignity. (2018). *Five wishes.* Retrieved from https://fivewishes.org

Bednash, G.P., Cronenwett, L., & Dolansky, M.A. (2013). QSEN transforming education. *Journal of Professional Nursing, 29*(2), 66-67.

Benner, P. (1985). Quality of life: A phenomenological perspective on explanation, prediction, and understanding in nursing science. *Advances in Nursing Science, 8*(1), 1-14.

Cronenwett L., Sherwood G., Barnsteiner J., Disch J., Johnson J., Mitchell P., ... Warren J. (2007). Quality and Safety Education for Nurses (QSEN). *Nursing Outlook, 55*(3), 122-131.

Dahlin, C. (2015). Palliative care: Delivering comprehensive oncology nursing care. *Seminars in Oncology Nursing, 31*(4), 327-337.

Dahlin, C., & Wittenberg, E. (2015). Communication in palliative care. In B.R. Ferrell, N. Coyle, & J. Paice (Eds.), *Oxford textbook of palliative nursing* (4th ed., pp. 81-100). New York, NY: Oxford University Press.

DiClemente, C.C., & Prochaska, J.O. (1998). Towards a comprehensive, transtheoretical model of change: Stages of change and addictive behaviors. In W.R. Miller & N. Heather (Eds.), *Applied clinical psychology. Treating addictive behaviors* (pp. 3-24). New York, NY: Plenum Press.

Empath Health. (2018). *Your experts in advance care planning.* Retrieved from http://empathchoicesforcare.org/choices-for-care/

Esposito, E.M., Rhodes, C.A., Besthoff, C.M., & Bonuel, N. (2016). Ambulatory care nurse-sensitive indicators series: Patient engagement as a nurse-sensitive indicator in ambulatory care. *Nursing Economic$, 34*(6), 303-306.

Fritz, E.A. (2017). Transition to practice in ambulatory care nursing. *Journal for Nurses in Professional Development, 33*(5), 257-258.

Glasgow, R.E., Funnell, M.M., Bonomi, A.E., Davis, C., Beckham, V., & Wagner, E.H. (2002). Self-management aspects of the improving chronic illness care breakthrough series: Implementation with diabetes and heart failure teams. *Annals of Behavioral Medicine, 24*(3), 80-87.

Guglielmi, C., Stratton, M., Healy, G.B., Shapiro, D., Duffy, W.J., Dean, B.L., & Groah, L.K. (2014). The growing role of patient engagement: Relationship-based care in a changing health care system. *AORN Journal, 99*(4), 517-528.

Halldorsdottir, S. (2008). The dynamics of the nurse-patient relationship: Introduction of a synthesized theory from the patient's perspective. *Scandinavian Journal of Caring Sciences, 22*(4), 643-652. doi:10.1111/j.1471-6712.2007.00568x

Horton, R., Rocker, G., Dale, A., Young, J., Hernandez, P., & Sinuff, T. (2013). Implementing a palliative care trial in advanced COPD: A feasibility assessment (the COPD IMPACT study). *Journal of Palliative Medicine, 16*(1), 67-73.

Interprofessional Education Collaborative (IPEC). (2016). *Core competencies for interprofessional collaborative practice.* Retrieved from https://www.aacom.org/docs/default-source/insideome/ccrpt05-10-11.pdf?sfvrsn=77937f97_2

Izumi, S. (2017). Advance care planning: The nurse's role. *The American Journal of Nursing, 117*(6), 56-61.

Krimshtein, N.S., Luhrs, C.A., Puntillo, K.A., Cortez, T.B., Livote, E.E., Penrod, J.D., & Nelson, J.E. (2011). Training nurses for interdisciplinary communication with families in the intensive care unit: An intervention. *Journal of Palliative Medicine, 14*(12), 1325-1332.

Mallisham, S.L., & Sherrod, B. (2017). The spirit and intent of motivational interviewing. *Perspectives in Psychiatric Care, 53*(4), 226-233.

Miller, N.H. (2010). Motivational interviewing as a prelude to coaching in healthcare settings. *Journal of Cardiovascular Nursing, 25*(3), 247-251.

National Consensus Project for Quality Palliative Care. (2013). *Clinical practice guidelines for quality palliative care.* Pittsburgh, PA: Author.

National Healthcare Decisions Day. (2018). *Advance care planning.* Retrieved https://www.nhdd.org/public-resources/

National Hospice and Palliative Care Organization. (2018). *Download your state's advance directives.* Retrieved from http://www.caringinfo.org/i4a/pages/index.cfm?pageid=3289

Olsen, J.M. (2014). Health coaching: A concept analysis. *Nursing Forum, 49*(1), 18-29.

Östlund, A.S., Wadensten, B., Kristofferzon, M.L., & Häggström, E. (2015). Motivational interviewing: Experiences of primary care nurses trained in the method. *Nurse Education in Practice, 15*(2), 111-118

Quill, T.E., & Abernethy, A.P. (2013). Generalist plus specialist palliative care – Creating a more sustainable model. *New England Journal of Medicine, 368*(13), 1173-1175.

Ridosh, M.M., Roux, G., Meehan, M., & Penckofer, S. (2017). Barriers to self-management in depressed women with type 2 diabetes. *Canadian Journal of Nursing Research, 49*(4), 160-169.

Swoboda, C.M., Miller, C.K., & Wills, C.E. (2017). Impact of a goal setting and decision support telephone coaching intervention on diet, psychosocial, and decision outcomes among people with type 2 diabetes. *Patient Education and Counseling, 100*(7), 1367-1373.

Temel, J.S., Greer, J.A., Muzikansky, A., Gallagher, E.R., Admane, S., Jackson, V.A., ... Lynch, T.J. (2010). Early palliative care for patients with metastatic non-small-cell lung cancer. *New England Journal of Medicine, 363*(8), 733-742.

The Conversation Project. (2018). *Overview.* Retrieved from https://theconversationproject.org

The Regents of the University of California. (2017). *The Integrating Multidisciplinary Palliative Care into the ICU (IMPACT-ICU) Project.* Retrieved from http://vitaltalk.org/resources/impact-icu/

VanBuskirk, K.A., & Wetherell, J.L. (2014). Motivational interviewing with primary care populations: A systematic review and meta-analysis. *Journal of Behavioral Medicine, 37*(4), 768-780.

Vermylen, J.H., Szmuilowicz, E., & Kalhan, R. (2015). Palliative care in COPD: An unmet area for quality improvement. *International Journal of Chronic Obstructive Pulmonary Disease, 10,* 1543-1551.

Weissman, D.E., & Meier, D.E. (2011). Identifying patients in need of a palliative care assessment in the hospital setting: A consensus report from the Center to Advance Palliative Care. *Journal of Palliative Medicine, 14*(1), 17-23.

World Health Organization. (2017). *WHO definition of palliative care.* Retrieved from http://www.who.int/cancer/palliative/definition/en/

Chapter 5

Person-Centered Care Planning

Instructions for Continuing Nursing Education Contact Hours
Continuing nursing education credit can be earned for completing the learning activity associated with this chapter. Instructions can be found at aaacn.org/CCTMCoreCNE

Carol A. Newman, DNP, MSED, MSN, RN, CPNP-PC
Dawn M. Gerz, MSN, MBA, RN, NEA-BC, RN-BC
Judith Toth-West, PhD, RN, CCTM, CCM, CPHQ
Jayme M. Speight, MSN, RN-BC

Learning Outcome Statement

After completing this learning activity, the learner will be able to demonstrate the ability to develop, implement, and provide ongoing management of a comprehensive, evidence-based, coordinated, person-centered plan of care focused on the individual's values, preferences, and health care needs in partnership with the primary care provider and interprofessional care team.

Learning Objectives

After reading this chapter, the Care Coordination and Transition Management registered nurse (CCTM® RN) will be able to:
- Perform a comprehensive person-centered needs assessment focusing on the adult and pediatric individual's health care needs to optimize the delivery of quality and safe care.
- Identify gaps in coordinated health care delivery and individualize the plan of care focus through proactive pre-encounter planning.
- Describe the process for the identification of high-risk populations and identification of risk factors.
- Utilize motivational interviewing as a communication method to guide the individual, family, and/or legal guardian planning to foster positive behavior changes to improve health.
- Develop a plan of care utilizing input from individual, family, legal guardian, and interprofessional team members.
- Design clinical interventions supported by evidence-based practice guidelines.
- Demonstrate the knowledge, skills, and attitudes required for the person-centered care planning dimension (see Table 5-1 on page 104).
- Demonstrate competency for the following Standards of Practice for Registered Nurses in Care

AAACN Care Coordination and Transition Management Standards
Standard 1. Assessment
Standard 3. Outcomes Identification
Standard 4. Planning
Standard 5. Implementation
Standard 9. Research and Evidence-Based Practice
Standard 11. Communication
Standard 13. Collaboration

Source: AAACN, 2016.

Competency Definition
"Recognize the patient or designee as the source of control and full partner in providing compassionate and coordinated care based on respect for patient's preferences, values, and needs" (Cronenwett et al., 2007, p. 123).

In designing the plan of care, the registered nurse (RN) engaged in Care Coordination and Transition Management (CCTM®) recognizes the integral role individuals, families, legal guardians, and caregivers have in ensuring the health and well-being of individuals. The CCTM RN acknowledges that emotional, social, and developmental support are critical components in the delivery of health care (Institute for Patient- and Family-Centered Care, 2014). Engaging individuals and their designees in care plan development supports improved patient outcomes, increases individual and family satisfaction, restores dignity and control, and contributes to financial stewardship in the allocation of resources. Core concepts for person-centered care planning include (a) respect and dignity: honor perspectives, choices, values, beliefs, and cultural backgrounds; (b) information sharing: timely, accurate, transparent, and complete communication; (c) participation: engagement and participation of individuals and families in care and decision-making; and (d) collaboration: inclusion of individuals and families in program design, implementation, policy development, and professional education (The Institute for Patient- and Family-Centered Care, 2014). The degree of inclusion is determined by the individual and does not preclude the individual making care decisions independently if he or she is competent to do so (Institute for Patient- and Family-Centered Care, 2014).

I. **Comprehensive Needs Assessment**

A. Patient Health Questionnaire: Patient Health Questionnaire, with two or nine questions (PHQ-2 or 9), is a validated tool to assess for signs and symptoms of depression (Manea, Gilbody, & McMillan, 2012; Seo & Park, 2015). The purpose of the PHQ-2 is not to establish final diagnosis or to monitor depression severity, but rather to screen for depression in a first-step approach (Horton & Perry, 2016). A score of 3 or more requires further inquiry using the PHQ-9 Questionnaire. The Patient Health Questionnaire-9 is a depression rating scale frequently utilized both in primary care and psychiatry clinics (Torous et al., 2015). Both questionnaires focus on the individual's health during the previous 2 weeks.
   1. It is scored by the primary care provider or another member of the team.
   2. A positive screen PHQ-9 is further assessed for presence and duration of suicide ideation.
   3. The questionnaire can be repeated at each visit to reflect improvement or worsening of depression and response to treatment.
   4. Notify primary care provider for worsening signs and symptoms.
   5. Emergent intervention when active suicidal intent is present.

B. Functional assessment: Katz Index of Independence in Activities of Daily Living (IADL) is the most appropriate instrument to use in assessing functional status when measuring an individual's ability to perform activities of daily living independently (Katz, Down, Cash, & Grotz, 1970). The Katz IADL scale assesses basic personal activities of daily living (ADLs) and ranks capability of performance in six functions: bathing, dressing, toileting, transferring, continence, and feeding (Mlinac & Feng, 2016).
   1. Tool is used to detect problems in performing ADLs.
   2. CCTM RNs should plan for increased services such as physical therapy, occupational therapy, and visiting nurse or aide services for individuals who have difficulties with ADLs.

C. CAGE and CAGE-AID: CAGE-AID is a questionnaire that focuses on both drug and alcohol abuse. The CAGE is used primarily for the detection of alcohol use (Williams, 2014). The CAGE-AID is a conjoint questionnaire in which the focus of each item of the CAGE questionnaire was expanded from alcohol alone to include other drugs (Basu, Ghosh, Hazari, & Parakh, 2016; Brown & Rounds, 1995). There are four questions to be completed by the individual. One or more *yes* responses is regarded to be a positive screen.
   1. Positive screen requires follow-up with primary care provider about drug and alcohol rehabilitation.
   2. Behavior medicine or behavioral health consult as needed.
   3. Monitor at each visit to promote dialogue about the problem.
   4. Recommend referral to Alcoholics Anonymous.
   5. Recommend referral to other drug or alcohol treatment programs in the area.

D. The Mini-Cog – Mental Status Assessment of Older Adults: Researchers estimate dementia affects between 2.4 million and 5.5 million Americans. Ideally, early identification of cognitive impairment would allow individuals and their families to receive care at an earlier stage in the disease process, which could lead to improved prognosis and decreased morbidity (Lin, O'Connor, Rossom, Perdue, & Eckstrom, 2013; Tsoi, Chan, Hirai, Wong, & Kwok, 2015).
   1. The Mini-Cog is a simple screening tool that takes 3 minutes to administer.
   2. Effective triage tool to identify individuals in need of further evaluation by a neurologist.
   3. Clock Drawing Test (CDT) is scored as normal or abnormal.
   4. CDT is considered normal if all numbers are present in correct sequence and position; hands are readably displayed at the correct time. (Length of hands is not a factor.)
   5. Instruct individual to remember three words such as table, pencil, and apple.
   6. Next, ask the individual to draw a clock showing the time of 11:15.
   7. Next, ask the individual to state the three recalled words.
   8. Award 1 point for each recalled word and 2 points for correct CDT.
   9. Score 0-2 is considered positive screen for dementia and requires prompt evaluation.

Chapter 5

   10. Early identification and intervention should lead to better outcomes.
E. Modified Caregiver Strain Index (MCSI): MCSI is a validated tool used to assess severity of caregiver strain (Jennings et al., 2015). "Caregivers may be prone to depression, grief, fatigue, financial hardship, and changes in social relationships. Screening tools are useful to identify families who would benefit from a more comprehensive assessment of the care giving experience" (Onega, 2018, p. 1).
   1. Thirteen-question tool that measures strain related to care provision.
   2. Covers five domains: financial, physical, psychological, social, and personal.
   3. Higher the score, higher the strain.
   4. Self-administered instrument by the client/caregiver.
   5. Appropriate interventions are needed to help the caregiver.
   6. Further assessment of the caregiver by his or her primary care provider.
   7. Early intervention could prevent further deterioration in the individual and caregiver.
F. Get Up and Go Test: "The timed Get Up and Go Test is a measurement of mobility. It includes a number of tasks such as standing from a seating position, walking, turning, stopping, and sitting down which are all important tasks needed for a person to be independently mobile" (Mathias, Nayak, & Isaacs, 1986, p. 387). Researchers have recently studied the validity of the Get Up and Go Test and have found it valid for both young and older adults (Alfonso-Mora, 2017; Tamura, Kocher, Finer, Murata, & Stickley, 2018).
   1. Test is performed when an individual is wearing regular footwear, using usual walking aid, and sitting in chair with an armrest.
   2. On the word "go," individual is asked to get up, walk 3 meters, turn, walk back to chair, and sit down.
   3. Time the second effort only.
   4. Observe individual for postural stability, step pace, stride length, and sway.
   5. Normal scoring is ≤ 10 seconds.
   6. Low score indicates good functional independence.
   7. High score indicates need for physical therapy consult for fall risk.
   8. Baseline should be done annually and repeated when any changes occur.
G. Patient Activation Measure: "The Patient Activation Measure (PAM) assessment gauges the knowledge, skills, and confidence essential to managing one's own health and health care. The PAM assessment segments consumers into one of four progressively higher activation levels. Each level addresses a broad array of self-care behaviors and offers deep insight into the characteristics that drive health activation. A PAM score can also predict health care outcomes including medication adherence, ER utilization, and hospitalization" (South Carolina Department of Health and Human Services, 2014, para. 2). The PAM tool is a proprietary tool. For pricing, visit the Insignia Health website at: https://www.insigniahealth.com/pam-license/commercial-pam-license
   1. Level 1: No confidence in their ability to change.
   2. Level 2: Lack confidence or understanding of their health.
   3. Level 3: Have knowledge and may begin to develop confidence.
   4. Level 4: Adopted new behaviors to effect change in their health status.
   5. Engaged individuals are more able to make positive changes in their health outcomes.
H. Comprehensive Geriatric Assessment: "Comprehensive geriatric assessment (CGA) is defined as a multidisciplinary diagnostic and treatment process that identifies medical, psychosocial, and functional limitations of a frail older person in order to develop a coordinated plan to maximize overall health with aging" (Ward & Reuben, 2018, para. 5). The CGA is the most researched model for health care delivery for frail older individuals (Welsh, Gordon, & Gladman, 2013). The geriatric individual presents many challenges such as polypharmacy and multimorbidity, as well as difficulties with psychosocial and functional status. An acute hospitalization can cause even more decline. "Within 6 months following an acute hospitalization, 30% to 50% of older patients experience a loss of activities of daily living (ADLs), 20% to 30% are readmitted and 20% to 30% die" (Buurman et al., 2016, p. 302).
   1. CGA informs a process by which to manage the geriatric individual.
   2. CGA is multidimensional and interprofessional.
   3. CGA identifies problems and goal-driven interventions.
   4. Ultimately provides and coordinates an integrated plan for treatment, rehabilitation, support, and long-term care (Welsh et al., 2013).
   5. Domains of the CGA include: physical medical conditions including comorbid conditions and disease severity, medication review, nutritional status, problem list;

mental health conditions including cognition, mood, and anxiety, fears; functional status such as mobility and balance, ADLs, life roles important to the individual; social circumstances including social networks, informal support available from family, network of friends, and contacts, and statutory care, financial needs; environment including housing, comfort, facilities and safety, transport facilities, potential for telehealth use, and accessibility to local resources (Welsh et al., 2013).
   6. Interprofessional team of the CGA includes medical doctor, pharmacist, care coordination transition management nurse, case manager, social worker, and other team members as needs are identified.
   7. CGA is an ongoing process, responsive to the individual's changing needs.
I. Pediatric considerations: When assessing for pediatric needs, Bright Futures, "a national health promotion and prevention initiative, led by the American Academy of Pediatrics and supported, in part, by the US Department of Health and Human Services, Health Resources and Services Administration (HRSA), Maternal and Child Health Bureau (MCHB)" provides a comprehensive list of assessment tools based on developmental stages of the pediatric population (American Academy of Pediatrics, 2018, para. 1).

II. **Pre-Encounter Chart Review and Visit Planning to Identify Gaps in Care and Individualize the Plan Focus**

A. Pre-encounter chart review may be completed by licensed or unlicensed health care personnel who are trained and competent to follow existing protocols (e.g. RN, LPN, medical assistants, health coaches, patient navigators) (Bodenheimer, 2015).
B. The individual's medical record or electronic health record is a useful tool in the early phase of individual assessment. Questions to be posed are:
   1. When was the individual last seen by his or her primary care provider (PCP)?
   2. Has he or she missed several appointments?
   3. Has it been over 13 months since his or her last preventive care visit?
   4. Are the individual's recommended preventive care guidelines up to date?
   5. Has the individual had a hemoglobin A1c (HbA1c) that is less than 7% in the last 6 months?
   6. What is the individual's most recent biometric data?
   7. What is the individual's body mass index (BMI)?
   8. Are medications up to date (expired or need refill)?
C. The U.S. Preventive Services Task Force (USPSTF) "is an independent panel of experts in primary care and prevention who systematically reviews the evidence of effectiveness and develops recommendations for clinical preventive services" (USPSTF, 2018, para. 1).
   1. Pre-encounter chart review: Examine individual's chart 24 to 48 hours before visit with PCP.
      a. Based on individual's age and sex, what are the recommended screenings and tests completed (e.g., colorectal screening ages 50-75)?
      b. Based on above, what screenings and/or tests are outstanding (missing screening such as Pap test)?
      c. Based on above, are there currently any pending orders for these tests (orders for screen pending)?
      d. Vaccination history and recommended vaccines needed at this appointment (e.g., flu vaccine during flu season)?
      e. Specialist appointments needed (e.g., yearly dilated eye exam for all diabetics related to diabetic retinopathy)?
      f. Abnormal lab work or test results to review with PCP?
      g. Is there a pattern of routinely missed appointments?
      h. Presence/absence of life-planning resources such as advanced directives, health care proxy/durable power of attorney for health care?
      i. Meaningful use core objectives as outlined by Centers for Medicare & Medicaid Services (CMS) (2018) should be included in chart review as indicated (e.g., smoking status for all individuals 13 years or older).
      j. Psychosocial information such as need for caregiver, housing assistance?
   2. Encounter planning: It is necessary to plan for the individual encounter in advance so outstanding test results, recommended preventive care, and PCP orders are obtained before encounter.
      a. Identify missing lab results obtained from outside lab (need to record results from outside lab into medical record).

b. Reports from outside ophthalmologist, endocrinologist, and discharge summary from hospital or emergency department (ED); dentist and pharmacy information should be obtained and updated in individual's chart.
   c. Review missing labs, X-rays, and immunizations with PCP before visit, so orders can be obtained.
   d. Notify individual (or caregiver) of any outstanding lab results, X-rays, etc.; schedule these tests before appointment with PCP. May utilize technology for individual contact (e.g., MyChart or email) in addition to telephone.
   e. Print life-planning resource documents for individual and caregiver (if applicable) to review during encounter.
   f. Print screening tools to be used during an encounter (e.g., PHQ-2 or 9).
3. Gaps in care: If any gaps in care are noticed, be sure to review with PCP before appointment, so these issues can be addressed at time of appointment.
   a. Missed appointments.
      (1) Ascertain with individual why he or she missed appointment.
   b. No recent lab work (routine labs to check progression of chronic disease).
   c. Discharge and pharmacy.
      (1) Meet with interprofessional team throughout discharge process.
      (2) Ensure inpatient case management and social work are included in plan.
      (3) Ensure PCP is aware of discharge plan through electronic or face-to-face communication.
      (4) Family and caregivers are aware and understand care plan.
      (5) Care plan is easily accessible to all stakeholders.
      (6) Care plan is updated as needed.

III. **Risk Stratification**

"One quarter (24%) of Americans have two or more chronic conditions. Their health care is often fragmented, low-quality, inefficient and unsatisfactory to them and their physicians. The Institute of Medicine has described chronic care in America as a 'nightmare to navigate.' People with multi-morbidity are also at high risk for generating high health care expenditures: 96% of the Medicare budget is spent on beneficiaries with multiple chronic conditions" (Boult et al., 2013, p. 412). Risk stratification is the process to proactively identify and outreach to at-risk individuals to develop person-centered care planning. In addition, the Advisory Board (2017) states that "a holistic approach starts with identifying which patients are at risk, and then prioritizing patients that are willing and will most likely benefit from planned interventions" (p. 5).

A. Different ways to identify individuals at risk:
   1. Predictive modeling software, such as Athena Clarity, IBM Premier, and Optum.
   2. Chronic disease-based models (e.g., such as diabetes, chronic obstructive pulmonary disease [COPD], hypertension, or congestive heart failure [CHF]).
   3. Age-specific models, chronic disease registries, and risk scoring using different methodologies (e.g., LACE Index, Interact, BOOST Tools) to predict re-admission risk.
   4. Once identified as a high-risk individual, one can be further risk stratified as high, moderate, and low risk. A common model is to focus on high-risk such as individuals with diabetes with HbA1c ranges greater than 8.0 with two or more co-morbidities.
   5. High-risk populations include recently discharged individuals from any site including acute care and post-acute care.
   6. Individuals in transition are at risk especially if they have multiple chronic diseases, polypharmacy, limited social support, age greater than 65, and decline in functional status after lengthy hospitalization (Le Berre, Maimon, Sourial, Guériton, & Vedel, 2017).
   7. Example of chronic disease risk stratification model of care (see Table 5-2).
B. High-risk individuals are identified through comprehensive chart review, consultation with PCP, and individual agreement. The CCTM RN assesses the following to develop foundation for care planning.
   1. Chart review.
      a. Does the individual meet high-risk criteria?
         (1) Individual is unstable.
         (2) Individual needs psychosocial support.
         (3) Individual does not have access to medications prescribed.
         (4) Individual has increased utilization of hospital and ED services.
         (5) Home situation has recently deteriorated. Examples could be:
            (a) Change in vision/hearing.
            (b) Change in living situation.
            (c) Change in social support.

Table 5-2.
Chronic Disease Risk Stratification Tool

Low (8-12 visits)	High (18-24 visits)
• Chronic renal failure (CRF) stage 1-2 with glomerular filtration rate (GFR) 60 or greater • A1C > or = 7.0 • Positive tobacco use • Controlled HTN <BP 140/90 • No appointment with PCP within 1 year • One ED visit and/or hospitalization in preceding 12 months	• CRF stages 4 or 5 GFR less than 29 • A1C > 8.0 • HTN stage 2:2 or ≥ 160; or ≥ 100 • History of CAD • Prescribed eight or more medications • Re-admission within 30 days • Mental health diagnosis • Age greater than 80 • Greater than one ED visit and/or hospitalization in preceding 3 months
Moderate (12-18 visits)	**Variances**
• CRF stage 3 GFR 30-59 • AIC > 7-8 • Uncontrolled HTN 2 or more readings > 140-159; or 90-99 • History of CAD • Prescribed eight or more medications • One ED visit and/or hospitalization in preceding 6 months	• Co-morbid disease exacerbation requiring medication initiation/titration • Cognitively impaired with caregiver support • Cognitively impaired without caregiver support • ED or inpatient re-admission after program initiation • Established adherence with program goals met • Established history of nonadherence • Identified barrier to learning • Mental health diagnosis, undertreated or unstable • New diagnosis • Reinforcement of treatment plan objectives needed • Risk stratification classification change to more complicated level

Source: Lahey Hospital & Medical Center, Burlington, MA. Reprinted with permission.

        (d) Change in cognition (Ward & Reuben, 2018).
   b. The individual meets high-risk criteria, but all needs are already met.
   c. Individual has additional care needs that require coordination.
        (1) Caregiver support.
        (2) Community resources or ancillary services.
        (3) Primary care and specialty medical management.
        (4) Psychosocial support.
        (5) Pharmacist support to optimize medication management (Improving Primary Care, 2018).
C. Review individual list with PCP.
   1. Provider feels individual would not benefit from interventions.
   2. Provider knows individual is moving out of state in the next few months.
   3. Provider knows individual, physically and mentally well.
   4. Provider recommends additional individuals not on registry.
   5. Individuals are actively using ED and inpatient services.
   6. History of non-adherence to hospital follow-up appointments.
   7. Frequent calls to the practice with minor complaints.
D. Individual engagement: Once the individual is identified as high-risk, next step is to contact the patient and/or caregiver for intake and assessment.
   1. Send an introductory letter explaining the program and identify individual's PCP.
   2. Meet the individual at an upcoming appointment.
   3. Meet the individual when he or she is admitted to the hospital.
   4. Assign a team member to do outreach calls when available.
      a. State you work with PCP _____, and he or she requested you set up an appointment.
      b. Explain you are available to help with transportation, medications, disease-specific questions, and to coordinate care overall.
      c. Keep conversations simple.
      d. If individual is not responding to calls, engage team members to assist with outreach individual activation. Outreach

to individual's caregiver or family may be necessary (e.g., geriatric population or individuals with dementia).
5. Before calling individual, spend 5 to 10 minutes to do chart review.
   a. Focus on missed appointments, history, and behavioral health history.
   b. Medications.
   c. Symptoms/diagnoses.
   d. Actively listen.
   e. Assess areas you may be able to assist with.
E. Barriers to individual engagement.
   1. Psychosocial or mental illness.
   2. Low motivation.
   3. Time constraints for providers.
   4. Not ready to change.
   5. Insufficient orientation and training of RN in new CCTM role.
   6. Illness or pain.
   7. Functional deficits.
   8. Substance abuse.
   9. Low health literacy (education).
   10. Religious beliefs.
   11. Culture differences.

IV. **Motivational Interviewing (MI)**

A skillful clinical communication style for eliciting from individuals their own motivations for making behavior changes in the interest of their health (Rollnick, Miller, & Butler, 2007). Motivational interviewing provides a practical method to achieve person-centered care in the situations where evidence supports behavior change and action is dependent on personal preferences (Elwyn et al., 2014).

A. MI is described as a form of collaborative conversation for strengthening an individual's own motivation and commitment to change. It is a person-centered counseling style for addressing the common problem of ambivalence about change by paying particular attention to the language of change.
B. MI is designed to strengthen an individual's motivation for and movement toward a specific goal by eliciting and exploring the individual's own reasons for change within an atmosphere of acceptance and compassion (Motivational Interviewing Network of Trainers, 2014).
C. MI is characterized as collaborative, evocative, and supporting of an individual's autonomy.
D. Utilize the four guiding principles of MI: acronym RULE (Rollnick et al., 2007).
   1. Resist the righting reflex.
   2. Understand and explore the individual's own motivations.
   3. Listen with empathy.
   4. Empower the individual, encouraging hope and optimism.
E. Key listening skills.
   1. Listen in an empathetic, attentive, nonjudgmental, warm, and supportive way. Good listening begins with following. Following the individual's lead at the beginning of a conversation allows for understanding of the individual's symptoms and how these fit into the larger picture of his or her life and health (Rollnick et al., 2007).
   2. Summarize what the individual said. This is key to demonstrate to the individual you are listening while verifying you understood correctly. Offer periodic brief summaries to highlight the "pearls."
F. Pediatric considerations: Developmental milestones should always be considered when using MI in pediatric settings (Barnes & Gold, 2012). MI can be used at any age with the use of developmentally appropriate modifications in congruence with using caregivers as the agent of change for very young children or pre-verbal children (Barnes & Gold, 2012).

V. **Keys to Successful MI**

A. Build rapport: 20% of conversation time is spent on building rapport.
   1. Engage the individual and invest in the beginning.
   2. The relationship is the most powerful tool in MI.
   3. The interaction between provider and individual powerfully influences the individual's resistance, compliance, and change.
   4. Ask mainly open-ended questions: "Tell me more about…"
   5. Use agenda setting to give the individual as much decision-making freedom as possible (Rollnick et al., 2007). A useful tool to achieve this is the bubble sheet, in which several relevant topics are outlined and the individual chooses which one to focus on. This brief conversation takes about 1 minute.
B. Resist the urge to "fix" things. This gets in the way of change.
C. Informing: Knowledge about the risks and benefits is an important element in deciding to change. Provide personal feedback, advice, and/or education in a neutral manner (Rollnick et al., 2007). When informing, it is important to resist the "righting reflex." The righting reflex is the compulsion to immediately point out risks or problems with the individual's behavior or plan (Salvo & Cannon-Breland, 2015).

D. Stages of change: Recognize individuals may relapse and progress through the stages several times before successfully maintaining the change; individuals may not move through the stages in a linear fashion; stages may be skipped or they may revert to an earlier stage (Levensky, Forcehimes, O'Donohue, & Beitz, 2007).
E. "Change talk:" Individuals who express motivation to change (change talk) are more likely to change; those who argue against change (sustained talk) are less likely to change.
   1. Listen for change talk. One of the first steps in helping individuals make the arguments for change is being able to recognize change talk (Rollnick et al., 2007).
F. Resistance: An observable behavior, it is not a trait of the individual.
G. Explore, offer, and explore.
   1. Explore: Ask what the individual knows or what he or she would like to know.
   2. Offer: Offer information in a neutral and nonjudgmental manner.
   3. Explore: Ask about the individual's thoughts, feelings, and reactions.
H. Next steps: Individuals who set goals for themselves are more likely to achieve behavior change than those who do not. In MI, this is called "next steps."
I. Becoming proficient in MI.
   1. Utilize a provider who is proficient in MI as a mentor.
   2. Practice in short blocks of time with an expert coach if possible.
   3. Attend a formal training. When practicing with individuals, pay attention to clues from them as to how you are doing.
   4. Understand it takes time and practice to be proficient in MI (Rollnick et al., 2007).
J. Pediatric considerations: When using MI in a pediatric setting, recognize the family must also be included in the process (Barnes & Gold, 2012). Avoid talking about the child during MI and focus on talking to or with the child as well as the caregivers to establish trust with the child (Barnes & Gold, 2012). Pediatric individuals are very open to sincerity and affirmative statements that compliment behavior (Barnes & Gold, 2012).

VI. **Plan of Care**

A. "Planning is the third part of the nursing process" (Nettina, 1996, p. 5). Planning is the development of goals and a plan of care designed to assist the individual in resolving the nursing diagnosis.
B. Care plans are developed based on mutually agreed upon goals, founded on evidence-based guidelines and begin and end with the individual.
   1. Care planning activities transcend barriers/transitions, keep the individual at the center, and provide individuals and caregivers with information necessary to prevent redundant care, and ensure quality care across care settings.
   2. When the CCTM RN meets with the individual and/or caregiver, he or she performs a complete clinical and psychosocial assessment. Based on the assessment, chart reviews, and provider input, the CCTM RN establishes small, incremental goals with the individual and/or caregiver.
C. Assessment: Start with a complete nursing assessment.
   1. Vital signs.
   2. Height, weight, BMI, birth history, and any past medical and/or surgical history.
      a. For pediatric individuals, growth chart comparison at this stage is key.
   3. Pain score.
   4. Risk assessments: Individual safety, fall risk, functional status, Mini-Cog exam, Patient Health Questionnaire-2 or -9, CAGE or CAGE-AID, Get Up and Go Test, tobacco history, sexual history, caregiver strain index, abuse, or neglect.
   5. Medication review and reconciliation including all over-the-counter and herbals.
   6. All care devices used and current readings including glucometers, peak flow devices, scales, blood pressure monitors.
   7. Special diet or restrictions.
   8. Current complaints or concerns.
   9. Psychosocial assessment, living situation, community services currently used, exercise or activity, sleep routine, trouble voiding or moving bowels, dental issues, swallowing issues.
   10. Advanced directives or life-planning documents.
   11. Immunization history, vaccines needed based on preventive care guidelines.
   12. Any support groups involved.
   13. Referrals to specialists needed.
D. Goal setting: Based on assessment, discuss goals that are agreeable to the individual and/or caregiver. The care plan is person-driven and all goals are person-centered, not provider-centered. Examples of goals:
   1. I will become more active by _____.

2. I will obtain my provider's approval before beginning an exercise program.
3. I will check my feet and skin after exercise.
E. Individual communication with providers, family, and friends.
1. I will organize my questions in advance before I see my provider. It may help for me to write them down and bring the list with me.
2. I will be assertive and not afraid to ask questions about my care.
3. I will communicate my needs to my provider and nurse.
4. I will contact my provider with questions, concerns, and issues that arise between visits.
F. Individual coping and relaxation.
1. I will identify a support person in my life.
2. I will work on stress management and relaxation.
3. I will seek help from a behavioral health specialist.
4. I will add relaxation techniques into my daily routine.
G. Individual healthy eating and weight management.
1. I will reduce my portion sizes.
2. I will add more fruits and vegetables to my diet.
3. I will add more fiber to my diet.
4. I will read food labels to identify serving size and total carbohydrates.
5. I will keep a food log.
H. Individual medication management.
1. I will carry a complete medication list with me at all times.
2. I will take all medications at the prescribed dosage with appropriate timing and frequency.
3. I will wear a medical alert bracelet/necklace.
4. I will refill my medications on time.
I. Individual pain, fatigue, and sleep goals.
1. I will treat my acute pain aggressively to prevent chronic pain.
2. I will identify and address the cause of my pain.
3. I will participate in a pain management program.
4. I will limit caffeine and reduce environmental stimuli 2-4 hours before sleep.
J. Individual personal safety.
1. I will look for opportunities to prevent accidents, falls, and injuries in my home.
2. I will use a cane, walker, or other device when walking short distances to prevent potential falls.
3. I will transition slowly between sitting/standing in case of dizziness or loss of balance.
4. I will report any bleeding or bruising to my provider while taking warfarin.
K. Individual problem solving.
1. I will notify my provider for any changes in my blood sugar readings, weight changes, blood pressure changes, or peak flow readings.
2. I will follow up on life-planning resources.
3. I will engage in activities to remedy or reduce financial concerns.
4. I will manage my home equipment issues by _____.
L. Individual self-monitoring.
1. I will check my blood sugar first thing in the morning.
2. I will check my weight daily.
3. I will check my feet regularly for signs of breakdown.
4. I will check my blood pressure _____ times per week.
M. Education: Once the goals have been determined, the individual and CCTM RN agree on a specified date and time for follow up. The individual leaves with an action plan outlining goals, recommended referrals, educational materials illness, and educational needs.
1. Individual will have action plan before leaving the office.
2. Individual will have follow-up appointments booked.
3. Individual will have culturally specific, literacy-based education material to review.
4. Individual will understand who to call with questions.
5. Individual will get follow-up community services discussed during the visit.
6. Individual will call the case manager before going to the ED or hospital.
7. Individual will have medication list updated.
8. Individual will have all prescriptions filled on time.
9. Individual will "teach back" all new learning.
10. CCTM RN will document individual's understanding through teach back and any areas of need for review.
N. Transitional Care Management (TCM) Services.
1. Performed when transitioning from the acute care setting back into the community.
2. The PCP accepts care of the individual from the acute facility with no gaps in care.
3. TCM must occur within the 30-day period after the individual is discharged from the acute care setting.

4. This is a billable service by the provider when all criteria are met.
5. Services may be provided by physician, certified nurse midwives, clinical nurse specialists, physician assistants, or nurse practitioners.
6. Some services can be provided by a non-provider under the direction of the provider.
    a. Identification of available community resources.
    b. Education to the individual and caregiver to encourage activation and self-care.
    c. Coaching for compliance of medication regimen.
    d. Assistance in accessing needed services and care (Centers for Medicare & Medicaid Services, U.S. Department of Health and Human Services, & Medicare Learning Network, 2016).
O. Geriatric and dementia considerations.
    1. Encourage individual Annual Wellness Visits (AWV) in the Medicare eligible population.
        a. Preventative focused.
        b. Includes a person-centered health risk assessment to improve health outcomes.
        c. Intended to keep the individual healthy or become healthier (CMS, 2017).
        d. Identifies any gaps in care.
    2. "Geriatric patients are a highly vulnerable population for hospital admission and readmission due to frailty, polypharmacy, comorbidities, cognition, and function decline" (Deniger, Troller, & Kennelty, 2015, p. 248).
    3. Interprofessional care team helps to assure individual needs are met. Effective communication is the key to successful transitions of care.
    4. CCTM RN performs a comprehensive geriatric assessment to ascertain specific needs of the individual, family, and caregiver(s).
    5. Depression can be common therefore a psychosocial needs assessment and screening for depression are important in this population.
    6. CCTM RN assesses caregiver needs and concerns.
    7. Recommendation of community resources to promote and encourage independence.
P. Dementia considerations.
    1. Components of a good transition of care for an individual with dementia should involve three components:
        a. Attempts to support adaptation to a new environment or maintaining the current environment.
        b. Caregiver involvement and support in the person-centered care plan.
        c. Support for managing challenging behaviors (Ray, Ingram, & Cohen-Mansfield, 2015).
    2. Comprehensive assessment of the individual (including the Mini-Cog exam, PHQ-2 or -9, and the Caregiver Strain index).
    3. Evaluate and understand baseline status of individual.
    4. Home safety assessment; address any gaps in plan of care.
    5. Assess needs of caregiver. Caring for those with dementia can have both an emotional and physical toll. Assist planning for respite care as needed.
    6. Recommend community resources available for both the individual and caregiver.
    7. Educate and coach caregiver to ensure individual medication adherence.

VII. Interprofessional Team Approach

Patterns of health care delivery have changed in a time of an aging population and the need to reduce hospital readmissions in the context of limited resources and a shortage of physicians and allied health professionals. Subsequently, the distribution of, and collaboration between, health care professionals must be viewed critically (Supper et al., 2015).

A. Interprofessional team members communicate regularly to discuss care focusing on the unique needs and desires of the individual. This communication may take place as rounds, regular huddles, or formal care conferences. The CCTM RN is instrumental in assessing for needs and facilitating the care conferences and other communication with the health care team. Effective interprofessional communication within teams includes information systems and communication technologies and "avoids discipline-specific terminology" (Interprofessional Education Collaborative [IPEC], 2016, p.13). Interprofessional collaboration can improve professional effectiveness and quality of practice for individuals. Interprofessional collaboration can be "defined as an integrative cooperation of different health professionals, blending complementary competences and skills, making possible the best use of resources"

(Supper et al., 2015, p. 716). Members of an interprofessional team may include:
1. Pharmacists working alongside clinicians can educate individuals and provide medication management in addition to the traditional role of dispensing medications.
2. Mental health providers address mental health needs in real time when working alongside other health care providers in the health care team.
3. Dieticians working as part of the health care team can educate and provide nutrition counseling for individuals.
4. Health coaches provide ongoing support and education for individuals struggling with barriers to health such as weight loss or tobacco cessation.
5. Social workers help individuals overcome barriers to care such as help with housing, transportation, or other needs.
6. Community health navigators connect individuals to resources in the community.

B. IPEC provides operational definitions for an interprofessional team approach.
1. Interprofessional education: "When students from two or more professions learn about, from and with each other to enable effective collaboration and improve health outcomes" (WHO, 2010, as cited in IPEC, 2016, p. 8).
2. Interprofessional collaborative practice: "When multiple health workers from different professional backgrounds work together with patients, families, [careers], and communities to deliver the highest quality of care" (WHO, 2010, as cited in IPEC, 2016, p. 8).
3. Interprofessional teamwork: "The levels of cooperation, coordination and collaboration characterizing the relationships between professions in delivering patient-centered care" (IPEC, 2016, p. 8).
4. Interprofessional team-based care: "Care delivered by intentionally created, usually relatively small work groups in health care who are recognized by others as well as by themselves as having a collective identity and shared responsibility for a patient or group of patients (e.g., rapid response team, palliative care team, primary care team, and operating room team)" (IPEC, 2016, p. 8).
5. Professional competencies in health care: "Integrated enactment of knowledge, skills, values, and attitudes that define the areas of work of a particular health profession applied in specific care contexts" (IPEC, 2016, p. 8).
6. Interprofessional competencies in health care: "Integrated enactment of knowledge, skills, values, and attitudes that define working together across the professions, with other health care workers, and with patients, along with families and communities, as appropriate to improve health outcomes in specific care contexts" (IPEC, 2016, p. 8).

C. An effective interprofessional team demonstrates the following four core competencies:
1. "Work with individuals of other professions to maintain a climate of mutual respect and shared values" (IPEC, 2016, p. 10).
2. "Use the knowledge of one's own role and those of other professions to appropriately assess and address the health care needs of patients and to promote and advance the health of populations" (IPEC, 2016, p. 10).
3. "Communicate with patients, families, communities, and professionals in health and other fields in a responsive and responsible manner that supports a team approach to the promotion and maintenance of health and the prevention and treatment of disease" (IPEC, 2016, p. 10).
4. "Apply relationship-building values and the principles of team dynamics to perform effectively in different team roles to plan, deliver, and evaluate patient/population centered care and population health programs and policies that are safe, timely, efficient, effective, and equitable" (IPEC, 2016, p. 10).

D. Research demonstrates individuals want to be partners in their own health care (Bernabeo & Holmboe, 2013). A critical aspect of partnering with individuals and families is shared decision-making. In this model, the clinician and the person, or family, make health-related decisions collaboratively, based on both the best available evidence and the person's values, beliefs, and preferences (Bernabeo & Holmboe, 2013). Shared decision-making in addition to other practices such as bedside shift report, shared medical records, teach back, care partner programs, and collaborative goal setting have been shown to promote person and family especially if they are utilized at key individual touchpoints before, during, and after a care episode (Frampton et al., 2017).

E. The development of an interprofessional care plan requires the following guiding principles (Jones, Jamerson, & Pike, 2012).
1. Individual problems linked to mutual goals.

2. Individual-stated goals with outlined expectations.
3. Outcomes (indicators) that document individual progress toward the goal.
4. Evidence-based interventions that align with assessment and treatments.
5. Education to prepare the individual and family for transitions in care.

VIII. Evidence-Based Care Resources

Evidence-based practice (EBP) is based on the translation of the best available research evidence to optimize clinical practice with consideration of the person's values and preferences to improve clinical outcomes. Evidence-based guidelines provide practice recommendations based on the systematic review of the best clinical practice evidence (Melnyk & Fineout-Overholt, 2015).

Multiple resources are available that promote the application of evidence-based care.

A. Evidence-based resources guide the CCTM process.
   1. Government-sponsored sites.
      a. Administration on Aging (AOA) (www.aoa.gov).
      b. Agency for Healthcare Research and Quality (AHRQ) (www.AHRQ.gov).
         (1) *Patient Safety and Quality: An Evidence-Based Handbook for Nurses.* This book is available online at the AHRQ website at http://www.ahrq.gov/qual/nurseshdbk/
         (2) Evidence-Based Reports https://www.ahrq.gov/research/findings/evidence-based-reports/search.html
      c. Centers for Disease Control and Prevention (CDC) (www.CDC.gov).
   2. Non-governmental sponsored sites.
      a. American Academy of Pediatrics (AAP) (www.academicpeds.org).
      b. American Academy of Medical-Surgical Nurses (AMSN) (www.AMSN.org).
      c. American Nurses Association (ANA) (www.ANA.org).
      d. American Geriatric Society (AGS) (www.americangeriatric.org).
      e. Hartford Institute for Geriatric Nursing (HIGN) (www.hartford.org).
      f. Institute for Healthcare Improvement (IHI) (www.IHI.org).
      g. National Council of State Boards of Nursing (NCSBN) (www.NCSBN.org).
      h. Nurses Improving Care for Health System Elders (NICHE) (www.NICHE.org).
      i. Society of Pediatric Nurses (SPN) (www.pedsnurses.org).
      j. The Patient-Centered Primary Care Collaborative (PCPCC) (https://www.pcpcc.org).
   3. Online libraries/databases.
      a. Cumulative Index to Nursing and Allied Health Literature (CINAHL) Complete (https://www.ebscohost.com/nursing/products/cinahl-databases/cinahl-complete).
      b. Cochrane Library (https://www.cochranelibrary.com).
      c. Joanna Briggs Institute (JBI) (http://joannabriggs.org).
      d. PubMed for Nurses (https://www.ncbi.nlm.nih.gov/pubmed).
      e. Virginia Henderson Global Nursing e-Repository (https://www.nursingrepository.org).
   4. Interventions to facilitate utilization of evidence-based knowledge afford continuous professional mentoring opportunities (Fritz, 2017).
      a. Journal clubs.
      b. Evidence-based practice presentations to colleagues.

IX. Monitoring and Measuring Individuals for Progress and Early Signs of Exacerbation/Increased Facility Utilization

A. Periodic reassessment of the individual's "needs for care and for coordination, including physical, emotional and psychological health; functional status; current health and health history; self-management knowledge and behaviors; current treatment recommendations, including prescribed medications; and need for support services" (AHRQ, 2010, p. 22). Partnering with the individual, the CCTM RN identifies incremental individual-improvement measures, including medication adherence.
B. CCTM RN revises and refines care plans as needed to accommodate new information or circumstances and to address failures (AHRQ, 2010).
C. Common "red flags" when monitoring an individual's progress include:
   1. Hospital re-admissions including all-cause 30-day re-admissions.
   2. Increased complications associated with disease process (e.g., new kidney disease associated with uncontrolled diabetes).
   3. Missed appointments (e.g., hospital follow-up appointments with specialist after new diagnosis of heart failure).

4. Underutilized prescriptions including missed refills.
5. Frequent ED visits.
6. Frequent falls.

X. **Quality Measures and Outcomes**

A. Measures of effectiveness (MOE) and Measures of performance (MOP) are often utilized to assess the effectiveness and efficiencies of health programs and clinical interventions. Data define health determinants that provide visualization of trends and afford the opportunity to identify leading practices and opportunities for improvement that require additional intervention. The delivery of quality health care is supported through the application of evidence-based medicine and utilization of decision-science tools that provide data to foster individual quality and safety (AHRQ, 2018a).

B. Several data sources are available to guide practice:
   1. AHRQ (www.AHRQ.gov) offers a variety of databases related to the delivery of health care to include utilization, cost, health care trends, insurance, individual satisfaction, experience of care, and accessibility. Pediatric and state-specific databases are additionally available.
   2. CDC (www.CDC.gov) provides a national center for health statistics to guide a nationwide *Healthy People 2020* health improvement effort. Measurable objectives and goals are based on evidence-based practice and provide a framework to focus clinical interventions on healthy lifestyle.
   3. The National Committee for Quality Assurance (NCQA) (www.NCQA.org) defines Health Effectiveness Data Information Set (HEDIS) performance measures. The standardized performance measures guide wellness, health promotion, and disease management. Examples include asthma medication use, cervical cancer screening, controlling high blood pressure, comprehensive diabetes care, breast cancer screening, childhood and adolescent immunization status, child and adult weight/BMI assessment, prenatal and postpartum care, and all-cause readmissions. The Quality Compass is an interactive, web-based comparison tool that affords the opportunity for comparative analysis of health plan performance.

C. CCTM RN is in a unique position to apply the CCTM process to lead and optimize person-centered health outcome improvements through the development of data-driven, coordinated, and comprehensive care. Person-centered goals and monitoring of progress are documented in the electronic medical record (EMR).

XI. **Communicating the Plan of Care**

A. Effective communication of an individualized, person-centered plan of care that achieves a mutual understanding between the person and interprofessional team improves health outcomes and promotes the delivery of safe and quality care. Health literacy is a factor that influences the comprehension of the plan of care (AHRQ, 2018b; Cartwright-Vanzant, 2017). AHRQ offers a Health Literacy Universal Precautions Tool Kit to guide the individual's understanding of the plan of care. The developmental age of the individual also impacts the individual's understanding of the plan of care.

B. The EMR provides a longitudinal clinical reference for the interprofessional team to develop a comprehensive and fully integrated plan of care. Additionally, verbal communication among the clinical team members is an important mechanism to share individual information in support of a quality hand-off of care during the transition process (Rosenthal, Okumura, Hernandez, Li, & Rehm, 2016). It is recommended the individual, family, and/or legal guardian possess a copy or have access through a patient portal to the current EMR plan of care to foster individual activation and engagement (Coughlin et al., 2017; Hibbard & Greene, 2013). Educational pamphlets addressing the transitions of care that are focused on the individual and family improve continuity of care, ensure confidence and decrease anxiety related to the transition process (Manente, McCluskey, & Shaw, 2017).

C. CCTM RN plays an integral role in communicating the coordinated plan of care and educating the person, family, and/or legal guardian. The CCTM RN is often the primary person to communicate the final plan during the transition process.

Chapter 5

Table 5-1.
Person-Centered Care Planning: Knowledge, Skills, and Attitudes for Competency

Knowledge	Skills	Attitudes	Sources
Integrate understanding of multiple dimensions of person-centered care: • Person/family/community preferences, values • Coordination and integration of care • Information, communication, and education • Physical comfort and emotional support • Involvement of family and friends • Transition and continuity Describe how diverse cultural, ethnic, and social backgrounds function as sources of individual, family, and community values.	Elicit individual values, preferences, and expressed needs as part of clinical interview, implementation of care plan, and evaluation of care. Communicate individual values, preferences, and expressed needs to other members of health care team. Provide person-centered care with sensitivity and respect for the diversity of human experience.	Value seeing health care situations "through individuals' eyes.' Respect and encourage individual expression of individual values, preferences, and expressed needs. Value the person's expertise with own health and symptoms. Seek learning opportunities with individuals who represent all aspects of human diversity. Recognize personally held attitudes about working with individuals from different ethnic, cultural, and social backgrounds. Willingly support person-centered care for individuals and groups whose values differ from own.	Cronenwett et al., 2007 Lor, Crooks, & Tluczek, 2016
Demonstrate comprehensive understanding of the concepts of pain and suffering, including physiologic models of pain and comfort.	Assess presence and extent of pain and suffering. Assess levels of physical and emotional comfort. Elicit expectations of individual and family for relief of pain, discomfort, or suffering. Initiate effective treatments to relieve pain and suffering in light of individual values, preferences, and expressed needs.	Recognize personally held values and beliefs about the management of pain or suffering. Appreciate the role of the nurse in relief of all types and sources of pain or suffering. Recognize that individual expectations influence outcomes in management of pain or suffering.	Cronenwett et al., 2007
Examine how the safety, quality, and cost effectiveness of health care can be improved through the active involvement of individuals and families. Examine common barriers to active involvement of individuals in their own health care processes. Describe strategies to empower individuals or families in all aspects of the health care process.	Remove barriers to presence of families and other designated surrogates based on individuals' preferences. Assess level of individual's decisional conflict and provide access to resources. Engage individuals or designated surrogates in active partnerships that promote health, safety and well-being, and self-care management.	Value active partnership with individual or designated surrogates in planning, implementing, and evaluating care. Respect individual preferences for degree of active engagement in care process. Respect individual's right to access personal health records.	Cronenwett et al., 2007 AHRQ, 2017 CDC, 2017 NCQA, 2018

continued on next page

**Table 5-1. (continued)
Person-Centered Care Planning: Knowledge, Skills, and Attitudes for Competency**

Knowledge	Skills	Attitudes	Sources
Explore ethical and legal implications of person-centered care. Describe the limits and boundaries of therapeutic person-centered care.	Recognize the boundaries of therapeutic relationships. Facilitate informed person consent for care.	Acknowledge the tension that may exist between individual rights and the organizational responsibility for professional, ethical care. Appreciate shared decision making with empowered individuals and families, even when conflicts occur.	Cronenwett et al., 2007 Lor et al., 2016
Discuss principles of effective communication. Describe basic principles of consensus building and conflict resolution. Examine nursing roles in assuring coordination, integration, and continuity of care.	Assess own level of communication skill in encounters with individuals and families. Participate in building consensus or resolving conflict in the context of individual care. Communicate care provided and needed at each transition in care.	Value continuous improvement of own communication and conflict resolution skills.	Cronenwett et al., 2007 Nancarrow et al., 2013 Lor et al., 2016
Describe strategies for learning about the outcomes of care in the setting in which one is engaged in clinical practice.	Seek information about outcomes of care for populations served in care setting. Seek information about quality improvement projects in the care setting.	Appreciate that continuous quality improvement is an essential part of the daily work of all health professionals.	Cronenwett et al., 2007
Recognize that nursing and other health profession students are parts of systems of care and care processes that affect outcomes for individuals and families. Give examples of the tension between professional anatomy and system functioning.	Use tools (such as flow charts, cause-effect diagrams) to make processes of care explicit. Participate in a root cause analysis of a sentinel event. Use quality measures to understand performance.	Value own and others' contributions to outcomes of care in local care settings.	Cronenwett et al., 2007 Nancarrow et al., 2013
Explain the importance of variation and measurement in assessing quality of care.	Use tools (such as control charts and run charts) that are helpful for understanding variation.	Appreciate how unwanted variation affects care. Value measurement and its role in good individual care.	Cronenwett et al., 2007 AHRQ, 2017 CDC, 2017 NCQA, 2018
Describe approaches for changing processes of care.	Design a small test of change in daily work.	Exemplify the value of change to reflect improvement.	Cronenwett et al., 2007

continued on next page

Table 5-1. (continued)
Person-Centered Care Planning: Knowledge, Skills, and Attitudes for Competency

Knowledge	Skills	Attitudes	Sources
Assessment and Analytic Skills "1A1. Assess the health status and health literacy of individuals and families, including determinants of health, using multiple sources of data. 1A2a. Use an ecological perspective and epidemiological data to identify health risks for a population. 1A2b. Identify individual and family assets, needs, values, beliefs, resources and relevant environmental factors. 1A3. Select variables that measure health and public health conditions. 1A4. Use a data collection plan that incorporates valid and reliable methods and instruments for collection of qualitative and quantitative data to inform the service for individuals, families, and a community. 1A5. Interpret valid and reliable data that impacts the health of individuals, families, and communities to make comparisons that are understandable to all who were involved in the assessment process. 1A6. Compare appropriate data sources in a community. 1A8. Apply ethical, legal, and policy guidelines and principles in the collection, maintenance, use, and dissemination of data and information.	Utilize data for the development of person-centered action plans by applying evidence-based practice to inform decision-making and priorities of effort.	Appreciate the value of data in relation to population assessment and application for person-centered approach with health care delivery.	Quad Council Coalition, 2018, p. 13

continued on next page

Table 5-1. (continued)
Person-Centered Care Planning: Knowledge, Skills, and Attitudes for Competency

Knowledge	Skills	Attitudes	Sources
1A9. Use varied approaches in the identification of community needs (i.e., focus groups, multi-sector collaboration, SWOT analysis).			Quad Council Coalition, 2018, p. 14
1A10. Use information technology effectively to collect, analyze, store, and retrieve data related to public health nursing services for individuals, families, and groups.			
1A11. Use evidence-based strategies or promising practices from across disciplines to promote health in communities and populations.			Quad Council Coalition, 2018, p. 15
1A12. Use available data and resources related to the determinants of health when planning services for individuals, families, and groups."			
Communication Skills "3A1. Determine the health, literacy, and the health literacy of the population served to guide health promotion and disease prevention activities. 3A2. Apply critical thinking and cultural awareness to all communication modes (i.e., verbal, non-verbal, written & electronic) with individuals, the community, and stakeholders. 3A3. Use input from individuals, families, and groups when planning and delivering health care programs and services. 3A4. Use a variety of methods to disseminate public health information to individuals, families, and groups within a population.	Present person-centered demographics, health care assessment, and action plan complimented by supporting data and analysis to inform key stakeholders to include the person receiving health care and the health care team.	Value the importance of person-centered literacy and individual comprehension to promote a common understanding of health expectations and actions of the person receiving health care and the health care team.	Quad Council Coalition, 2018, p. 19

continued on next page

Table 5-1. (continued)
Person-Centered Care Planning: Knowledge, Skills, and Attitudes for Competency

Knowledge	Skills	Attitudes	Sources
3A6. Use communication models to communicate with individuals, families, and groups effectively and as a member of the interprofessional team(s) or interdisciplinary partnerships. 3A8. Apply communication techniques and models when interacting with peers and other healthcare team members including conflict management."			Quad Council Coalition, 2018, p. 20
Cultural Competency "4A1. Use determinants of health effectively when working with diverse individuals, families, and groups. 4A2. Use data, evidence and information technology to understand the impact of determinants of health on individuals, families, and groups. 4A5. Demonstrate the use of evidence-based cultural models in a work environment when providing services to individuals, families, and groups. Provide culturally responsive care coordination for individuals, families, and groups."	Demonstrate an understanding of the diverse health care needs of the individual person.	Acknowledge awareness of individual person diversity related to cultural background and competence.	Quad Council Coalition, 2018, p. 21. Quad Council Coalition, 2018, p. 22. Quad Council Coalition, 2018.
Community Dimensions of Practice Skills "5A1b. Assist individuals, families, and groups to identify and access necessary community resources or services through the referral and follow-up process.	Apply community determinants when assessing and developing person-centered care to facilitate comprehensive care coordination.	Realize the impact of community variables to optimize the delivery of person-centered care.	Quad Council Coalition, 2018, p. 23

continued on next page

Table 5-1. (continued)
Person-Centered Care Planning: Knowledge, Skills, and Attitudes for Competency

Knowledge	Skills	Attitudes	Sources
5A2. Use formal and informal relational networks among community organizations and systems conducive to improving the health of individuals, families, and groups within communities. 5A3b. Function effectively with key stakeholders in activities that facilitate community involvement and delivery of services to individuals, families, and groups. 5A4. Build stakeholder capacity to advocate for the health issues of individuals, families, and groups. 5A5. Use community assets and resources, including the government, private, and non-profit sectors, to promote health and to deliver services to individuals, families, and groups. 5A7a. Interview individuals, families, and groups to identify community resource preferences. 5A7b. Build preferences into public health services. 5A7c. Identify opportunities for individuals, families, and groups to link with advocacy organizations. 5A8. Identify evidence of the effectiveness of community engagement strategies on individuals, families, and groups."			Quad Council Coalition, 2018, p. 24

continued on next page

Table 5-1. (continued)
Person-Centered Care Planning: Knowledge, Skills, and Attitudes for Competency

Knowledge	Skills	Attitudes	Sources
Values/Ethics for Interprofessional Practice "Work with individuals of other professions to maintain a climate of mutual respect and shared values." (Values/Ethics for Interprofessional Practice)	"VE1. Place interests of patients and populations at center of interprofessional health care delivery and population health programs and policies, with the goal of promoting health and health equity across the life span. VE5. Work in cooperation with those who receive care, those who provide care, and others who contribute to or support the delivery of prevention and health services and programs. VE6. Develop a trusting relationship with patients, families, and other team members. VE7. Demonstrate high standards of ethical conduct and quality of care in contributions to team-based care. VE8. Manage ethical dilemmas specific to interprofessional patient/population centered care situations. VE9. Act with honesty and integrity in relationships with patients, families, communities, and other team members. VE10. Maintain competence in one's own profession appropriate to scope of practice."	"VE2. Respect the dignity and privacy of patients while maintaining confidentiality in the delivery of team-based care. VE3. Embrace the cultural diversity and individual differences that characterize patients, populations, and the health team. VE4. Respect the unique cultures, values, roles/responsibilities, and expertise of other health professions and the impact these factors can have on health outcomes."	IPEC, 2016, p. 10-11

continued on next page

Table 5-1. (continued)
Person-Centered Care Planning: Knowledge, Skills, and Attitudes for Competency

Knowledge	Skills	Attitudes	Sources
Roles and Responsibilities for Interprofessional Practice "Use the knowledge of one's own role and those of other professions to appropriately assess and address the healthcare needs of patients and to promote and advance the health populations." (Roles and Responsibilities)	"RR1. Communicate one's roles and responsibilities clearly to patients, families, community members, and other professionals. RR3. Engage diverse professionals who complement one's own professional expertise, as well as associated resources, to develop strategies to meet specific health and healthcare needs of patients and populations. RR4. Explain the roles and responsibilities of other providers and how the team works together to provide care, promote health, and prevent disease. RR5. Use the full scope of knowledge, skills, and abilities of professionals from health and other fields to provide care that is safe, timely, efficient, effective, and equitable. RR6. Communicate with team members to clarify each member's responsibility in executing components of a treatment plan or public health intervention. RR7. Forge interdependent relationships with other professions within and outside of the health system to improve care and advance learning. RR8. Engage in continuous professional and interprofessional development to enhance team performance and collaboration.	"RR2. Recognize one's limitations in skills, knowledge, and abilities."	IPEC, 2016, p. 10, 12

continued on next page

Table 5-1. (continued)
Person-Centered Care Planning: Knowledge, Skills, and Attitudes for Competency

Knowledge	Skills	Attitudes	Sources
	RR9. Use unique and complementary abilities of all members of the team to optimize health and patient care. RR10. Describe how professionals in health and other fields can collaborate and integrate clinical care and public health interventions to optimize population health."		
Interprofessional Communication "Communicate with patients, families, communities, and professionals in health and other fields in a responsive and responsible manner that supports a team approach to the promotion and maintenance of health and the prevention and treatment of disease." (Interprofessional Communication)	"CC1. Choose effective communication tools and techniques, including information systems and communication technologies, to facilitate discussions and interactions that enhance team function. CC2. Communicate information with patients, families, community members, and health team members in a form that is understandable, avoiding discipline-specific terminology when possible. CC4. Listen actively, and encourage ideas and opinions of other team members. CC5. Give timely, sensitive, instructive feedback to others about their performance on the team, responding respectfully as a team member to feedback from others. CC6. Use respectful language appropriate for a given difficult situation, crucial conversation, or conflict.	"CC3. Express one's knowledge and opinions to team members involved in patient care and population health improvement with confidence, clarity, and respect, working to ensure common understanding of information, treatment, care decisions, and population health programs and policies."	IPEC, 2016, p. 10, 13

continued on next page

Table 5-1. (continued)
Person-Centered Care Planning: Knowledge, Skills, and Attitudes for Competency

Knowledge	Skills	Attitudes	Sources
	CC7. Recognize how one's uniqueness (experience level, expertise, culture, power, and hierarchy within the health team) contributes to effective communication, conflict resolution, and positive interprofessional working relationships. CC8. Communicate the importance of teamwork in patient-centered care and population health programs and policies."		
Team and Teamwork "Apply relationship-building values and the principles of team dynamics to perform effectively in different team roles to plan, deliver, and evaluate patient/population-centered care and population health programs and policies that are safe, timely, efficient, effective, and equitable." (Teams and Teamwork)	"CC1. Choose effective communication tools and techniques, including information systems and communication technologies, to facilitate discussions and interactions that enhance team function. CC2. Communicate information with patients, families, community members, and health team members in a form that is understandable, avoiding discipline-specific terminology when possible. CC4. Listen actively, and encourage ideas and opinions of other team members. CC5. Give timely, sensitive, instructive feedback to others about their performance on the team, responding respectfully as a team member to feedback from others. CC6. Use respectful language appropriate for a given difficult situation, crucial conversation, or conflict.	"CC3. Express one's knowledge and opinions to team members involved in patient care and population health improvement with confidence, clarity, and respect, working to ensure common understanding of information, treatment, care decisions, and population health programs and policies."	IPEC, 2016, p. 10, 13

continued on next page

Table 5-1. (continued)
Person-Centered Care Planning: Knowledge, Skills, and Attitudes for Competency

Knowledge	Skills	Attitudes	Sources
	CC7. Recognize how one's uniqueness (experience level, expertise, culture, power, and hierarchy within the health team) contributes to effective communication, conflict resolution, and positive interprofessional working relationships (University of Toronto, 2008).		
	CC8. Communicate the importance of teamwork in patient-centered care and population health programs and policies."		

Source: Cronenwett et al. (2007). *Nursing Outlook, 55*(3), 122-131. Reprinted with permission from Elsevier.

Chapter 5

Case Study 5-1.
Pediatric Case Study

Introduction

Susie is a 5-year-old Hispanic female who is newly diagnosed with type 1 diabetes (juvenile diabetes). Her weight is above the 95th percentile and height is 10th percentile on her growth chart. She attends kindergarten at an inner-city public school. She rides the school bus to and from school each day and has been absent from school 5 days this past month. Her parents are divorced. She lives with her mother who is her sole provider in a fourth-floor studio apartment. She has a 16-year-old babysitter who provides after-school care during the week. Her grandmother provides childcare on the weekends while the mother is working her second job. Susie's caregivers are experiencing denial related to her diagnosis of diabetes.

Clinical Interaction

The CCTM® RN applies the technique of motivational interviewing (MI) with Susie and her caregivers.

Assessment of care needs: Susie's comprehensive nursing assessment includes addressing her person-centered health care status encompassing her psychosocial (e.g., developmental and single sibling status) and physical needs (e.g., maintenance of controlled diabetes).

MI technique: *Open-ended questions*. The CCTM RN starts the dialogue with an open-ended inquiry with the caregivers such as "Tell me how you are feeling about Susie being diagnosed with diabetes."

Prescribed Interventions

Diet, exercise, pharmaceutical treatment, and immunization status need to be addressed.

Initial follow up with the pediatrician is scheduled 1 week post-discharge.

MI technique: *Shared agenda setting/collaborative decision-making*. The CCTM RN inquires with Susie and the caregivers about their choices regarding Susie's favorite foods or preferred activities and includes these items in her person-centered care plan.

Clinical Implications

Required follow up: Coordination of follow-up instructions need to optimally include her mother, grandmother, and the babysitter due to the variability of caregivers.

The kindergarten teacher and school nurse also need to be informed and provided a copy of Susie's comprehensive care plan and medical points of contact to answer questions they may have regarding Susie's health care needs.

MI technique: *Shared agenda setting/collaborative decision-making*. The CCTM RN asks Susie's caregivers about their choice of follow-up appointment times to improve ownership of Susie's care and compliance with required follow-up appointments. Flexibility related to Susie's school schedule is considered so she does not experience excessive absences.

Nursing Considerations

Since Susie is newly diagnosed with type 1 diabetes, a person-centered diabetes education plan needs to be created that addresses Susie's developmental age and available caregiver support. Educational pamphlets and videos in both English and Spanish and face-to-face instruction complemented by the return demonstration of insulin administration to validate assimilation of knowledge are required. Play therapy may be utilized to assist Susie's understanding of her new chronic diagnosis of diabetes.

The person-centered care plan needs to address Susie's medication requirements and administration techniques (e.g., insulin), diet, daily activity, and action plan for variations in health status (e.g., sickness).

Enrollment in a pediatric-focused diabetes support group should be offered to assist Susie and her caregivers with coping with the chronic disease of diabetes and understanding of lifestyle modifications.

MI technique: *Reflective listening/hypothesis testing*. The CCTM RN demonstrates his/her understanding of Susie's diabetes diagnosis and asks the caregivers what diabetes means to them? The CCTM RN expresses a sympathetic understanding of the caregivers' coping mechanism of denial (feeling reflection).

Lifestyle and Cultural Issues

Lifestyle modifications are required due to the chronicity of the diabetes disease process and need to be communicated to the caregivers in an acceptable manner.

Susie has minimal exercise in her current lifestyle. Inclusion of a daily walk or time at the local playground with her caregiver after school is recommended.

Often times, the Hispanic diet is supported by the consumption of high carbohydrate foods. A nutrition care plan that is customized to her diabetes, age, and food preferences is required to ensure compliance with dietary habits.

MI technique: *Reflective listening/hypothesis testing*. The CCTM RN states his/her understanding of Susie's caregivers' concerns related to her required lifestyle modifications to promote living a healthier life (content reflection).

Significant/Other Involvement

Susie's caregivers need to possess an understanding of her disease process and care plan to include her mother, grandmother, babysitter, teacher, and school nurse. Each member needs to individually possess a copy of Susie's care plan and points of contact if a health emergency occurs.

MI technique: *Elicit change talk*. The CCTM RN asks Susie's caregivers how confident they are that they can change Susie's lifestyle (e.g., diet and activity). The RN reviews a list of the pros and cons of changing Susie's lifestyle with her caregivers.

continued on next page

**Case Study 5-1. (continued)
Pediatric Case Study**

Environmental Issues

The location of the fourth-floor apartment affords the daily opportunity to improve activity by walking up four flights of stairs instead of utilizing the elevator.

The caregivers are encouraged to have nutritious snacks available for Susie due to her living location.

MI technique: *Reflective listening/hypothesis testing*. The CCTM RN elicits the caregivers' understanding of Susie's treatment plan by reviewing the environmental compliments that are available to maximize Susie's healthy lifestyle.

Other

The financial support of Susie's health requires clarification. Does the mother have a comprehensive health plan that will sufficiently cover Susie's anticipated health care needs (e.g., doctor's appointments, insulin, immunizations, etc.)? If not, does she qualify for state or federal subsidized health care support (e.g., Women, Infant, and Children [WIC], Children's Health Insurance Program [CHIP], etc.).

MI technique: *Summarizing*. The CCTM RN reviews Susie's care plan with the caregivers and facilitates a mutual understanding of expectations.

Motivational Techniques

1. Open-ended questions.
2. Shared agenda setting/collaborative decision-making.
3. Reflective listening/hypothesis testing.
4. Eliciting change talk.
5. Summarizing.

Source: American Academy of Pediatrics, 2018.

Case Study 5-2.
Adult Case Study

Introduction

Mrs. Smith is a 60-year-old African-American female who was recently discharged from the local hospital where she was treated for an exacerbation of her COPD and CHF. She has been a long-standing patient of Dr. Wells who has been treating her for several comorbid conditions that include CHF, obesity, sleep apnea, and COPD. Mrs. Smith is known to Dr. Wells' practice to be non-adherent with her medication regimen and prescribed diet for weight loss. The individual has been married for 32 years. Her husband accompanies her to her appointments with Dr. Wells and is very supportive. The couple has two adult children who are independent but very supportive of their mother's needs. Mr. and Mrs. Smith live alone in a modest two-story home in rural Alabama.

Clinical Interaction

The CCTM® RN applies assessment skills to develop an appropriate plan of care for Mrs. Smith.

Assessment and Development of Person-Centered Plan of Care
Assessment: The CCTM RN contacts the individual post discharge to perform an assessment of Mrs. Smith's post-hospital needs. This assessment will include:
- Both physical and psychosocial needs.
- Review of daily weights and blood pressure since discharge.
- Complete review of medications. Discrepancies reported to Dr. Wells.
- Can Mrs. Smith afford her medications on a monthly basis?
- Does Mrs. Smith understand her:
  Diet and fluid restrictions.
  Home care devices (e.g. blood pressure cuff, CPAP).
- Are there any food insecurities?
- Does the individual's home have stairs, carpeting, area rugs, and other fall hazards?
- Is Mrs. Smith able to be mobile within her home? Is she able to navigate the stairs to her bedroom safely?
- Mrs. Smith states that a homecare nurse is coming twice a week to evaluate her progress and make sure that she is safe in the home.
- Is Mrs. Smith able to rest and is she sleeping well?
- Are there any other gaps in care such as financial or transportation issues (e.g. utility payments)?
- Do the Smith's feel safe in their home?
- Does Mrs. Smith or her husband have any specific questions or concerns?

Prescribed Interventions

The CCTM RN will develop a person-centered plan of care based on assessment of the individual. Mrs. Smith's plan of care will include reinstruction on the importance of daily weights and fluid intake management. Diet restrictions will be low sodium and additional diet prescribed by Dr. Wells for weight loss. The nurse realizes that Southern diets often include high fat and sodium content; therefore, motivational interviewing techniques and coaching are used to encourage and reeducate to her prescribed diet. The CCTM RN will use these same techniques to assure Mrs. Smith follows the prescribed medication regimen (medication affordability and right dosage). The CCTM RN assures the Smith's understanding and use of the blood pressure cuff and her CPAP machine. The Smiths should be instructed to work with the home care nurse to perform a safety check of their home and remove area rugs and items that may be a trip hazard. Mrs. Smith should be encouraged to increase her activity as tolerated and to maintain movement. The CCTM RN instructs the Smiths to call the office immediately if they notice weight gain, increased shortness of breath, decreased activity tolerance. The nurse also assures that the Smiths are aware of local support groups and community resources for her comorbid conditions.

Clinical Implications

Required follow up: The CCTM RN follows up weekly and more often as assessment dictates. This follow up should include Mr. Smith so he is included in the plan of care and has the opportunity to bring up questions and concerns. The CCTM RN may offer to speak to family members if there are questions and the Smiths approve of the contact. Ongoing assessment of psychosocial needs should continue. Education of the family of what to do if Mrs. Smith exhibits sudden changes (e.g., shortness of breath or rapid increase in weight). If such changes occur during office hours, the Smiths should attempt to call Dr. Wells or CCTM RN. During evening hours and on the weekend, Mrs. Smith should go to the emergency room immediately.

Nursing Considerations

Mrs. Smith is well known to Dr. Wells' practice. The nurse must remain aware of the individual's history of non-adherent behavior and be vigilant in follow up and reinforcement of treatment rationale. The nurse should investigate through coaching and motivational interviewing other possible reasons for non-adherent behavior and address those issues. Through interviewing techniques, the family's lifestyle and preferences will be realized (cultural, environmental). The CCTM RN assures that educational information is supplied to the family. The use of teach-back methodology can be used. The CCTM RN assists in family adaptation to lifestyle changes that may be needed due to the chronicity of Mrs. Smith's disease processes (e.g., activity intolerance may necessitate moving the bedroom to the first-floor of the home).

Chapter 5

References

Advisory Board. (2017). *Addressing the needs of your rising risk patients* (Executive summary). Retrieved from https://www.advisory.com/-/media/Advisory-com/Research/PHA/Research-Briefings/2018/Addressing-the-Needs-of-Your-Rising-Risk-Patients.pdf

Agency for Healthcare Research and Quality (AHRQ). (2010). *Care coordination measures atlas.* Rockville, MD: U.S. Department of Health and Human Services.

Agency for Healthcare Research and Quality (AHRQ). (2017). *Data resources.* Retrieved from https://www.ahrq.gov/research/data/dataresources/index.html

Agency for Healthcare Research and Quality (AHRQ). (2018a). *Defining the PCMH.* Retrieved from https://pcmh.ahrq.gov/page/defining-pcmh

Agency for Healthcare Research and Quality (AHRQ). (2018b). *AHRQ health literacy universal precautions toolkit: 2nd edition.* Retrieved from http://www.ahrq.gov/professionals/quality-patient-safety/quality-resources/tools/literacy-toolkit/index.html

Alfonso-Mora, M. (2017). Metric properties of the "timed get up and go-modified version" test, in risk assessment of falls in active women. *Columbia Mèdica, 48*(1), 19-24.

American Academy of Ambulatory Care Nursing (AAACN). (2016). *Scope and standards of practice for registered nurses in care coordination and transition management.* Pitman, NJ: Author.

American Academy of Pediatrics. (2018). *Bright futures.* Retrieved from https://brightfutures.aap.org/Pages/default.aspx

American Academy of Pediatrics. (2018). *Mental health initiatives: Motivational interviewing.* Retrieved from https://www.aap.org/en-us/advocacy-and-policy/aap-health-initiatives/Mental-Health/Pages/motivational-interviewing.aspx

Barnes, A.J., & Gold, M.A. (2012). Promoting healthy behaviors in pediatrics. *Pediatrics in Review, 33*(9). doi:10.1542/pir.33-9-e57

Basu, D., Ghosh, A., Hazari, N., & Parakh, P. (2016). Use of family CAGE-AID questionnaire to screen the family members for diagnosis of substance dependence. *The Indian Journal of Medical Research, 143*(6), 722-730. doi:10.4103/0971-5916.191931

Bernabeo, E., & Holmboe, E.S. (2013). Patients, providers, and systems need to acquire a specific set of competencies to achieve truly patient-centered care. *Health Affairs, 32*(2), 250-258. doi:10.1377/hlthaff.2012.1120

Bodenheimer, T. (2015). Unlicensed health care personnel and patient outcomes. *Journal of General Internal Medicine, 30*(7), 873-875. doi:10.1007/s11606-015-3274-x

Boult, C., Leff, B., Boyd, C.M., Wolff, J.L., Marsteller, J.A., Frick, K.D., ... Scharfstein, D.O. (2013). A matched-pair cluster-randomized trial of guided care for high-risk older patients. *Journal of General Internal Medicine, 28*(5), 612-621. doi:10.1007/s11606-012-2287-y

Buurman, B. M., Parlevliet, J. L., Allore, H.G., Blok, W., van Deelen, B.A.J., Moll van Charante, E., ... de Rooij, S.E. (2016). Comprehensive geriatric assessment and transitional care in acutely hospitalized patients: The transitional care bridge randomized clinical trial. *JAMA Internal Medicine,176*(3) 302-309. doi:10.1001/jamainternmed.2015.8042

Brown, R.L., & Rounds, L.A. (1995). Conjoint screening questionnaires for alcohol and other drug abuse: Criterion validity in a primary care practice. *Wisconsin Medical Journal, 94*(3), 135-140.

Cartwright-Vanzant, R. (2017). Identify and address health literacy needs to establish relevant goals and strategies for the life care plan. *Journal of Nurse Life Care Planning, 17*(2), 22-28.

Centers for Disease Control and Prevention. (2017). *National center for health statistics: Healthy people.* Retrieved from https://www.cdc.gov/nchs/healthy_people/index.htm

Centers for Medicare & Medicaid Services (CMS). (2017). *The ABCs of the annual wellness visit (AWV).* Retrieved from http://depts.washington.edu/fammed/wp-content/uploads/2017/10/AWV-Checklist-Billing-Medicare.pdf

Centers for Medicare & Medicaid Services. (2018). *Promoting interoperability (PI).* Retrieved from www.cms.gov/EHR incentivePrograms

Centers for Medicare & Medicaid Services, U.S. Department of Health and Human Services, & Medicare Learning Network. (2016). *Transitional care management services.* Retrieved from https://www.cms.gov/Outreach-and-Education/Medicare-Learning-Network-MLN/MLNProducts/Downloads/Transitional-Care-Management-Services-Fact-Sheet-ICN908628.pdf

Coughlin, S.S., Prochaska, J.J., Williams, L.B., Besenyi, G.M., Heboyan, V., Goggans, D.S. ... De Leo, G. (2017). Patient web portals, disease management, and primary prevention. *Risk Management and Healthcare Policy, 10*, 33-40. doi:10.2147/RMHP.S130431

Cronenwett, L., Sherwood, G., Barnsteiner, J., Disch, J., Johnson, J., Mitchell, P., ... Warren, J. (2007). Quality and safety education for nurses. *Nursing Outlook, 55*(3), 122-131. doi:10.1016/j.outlook.2007.02.006

Deniger, A., Troller, P., & Kennelty, K.A. (2015). Geriatric transitional care and readmissions review. *Journal for Nurse Practitioners, 11*(2), 248-252. doi:10.1016/j.nurpra.2014.08.014

Elwyn, G., Dehlendorf, C., Epstein, R., Marrin, K., White, J. & Frosch, D.L. (2014). Shared decision making and motivational interviewing: Achieving patient-centered care across the spectrum of health care problems. *Annals of Family Medicine, 12*(3), 270-275. doi:10.1370/afm.1615

Frampton, S. B., Guastello, S., Hoy, L., Naylor, M., Sheridan, S., & Johnston-Fleece, M. (2017). *Harnessing evidence and experience to change culture: A guiding framework for patient and family engaged care* (Discussion paper). Washington, DC: National Academy of Medicine. doi:10.31478/201701f

Fritz, E. (2017). Interventions to increase use of evidence-based practice by ambulatory care nurses. *ViewPoint, 39*(4), 4-7. Pitman, NJ: American Academy of Ambulatory Care Nursing.

Hibbard, J.H., & Greene, J. (2013). What the evidence shows about patient activation: Better health outcomes and care experiences; fewer data on costs. *Health Affairs, 32*(2), 207-214. doi:10.1377/hlthaff.2012.1061.

Horton, M., & Perry, A.E. (2016). Screening for depression in primary care: A Rasch analysis of the PHQ-9. *British Journal of Psychiatry, 40*(5), 237-243. doi:10.1192/pb.bp.114.050294

Improving Primary Care. (2018). *Primary care team guide: The clinical pharmacist.* Retrieved from http://www.improvingprimarycare.org/team/clinical-pharmacist

Institute for Patient- and Family-Centered Care. (2014). *Patient- and family-centered care.* Retrieved from http://www.ipfcc.org/about/pfcc.html

Interprofessional Education Collaborative (IPEC). (2016). *Core competencies for interprofessional collaborative practice: 2016 update.* Retrieved from https://nebula.wsimg.com/2f68a39520b03336b41038c370497473?AccessKeyId=DC06780E69ED19E2B3A5&disposition=0&alloworigin=1

Jennings, L.A., Reuben, D.B., Evertson, L.C., Serrano, K.S., Ercoli, L., Grill, J., ... Wenger, N.S. (2015). Unmet needs of caregivers of individuals referred to a dementia care program. *Journal of the American Geriatrics Society, 63*(2), 282-289. doi:10.1111/jgs.13251

Jones, K.L., Jamerson, C., & Pike, S. (2012). The journey to electronic interdisciplinary care plans. *Nursing Management, 43*(12), 9-12. doi:10.1097/01.NUMA.0000422896.29829.03

Katz, S., Down, T.D., Cash, H.R., & Grotz, R.C. (1970). Progress in development of the index of ADL. *The Gerontologist, 10*(1), 20-30. doi:10.1093/geront/10.1_Part_1.20

Le Berre, M., Maimon, G., Sourial, N., Guériton, M., & Vedel, I. (2017). Impact of transitional care services for chronically ill older patients: A systematic evidence review. *Journal of the American Geriatrics Society, 65*(7), 1597-1608. doi:10.1111.jgs.14828

Levensky, E.R., Forcehimes, A., O'Donohue, W.T., & Beitz, K. (2007). Motivational interviewing: An evidence-based approach to counseling helps patients follow treatment recommendations. *American Journal of Nursing, 107*(10), 50-58. doi:10.1097/01.NAJ.0000292202.06571.24

Lin, J.S., O'Connor, E., Rossom, R. C., Perdue, L. A., & Eckstrom, E. (2013). Screening for cognitive impairment in older adults: A systematic review for the U.S. Preventive Services Task Force. *Annals of Internal Medicine, 159*(9), 601-612. doi:10.7326/0003-4819-159-9-201311050-00730

Chapter 5

Lor, M., Crooks, N., & Tluczek, A. (2016). A proposed model of person-, family-, and culture-centered nursing care. *Nursing Outlook, 64*(4), 352-366. doi:10.1016/j.outlook.2016.02.006

Manea, L., Gilbody, S., & McMillan, D. (2012). Optimal cut-off score for diagnosing depression with the patient health questionnaire (PHQ-9): A meta-analysis. *Canadian Medical Association Journal, 184*(3), E191-E196. doi:10.1503/cmaj.110829\

Manente, L., McCluskey, T., & Shaw, R. (2017). Transitioning patients from the intensive care unit to the general pediatric unit: A piece of the puzzle in family-centered care. *Pediatric Nursing, 43*(2), 77-82.

Mathias, S., Nayak, U.S., & Isaacs, B. (1986). Balance in elderly patients: The "get-up and go" test. *Archives Physical Medicine and Rehabilitation, 67*(6), 387-389.

Melnyk, B.M., & Fineout-Overholt, E. (2015). *Evidence-based practice in nursing & healthcare: A guide to best practice* (3rd ed.). Philadelphia, PA: Wolters Kluwer Health

Mlinac, M.E., & Feng, M.C. (2016). Assessment of activities of daily living, self-care, and independence. *Archives of Clinical Neuropsychology, 31*(6), 506–516. doi:10.1093/arclin/acw049

Motivational Interviewing Network of Trainers. (2014). *Motivational interviewing training new trainers manual.* Retrieved from http://www.motivationalinterviewing.org/sites/default/files/tnt_manual_2014_d10_20150205.pdf

Nancarrow, S. A., Booth, A., Ariss, S., Smith, T., Enderby, P., & Roots, A. (2013). Ten principles of good interdisciplinary team work. *Human Resources for Health, 11,* 19. doi:10.1186/1478-4491-11-19

National Committee for Quality Assurance (NCQA). (2018). *HEDIS measures.* Retrieved from http://www.ncqa.org/hedis-quality-measurement/hedis-measures

Nettina, S.M. (1996). *The Lippincott manual of nursing practice* (6th ed). Philadelphia, PA: Lippincott Williams & Wilkins.

Onega, L. L. (2018). *The modified caregiver strain index (MCSI).* New York, NY: The Hartford Institute for Geriatric Nursing, NYU Rory Meyers College of Nursing.

Quad Council Coalition. (2018). *Community/public health nursing [C/PHN] competencies.* Retrieved from http://www.quadcouncilphn.org/documents-3/2018-qcc-competencies/

Ray, C.A., Ingram, V., & Cohen-Mansfield, J. (2015). Systematic review of planned care transitions for persons with dementia. *Neurodegenerative Disease Management, 5*(4), 317-331. doi:10.2217/nmt.15.23

Rollnick, S., Miller, W.R., & Butler, C.C. (2007). *Motivational interviewing in health care: Helping patients change behavior.* New York, NY: The Guilford Press.

Rosenthal, J.L., Okumura, M.J., Hernandez, L., Li, S.T., & Rehm, R.S. (2016). Interfacility transfers to general pediatric floors: A qualitative study exploring the role of communication. *Academic Pediatrics, 16*(7), 692-699. doi:10.1016/j.acap.2016.04.003

Salvo, M.C., & Cannon-Breland, M.L. (2015). Motivational interviewing for medication adherence. *Journal of the American Pharmacists Association, 55*(4), 354-361. doi:10.1331/JAPhA.2015.15532.

Seo, J., & Park, S. (2015). Validation of the patient health questionnaire-9 (PHQ-9) and PHQ-2 in patients with migraine. *The Journal of Headache and Pain,* 65(16). doi:10.1186/s10194-015-0552-2

South Carolina Department of Health and Human Services. (2014). *Social determinants of health tool.* Retrieved from https://msp.scdhhs.gov/proviso/site-page/social-determinants-health-tool

Supper, I., Catala, O., Lustman, M., Chemla, C., Bourgueil, Y., & Letrilliart, L. (2015). Interprofessional collaboration in primary health care: A review of facilitators and barriers perceived by involved actors. *Journal of Public Health, 37*(4), 716-727. doi:10.1093/pubmed/fdu102

Tamura, K., Kocher, M., Finer, L., Murata, N., & Stickley, C. (2018). Reliability of clinically feasible dual-task tests: Expanded timed get up and go tests as a motor task on young healthy individuals. *Gait & Posture,* (60), 22-27.

Torous, J., Staples, P., Shanahan, M., Lin, C., Peck, P., Keshavan, M., & Onnela, J.P. (2015). Utilizing a personal smartphone custom app to assess the patient health questionnaire-9 (PHQ-9) depressive symptoms in patients with major depressive disorder. *JMIR Mental Health, 2*(1), e8. doi:10.2196/mental.3889

Tsoi, K.K., Chan, J.Y., Hirai, H.W., Wong, S.Y., & Kwok, T.C. (2015). Cognitive tests to detect dementia: A systematic review and meta-analysis. *JAMA Internal Medicine, 175*(9), 1450–1458. doi:10.1001/jamainternmed.2015.2152

U.S. Preventive Services Task Force (USPSTF). (2018). *Recommendations for primary care practice.* Retrieved from https://www.uspreventiveservicestaskforce.org/Page/Name/recommendations

Ward, K.T., & Reuben, D.B. (2018). *Comprehensive geriatric assessment.* Retrieved from https://www.uptodate.com/contents/comprehensive-geriatric-assessment

Welsh, T.J., Gordon, A.L., Gladman, J.R. (2013). Comprehensive geriatric assessment – A guide for the non-specialist. *The International Journal of Clinical Practice, 68*(3), 290-293. doi:10.1111/ijcp.12313

Williams, N. (2014). The CAGE questionnaire. *Occupational Medicine, 64*(6), 473-474. doi:10.1093/occmed/kqu058

Additional Readings

Centers for Medicare & Medicaid Services, & Medicare Learning Network. (2017). *The ABCs of the annual wellness visit (AWV).* Retrieved from https://www.cms.gov/Outreach-and-Education/Medicare-Learning-Network-MLN/MLNProducts/downloads/AWV_chart_ICN905706.pdf

Hughes, R.G. (2008). *Patient safety and quality: An evidence-based handbook for nurses.* Rockville, MD: Agency for Healthcare Research and Quality.

Motivational Interviewing Network of Trainers. (2018). *What is motivational interviewing?* Retrieved from http://www.motivationalinterviewing.org/

Quality and Safety Education for Nurses Institute. (2012). *Graduate QSEN competencies.* Retrieved from http://qsen.org/competencies/graduate-ksas/

Quality and Safety Education for Nurses Institute. (2012). *QSEN competencies.* Retrieved from http://qsen.org/competencies/pre-licensure-ksas/

Wasson, J.H., Godfrey, M.M., Nelson, E.C., Mohr, J.J., & Batalden, P. B. (2003). Microsystems in health care: Part 4. Planning patient-centered care. *Joint Commission Journal on Quality & Safety, 29*(5), 227-237.

Chapter 6

Support for Self-Management

Vanessa DeBiase, MSN, MEd, RN
Kathryn D. Swartwout, PhD, APRN, FNP-BC
Pa Choua Xiong, MSN, RN, CCCTM®

Instructions for Continuing Nursing Education Contact Hours
Continuing nursing education credit can be earned for completing the learning activity associated with this chapter. Instructions can be found at aaacn.org/CCTMCoreCNE

Learning Outcome Statement

After completing this learning activity, the learner will be able to articulate the primary components of self-management support, including the importance of a comprehensive needs assessment, common strategies for collaborative goal setting, and concepts important to self-management.

Learning Objectives

After reading this chapter, the Care Coordination and Transition Management registered nurse (CCTM® RN) will be able to:
- Describe the concepts associated with support of self-management by RNs who are providing care coordination and transition management within the CCTM Model including:
  - Knowledge and understanding of common symptoms of chronic condition(s).
  - Ability to positively impact health promotion and disease-prevention activities.
  - Recognition of the importance of social and lifestyle adaptation.
  - Support for development of self-regulation skills.
- Discuss the need for person-centered assessment and incorporation of values, goals, and preferences into planned care activities and approaches.
- Identify individual self-management skills and gaps or barriers often encountered by members of the health care team.
- Outline the importance of recognizing the individual and health care team as equal partners in managing chronic conditions with the CCTM RN focused on building the individual's and family's knowledge, skills, and attitudes for self-management.
- Demonstrate understanding of knowledge, skills, and attitudes required for the support for the self-management dimension (see Table 6-1 on page 130).

AAACN Care Coordination and Transition Management Standards

Standard 1. Assessment
Standard 2. Nursing Diagnosis
Standard 3. Outcomes Identification
Standard 4. Planning
Standard 5. Implementation
Standard 5a. Coordination of Care
Standard 5b. Health Teaching and Health Promotion
Standard 6. Evaluation
Standard 11. Communication
Standard 13. Collaboration
Standard 15. Resource Utilization

Source: AAACN, 2016.

Competency Definition

Self-management support is defined as the "systematic provision of education and supportive interventions by health care staff to increase patients' skills and confidence in managing their health problems, including regular assessment of progress and problems, goal setting, and problem-solving support" (Pearson, Mattke, Shaw, Ridgely, & Wiseman., 2007, p. 1). People self-manage by goal setting and adapting behaviors (or behaviors performed by their families) to manage their condition and maximize their health (Franklin, Lewis, Willis, Bourke-Taylor, & Smith, 2018). Not only do people need to be engaged and modify behaviors, but the more self-management support they have, the better their outcomes (Cunningham, 2016). For children and adolescents with chronic conditions, self-management is a transitional process where younger children might need more support and the adolescent might be more independent from his/her family. Additionally, children and adolescents might need more reinforcement of family self-management support in order to perform the activities and processes and meet their self-management goals (Chao, Whittemore, Minges, Murphy, & Grey, 2014). For some adults, decision-making activities may also be shared with significant others or become the responsibility of a designated decision-making surrogate.

Self-management support is an essential dimension of the role of the CCTM RN. Self-management support incorporates "activities provided by family, peers, community organizations and/or healthcare professionals in conjunction with patients. It includes patient education, goal-setting, problem solving and action planning" (Franklin et al., 2018, p. 2). In a comparative effectiveness review of studies related to outpatient case management for adults with complex care needs, the Agency for Healthcare Research and Quality (AHRQ) (2013) found evidence of successful interventions for a variety of chronic conditions included providing support of self-management. Self-management support recognizes, develops, and harnesses people's assets and empowers people to adopt a healthier lifestyle (Cockayne, Pattenden, Worthy, Richardson, & Lewin, 2014). Setting goals and engaging in healthy behaviors reduces health care utilization and cost by empowering individuals to better manage their conditions, which limits disease progression and avoids more intensive levels of support (Franklin et al., 2018). The means by which the health service can support individuals with long-term conditions to engage in self-management include: appropriate and accessible advice, health education, self-care skills training, and increasing self-monitoring via telehealth technologies.

Given all people are chronic disease self-managers, the role of the CCTM RN in self-management support is to positively impact how self-management occurs (van Hooft, Dwarswaard, Jedeloo, Bal, & van Staa, 2014). This process begins with an assessment of the individual's knowledge, skills, behaviors, and confidence in managing chronic conditions and maintaining health. The CCTM RN works directly with the individual, his/her family, and the health care team to develop a collaborative plan of care that is built around the individual's values and preferences. Another critical component of the assessment and plan are the key supports and resources required to address social and lifestyle needs. Finally, the CCTM RN helps the individual develop important self-regulatory skills to support critical self-management decisions. Self-management support occurs in a variety of settings and venues: individual or group, face-to-face, or utilizing an ever-expanding arsenal of telehealth tools.

I. **Support Knowledge and Understanding of Chronic Condition(s)**
    A. Perform comprehensive assessment of understanding of chronic condition(s) and initiate discussion of self-management techniques.
    B. Develop tailored education for the individual/family considering (Cramm & Nieboer, 2015):
        1. Health literacy.
        2. Educational level.
        3. Cognitive/developmental level.
        4. Language.
        5. Preferences.
        6. Family/significant other.
        7. Learning style.
        8. Adult learning principles.
        9. Readiness to learn.
            a. Information may need to be repeated.
            b. When the individual is ready to learn.
        10. Environment.
        11. Gender.
        12. Perceptions of disease.
    C. Emphasize self-management concepts.
        1. Cause of chronic condition: Often multiple causes and contributing factors (Tu et al., 2018).
            a. Heredity.
            b. Lifestyle (ever smoked, alcohol consumption).
            c. Environmental factors (e.g., secondhand smoke).
            d. Physiological changes.
        2. Individual expertise in living with chronic condition(s) and social situation.
        3. Symptoms and symptom management: Even though diseases may differ, symptoms may be similar. Understanding symptoms and self-management strategies is essential to improve quality of life. Assess and support individual's and family's problem solving around these common symptoms (Taylor et al., 2014).
            a. Fatigue: May be caused by the disease process, inactivity, poor nutrition, ineffective sleep, stress, or medications (Kos et al., 2015).
                (1) Increase physical activity.
                (2) Stress management.
                (3) Screen for depression.
                (4) Improve nutrition.
                (5) Improve sleep quality.

(6) Diet modifications.
(7) Pace daily activities.
b. Pain/physical discomfort: May be caused by the disease process, muscle tension, deconditioning, stress and emotional responses, and medications (Mann, Lefort, & Vandenkerkhof, 2013).
  (1) Chronic pain has a strong emotional component that can increase perceived pain levels.
  (2) Encourage stretching, increased aerobic and muscle strengthening activity.
  (3) Ice, heat, massage.
  (4) Integrative techniques: distraction, music, relaxation, etc.
  (5) Medication use.
  (6) Diet modifications.
  (7) Cognitive strategies.
c. Shortness of breath: May be caused by multiple disease processes that interfere with pulmonary or cardiac function, being overweight or obese, a deconditioned state or smoking (Centers for Disease Control and Prevention [CDC], 2017).
  (1) Teach breathing management techniques such as diaphragmatic or pursed-lip breathing, huffing, and positions that ease breathing.
  (2) Follow low-sodium diet.
  (3) Prop up with pillows to aid sleeping.
  (4) Monitor fluid retention and weight gain.
  (5) Encourage fluid intake unless restricted.
  (6) Eliminate smoke exposure.
  (7) Increase activity, if possible.
  (8) Reduce weight.
  (9) Proper use of medications.
  (10) Communicate with support system.
  (11) Manage depression.
d. Sleep disturbances: High-quality sleep is very important (Ramar & Olson, 2013).
  (1) Comfort positions in bed (pillows, head of bed).
  (2) Regular routine.
  (3) Depression management.
  (4) Safe environment: lighting, assistive devices.
  (5) Sleep hygiene.
    (a) Avoid alcohol and eating at bedtime.
    (b) Avoid caffeine late in the day.
    (c) Avoid stimulating activities near bedtime.
    (d) Avoid sleeping pills or diuretics at bedtime.
    (e) Comfortable bed and room temperature.
    (f) No pets.
  (6) Professional help for sleep apnea.
  (7) Sleep log.
e. Memory loss.
  (1) Professional help if memory loss interferes with life activities. See Chapter 4, *Coaching and Counseling of Individuals and Families*.
f. Itching (pruritus) – may be difficult to pinpoint cause.
  (1) Keep skin dry.
  (2) Wear comfortable clothes.
  (3) Soothing medications.
  (4) Stress management.
  (5) Minimize scratching.
g. Urinary incontinence: More common in women (Hersh & Salzman, 2013).
  (1) Use of pelvic floor exercises, bladder-emptying techniques, scheduled urination.
  (2) Consume fewer beverages at bedtimes, especially those that stimulate urine production.
  (3) Use of absorbent pads.
  (4) Weight reduction.
  (5) Pharmacologic therapy.

D. Impact of disease and treatment (Richardson et al., 2014).
  1. Physiological.
  2. Psychological.
  3. Social.
E. Disease trajectory (Grey, Schulman-Green, Knafl, & Reynolds, 2015).
  1. Full recovery often not possible.
  2. Disease pattern may be unpredictable.
  3. Symptoms can contribute to development of additional symptoms.
F. Set goals collaboratively (AHRQ, 2016).
  1. Individual as full partner.
  2. Health care team.
  3. Community providers.
  4. Incorporate end-of-life wishes.
  5. Action plans.
G. Train and develop skills (Galdas et al., 2015).
  1. Medication use.
  2. Monitoring and medication adjustment.
  3. Use of medical equipment.
  4. Adaptive devices and supports.

5. Lifestyle modifications.
6. Peer support.
H. Recognize acute symptoms and emergencies (Toukhsati, Driscoll, & Hare, 2015). Sick day plans.
   1. Collaborative plan for person-initiated activities to address symptom exacerbation.
   2. When and how to seek care.
I. Use medications safely (Mann et al., 2013).
   1. Use of reminder devices (e.g., blister packs, med-planners, reminder devices, and machines that dispense medication).
   2. Adherence.
J. Communicate effectively with health care team (CDC, 2018a).
   1. Effective communication strategies.
   2. Understanding who and how to contact regarding health care needs and questions.
K. Support transitions of care (Pollack et al., 2016).
   1. Update plan of care at transitions.
   2. Include individual goals for transition.
   3. Maintain communication between care team and individual and/or families.

II. Support Knowledge and Understanding of Health Promotion and Disease Prevention

A. Assess current health promotion and disease prevention knowledge and unmet preventive service needs.
B. Assess health behavior/lifestyle risks (Kemppainen, Tossavainen, & Turunen, 2013).
C. Advising/coaching regarding healthy behaviors/lifestyle (CDC, 2018b).
   1. Regular physical activity.
   2. Balanced diet.
   3. Fluid intake.
   4. Weight management.
   5. Adequate sleep and rest.
   6. Tobacco cessation.
   7. Alcohol consumption or mood-altering substances.
   8. Stress management.
   9. Medication adherence.
   10. Dental and oral health.
   11. Depression management.
D. Incorporate planned lifestyle changes into collaborative plan of care.
E. Encourage self-monitoring of behavior changes.

III. Support Social and Lifestyle Adaptations

A. Perform a comprehensive assessment of barriers to self-management including physical, psychological, cognitive, economic, social, and cultural barriers (Baumann & Dang, 2012).
   1. Physical barriers.
      a. Assess physical disabilities.
      b. Perform functional assessment (activities of daily living and instrumental activities of daily living) (Family Practice Notebook, 2018).
      c. Assess fall risk (Get Up and Go Test) (Family Practice Notebook, 2018).
      d. Assess for safety and accessibility of the living environment.
         (1) Narrow doorways.
         (2) Stairs.
         (3) Bathroom accessibility.
         (4) Kitchen/food preparation access.
         (5) Hazards such as clutter, throw rugs, and electrical cords.
      e. Assess need for assistive devices and/or durable medical equipment.
      f. Assess for transportation concerns.
         (1) Access to health care facilities.
         (2) Access to other necessary goods and services such as groceries.
      g. Assess for social support.
         (1) Assess family/significant other physical ability to support care.
         (2) Assess need for support services.
   2. Psychological barriers.
      a. Assess for history of psychological conditions that may interfere with self-management.
         (1) Depression, anxiety, or other emotional distress.
         (2) Post-traumatic stress disorder (PTSD).
         (3) Schizophrenia.
         (4) Substance abuse.
      b. Use standardized tools for screening and/or monitoring as indicated and as selected by your institution. See Chapter 5, "Person-Centered Care Planning."
         (1) Patient Health Questionnaire (PHQ-2 or PHQ-9).
         (2) Drug Abuse Screening Test (DAST).
         (3) Generalized Anxiety Scale (GAD-7).
      c. Assess for caregiver burden using standardized tools as selected for use by your institution.
         (1) Zarit Burden Interview (American Psychological Association [APA], 2018a).
         (2) Caregiver Reaction Scale (APA, 2018b).

d. Determine if social networks or peer support groups would be beneficial to the individual, family, or other caregivers.
3. Cognitive barriers.
   a. Assess for history of cognitive conditions or brain injuries that may interfere with self-management. See Chapter 2, "Advocacy."
      (1) Dementia.
      (2) Alzheimer's disease.
      (3) Delirium.
      (4) Traumatic brain injuries.
      (5) Stroke.
      (6) Developmental delays.
      (7) Other serious mental illnesses.
   b. Assess for medications with side effects that may interfere with cognition (National Institute on Aging [NIA], 2018a).
      (1) Antihistamines.
      (2) Antidepressants, antipsychotics, and antianxiety agents.
      (3) Sleep aids.
      (4) Muscle relaxants.
      (5) Pain medications.
      (6) Some medications used to treat urinary incontinence or gastrointestinal cramps.
   c. Perform cognitive assessment using standardized tools for screening and/or monitoring as indicated and as selected by your institution (NIA, 2018b).
      (1) Mini-Mental State Examination (MMSE).
      (2) Mini-Cog.
      (3) Montreal Cognitive Assessment (MoCA).
4. Economic barriers.
   a. When appropriate, assess for barriers to seek/maintain employment.
      (1) Chronic illness may impact employment.
         (a) Inability to drive a commercial vehicle (e.g., seizure disorders and insulin-dependent diabetes).
         (b) Physical disabilities (e.g., inability to lift or stand for long periods).
         (c) Mental illness.
         (d) Illness requiring frequent absences for medical care.
      (2) Inaccessible or unavailable transportation.
   b. Assess availability of homecare services.
      (1) Home health.
      (2) Home-based primary care.
      (3) Home telemonitoring.
   c. Assess insurance benefit coverage.
   d. Assess concerns about loss of income or benefits due to disability or premature death.
5. Social and cultural barriers.
   a. Assess individual and family cultural norms.
      (1) Beliefs about disease processes.
      (2) Religious beliefs.
      (3) Traditional practices.
      (4) Preferred language for both verbal and written communication.
   b. Assess support systems.
      (1) Family structure.
      (2) Religious community supports.
      (3) Availability of culturally specific services such as community-based health educators (e.g., Promotoras are lay community members who provide basic health education to Hispanic/Latino communities).
B. Provide CCTM interventions to support lifestyle adaptations for self-management.
1. Create a safe and accessible home environment.
   a. Assist with obtaining home adaptive devices such as walkers, wheelchairs, grab bars, raised toilet seats, and commodes.
   b. Assist with obtaining necessary medical equipment such as hospital bed, oxygen, CPAP, hearing, and vision aids.
   c. Assist with obtaining necessary home repairs such as installation of hand rails on stairs.
   d. Assist with obtaining home services such as home health nursing or aides, grocery delivery, home-delivered meals, respite care, palliative care, and home cleaning assistance.
   e. Work with individual and family to consider moving to a safer environment if necessary.
2. Maintain physical independence.
   a. Assist with connecting individual to medically prescribed physical therapy/occupational therapy/rehab services.
   b. Support condition-appropriate physical activities for increasing or maintaining physical function.
3. Assist with plans that support social interactions with relatives, friends, religious community, or other interest groups outside the home.

4. Assist with connecting caregiver to support groups.
5. Refer to social service staff to assist with identifying eligible benefits (e.g., social security disability).
6. Suggest that family review insurance policies and employee benefits that may be available to provide support.
7. Collaborate with or refer to other members of the interprofessional health care team when appropriate.
8. Utilize technology-based support such as telehealth (Hanlon et al., 2017), and consider use of social media and computer-based support.
9. Assess possibility of obtaining service animals (e.g., dogs) for interested individuals with disabilities (Invisible Disabilities Association, 2018); pets may be helpful in situations such as social isolation (Cherniack & Cherniak, 2014).

IV. **Support Development of Self-Management Skills**

A. Self-regulation.
   1. Emphasizes the individual's central role in managing his or her own health.
   2. Based in Social Cognitive Theory (Tougas, Hayden, McGrath, Huguet, & Rozario, 2015).
   3. Results from combined impacts of a person's cognitive processes, social and physical environment, and behavior to reach a goal.
   4. Developed by the individual and family, along with the support from the health care team.
   5. Involves development of the following skills (Tougas et al., 2015; Zahry, Cheng, & Peng, 2016).
      a. Goal setting and self-monitoring.
      b. Reflective thinking.
      c. Decision making.
      d. Development of an action plan and implementation.
      e. Self-evaluation and tailoring.
      f. Management of physical, emotional, and cognitive responses related to the behavior change.
B. Goal setting and self-monitoring by the individual and family.
   1. Five phases of goal setting (Herre, Graue, Kolltveit, & Gjengedal, 2016).
      a. Preparation.
         (1) Education, reflection, and topic identification.
      b. Formulation of goals (independently or collaboratively).
         (1) Specific goal(s) are written down.
      c. Formulation of action plan.
         (1) Explicit action plan identified and written down.
      d. Coping planning.
         (1) Identify barriers and strategies to overcome them, identify the action plan facilitator(s), and assess confidence.
      e. Follow-up.
         (1) Self-monitoring, providing support, and evaluation of progress.
   2. Self-care goals must be the goals of the individual and/or family, not those of the health care team.
   3. Develop goals that reflect the individual's own values and beliefs in collaboration with members of the health care team, directed toward positively influencing health outcomes (Lenzen, Daniëls, van Bokhoven, van der Weijden, & Beurskens, 2017).
   4. Types of individual and family goals may include:
      a. Learning goals.
      b. Goals to change behaviors, such as physical activity, diet, medication compliance, health promotion, or risk reduction.
      c. Clinical status goals, such as better control of glycemia or blood pressure.
   5. I-SMART goals (Lee, 2015).
      a. Important.
         (1) "What is most important for you (individual/family) to work on?"
         (2) "On a scale of 1-10, how important is this to you?"
      b. Specific.
         (1) "What will you do? Where? When?"
      c. Measurable.
         (1) "How much will you do? How often?"
      d. Achievable.
         (1) "What barriers might you face? How will you deal with them?"
         (2) "On a scale of 1-10, how confident are you that you can complete this specific plan?"
      e. Relevant.
         (1) "How will this step help you achieve your overall goal?"
      f. Time-specific.
         (1) "How long will you try this experiment?"

6. Self-monitoring.
   a. Success with solving problems and reaching goals leads to increased confidence in self-efficacy.
   b. Regular contact with the health care team assists the individual and family with removing barriers, modifying goals and strategies, and acknowledging accomplishments.
C. Reflective thinking by the individual and family.
   1. In considering self-management tasks and changes, individuals and families engage in self-reflection about readiness and ability to change beliefs and barriers.
   2. Self-efficacy: Personal confidence in own ability to perform specific actions necessary to achieve a desired goal (Finney Rutten et al., 2016).
      a. Is a continuum, not simply present or absent.
      b. Is task-specific.
      c. Enhanced by personal mastery, practice, interpretation of symptoms, and peer influence.
      d. Leads to improved behaviors, emotions, motivation, and thinking.
      e. Assesses individual's importance, readiness, and confidence levels.
   3. Five stages of readiness for change (Daoud et al., 2015).
      a. Pre-contemplation ("I'm not seriously thinking about quitting smoking").
      b. Contemplation ("I will quit smoking sometime in the next 6 months").
      c. Preparation ("I will quit in the next month").
      d. Action ("I have quit and am using nicotine replacement").
      e. Maintenance ("I have not smoked for more than 6 months").
   4. Health beliefs and attitudes (Lee, Stange, & Ahluwalia, 2015).
      a. Based on the Health Belief Model: An individual's use of health services is primarily due to the following factors:
         (1) Susceptibility.
            (a) The extent to which a person believes he or she is susceptible to the ill health condition ("Will smoking cause me to have heart or lung disease or cancer?").
         (2) Severity.
            (a) If he or she would develop it, how serious does the person believe the consequences will be in his or her life ("If I have cancer due to smoking, how sick will I be? Could I possibly die?").
         (3) Benefits and barriers.
            (a) The extent to which benefits to the person outweigh the barriers ("It is really hard to quit and I like smoking. Is it worth the effort?").
         (4) Cues to action and self-efficacy.
            (a) The sense of confidence that the person can perform the action ("I have quit before, but started again. Can I do it this time?").
D. Decision making by the individual and family.
   1. In collaboration with the health care team, the individual and family weigh priorities.
      a. Build on individualized assessment of strengths and weaknesses.
      b. Identify what is valued by the individual and family.
      c. Build on small incremental steps of change.
   2. Problem-solving skills (Palermo et al., 2016).
      a. Clearly identify the problem.
      b. Generate options of possible solutions.
         (1) Can base options on own prior experiences.
         (2) May seek input from health care team members.
         (3) May seek input from family members or friends.
         (4) Avail self of other resources online or in the community.
         (5) Evaluate options for decision-making.
      c. Implementation of solution.
      d. Evaluation of solution.
E. Development of an action plan and implementation (Herre et al., 2016).
   1. Collaborative plan identifies actions to be taken, person responsible, and time frame for review.
   2. Health care team takes responsibility for ordering of tests and treatments, support, and follow-up.
   3. Individual or family activities for self-management may include development of the following knowledge, skills, or abilities.
      a. Knowledge of condition(s).
      b. Knowledge of treatment(s).
      c. Ability to take medication.
      d. Ability to share in decisions.
      e. Ability to arrange appointments.
      f. Ability to attend appointments.

g. Understanding of monitoring and recording.
h. Ability to monitor and record.
i. Understanding of symptom management.
j. Ability to manage symptoms.
k. Ability to manage the physical impact.
l. Ability to manage the social impact.
m. Ability to manage the emotional impact.
n. Progress toward a healthy lifestyle.

F. Self-evaluation and tailoring by the individual and family
  1. Requires the individual and family to measure success against personalized goals (Lenzen et al., 2016).
     a. Success should not be measured strictly according to compliance or adherence to medical treatment plan.
     b. Frustration or perceptions of failure may indicate need to modify the goals and/or the action plan.
     c. Progress toward goals may not be appreciated by the individual and family; the health care team may provide valuable feedback and encouragement.
  2. Exacerbation or progression of the condition may require re-evaluation of current interventions and development of new goals to support care.

G. Management of physical, emotional, and cognitive responses related to the behavioral change by the individual and family.
  1. Individuals and families vary in their ability to incorporate management of chronic conditions into their routines.
  2. Studies have shown that most families view themselves as capable of managing the treatment regimen well and report positive benefits of caregiving (APA, 2018c).

H. Methods for supporting self-management.
  1. Motivational interviewing (Lee, 2015).
     a. Person-centered communication skill.
        (1) OARS: Open-ended questions, Affirmation, Reflection, Summarize using simple reflections.
        (2) Active listening, express empathy, use "change talk."
     b. Elicits concerns/barriers, identifies ambivalence, and motivates behavioral change.
     c. Requires development of partnership with individuals and exchange of information for informed decision making by that individual.
     d. Requires the clinician to be trained, to practice, and receive feedback in order to master the technique.
     e. Effective with some individual populations, but not others.
  2. Empowerment approach (Fitzgerald, O'Tuathaign, & Moran, 2015).
     a. Person-centered approach.
     b. Partnership between individual and health care provider.
     c. Self-awareness/self-motivation.
        (1) Designed to help individuals choose personally meaningful goals that result in behavioral changes that are internally motivated.
     d. Self-care/self-management.
        (1) Emphasizes autonomy, while helping individuals examine the social, cognitive, and emotional aspects of their lives and the influences on their decision-making.
     e. Problem solving.
     f. Reflection.
     g. Commonly used in individuals with type 2 diabetes, hypertension, and for weight management.
  3. Five A's Model (van Dillen, Noordman, van Dulmen, & Hiddink, 2015). See Chapter 4, "Coaching and Counseling of Individuals and Familes."
     a. Assess, advise, agree, assist, and arrange.
     b. Used to develop an individualized, collaborative plan to attain goals.
     c. Not a linear process; steps overlap.
     d. Has been applied successfully and in combination with other approaches with a variety of patient populations.
  4. Peer coaching (Best, Miller, Eng, & Routhier, 2016).
     a. Successful in lowering A1c in diabetic individuals and enhancing self-management.
     b. Peers function as educators, advocates, cultural translators, mentors, case managers, and/or group facilitators.
     c. Peers teach individuals and families to:
        (1) Communicate with providers.
        (2) Obtain resources.
        (3) Seek emotional support.
        (4) Set goals.
        (5) Make decisions.
        (6) Develop action plans.
        (7) Problem solve.

d. Training of peer counselors vary widely.
e. Stanford Chronic Disease Self-Management Program (Liddy, Johnston, Nash, Irving, & Davidson, 2016).
   (1) Structured 6-week group course with both a health professional and a trained peer leader.
   (2) Teach participants self-regulation skills.
   (3) Objectively measures participants' knowledge, skills, and abilities pre- and post-course and provides feedback tools.
   (4) Scientifically evaluated with a variety of chronic conditions for over 25 years.
5. Information and communication technologies (Wildevuur, Thomese, Ferguson, & Klink, 2017).
   a. Supports the partnership between individuals and their health care providers.
   b. Offers empowerment, exchange of information, and supports physical and psychosocial well-being.
      (1) Self-monitoring tools to inform decision-making.
      (2) In-home/remote monitoring.
      (3) Online diary with feedback.
   c. Individual education to enhance knowledge.
   d. Webinars (Moody et al., 2015).
   e. Applications can sometimes be designed without the individual in mind.
6. Traditional health coaching and counseling programs.
   a. Can be done individually with health professional or group.
   b. Disease-specific or general information about living with chronic conditions.
   c. Supports individual engagement using motivational interviewing techniques and goal setting.
   d. Variability exists in referral sources to programs, characteristics of the participants and health coaches, and in the counseling process itself.
   e. The Flinders Program™ (Sahafi, Smith, Georgiou, Krishnan, & Battersby, 2016).
      (1) Individual, person-centered assessment and care planning, using various tools incorporating motivational interactions.
      (2) Standardized tools and forms for individual self-assessment of capacity to change, guide for motivational interviewing, development and prioritization of goals, and construction of the self-management plan.
      (3) Addresses the behaviors necessary in both the individual and clinician to meet health goals.
I. Follow-up.
   1. Systematic follow-up improves behavioral changes, both in chronic condition self-management and risk factor reduction.
   2. Successful methods include:
      a. Follow-up appointments.
      b. Case management via telephone/teleconferencing.
      c. Home telemonitoring.
      d. Personalized reminders.
   3. Evaluation of outcomes vary widely.
      a. Can be classified as performance, perception, or evaluation-based.
      b. Enhanced if progress toward goals is monitored and barriers are addressed.
   4. National Standards for Diabetes Self-Management Education and Support: Ten standards that define quality diabetes self-management education (Beck et al., 2017).
      a. Collaboratively developed plan of care must include follow-up plan for ongoing self-management that supports:
         (1) Lack of knowledge or understanding.
         (2) Low health literacy.
         (3) Impairment of cognitive functioning.
         (4) Economic, social, and cultural barriers.
      b. Curriculum should include (as applicable) (Beck et al., 2017):
         (1) Diabetes pathophysiology and treatment options.
         (2) Diet management.
         (3) Physical activity plan.
         (4) Medication usage.
         (5) Monitoring blood sugars.
         (6) Preventing, detecting, and treating acute and chronic complications.
         (7) Address psychosocial issues.
         (8) Problem-solve to promote health and change behaviors.

Table 6-1.
Support for Self-Management: Knowledge, Skills, and Attitudes for Competency

Person-Centered Care			
The CCTM RN will provide comprehensive care that recognizes the individual and families as the source of control and full partner in providing compassionate and coordinated care based on respect for individual's preferences, values, and needs (Cronenwett et al., 2009).			
Knowledge	**Skills**	**Attitudes**	**Sources**
Demonstrate comprehensive knowledge about chronic conditions, including skills and techniques for monitoring and managing common symptoms.	Apply knowledge of chronic conditions in all individual interactions. Teach/demonstrate self-management techniques to individuals. Develop educational resources if needed. Understand references/resources for enhancing knowledge of chronic conditions. Assess individual and family understanding of chronic condition, causes, treatment options, and self-management requirements. Address identified needs and gaps in understanding through planned learning activities.	Understand knowledge limitations and utilizes resources effectively. Value resources of the interprofessional team to augment self-management support (e.g., MD, nurse practitioner, physician assistant, pharmacist, diabetes educator, dietitian, social worker). Value peer-provided support. Respect individual's values, preferences, and choices. Value team-based approach to individual care. Value individualized approach to address person-identified needs.	Lorig et al., 2012 Grady & Gough, 2014 AHRQ, 2017 Glasgow, Davis, Funnell, & Beck, 2003 Pearson, Mattke, Shaw, Ridgely, & Wiseman, 2007
Demonstrate knowledge regarding evidence-based standards or guidelines in the care of individuals with chronic conditions.	Critically seek and review evidence-based guidelines or standards of care and incorporates into care. Understand and apply theoretical models related to self-management support (e.g., social cognitive theory, transtheoretical model, adult learning theory, etc.).	Value the use of evidence-based approach to care. Commit to continuous learning and staying up-to-date on current standards and guidelines.	Battersby et al., 2010 Grady & Gough, 2014 Funnell et al., 2011 Pearson et al., 2007
Describe how the strength and relevance of available evidence influences the choice of interventions in provision of person-centered care.	Participate in structuring the work environment to facilitate integration of new evidence into standards of practice. Question rationale for routine approaches to care that result in less-than-desired outcomes or adverse events.	Value the need for continuous improvement in clinical practice based on new knowledge.	Cronenwett et al., 2007 Grady & Gough, 2014

continued on next page

Table 6-1. (continued)
Support for Self-Management: Knowledge, Skills, and Attitudes for Competency

Knowledge	Skills	Attitudes	Sources
Understand the importance of health promotion and prevention activities applicable to the individual.	Promote completion of appropriate health promotion and preventive services. Support the individual/family in understanding need for preventive care. Empower individuals/families by collaborating on goals and plan of care.	Value the importance of health-promoting activities. Confront any personal negative beliefs regarding lifestyle changes (smoking cessation, weight loss, etc.). Appreciate the value of integrative therapies as self-management approaches.	Lorig et al., 2012 Kemppainen et al., 2013 Grady & Gough, 2014 Ryan & Sawin, 2009
Identify potential barriers to self-care including physical, psychological, cognitive, economic, social, and cultural.	Perform comprehensive assessment of barriers to self-care. Provide coaching and identify resources to diminish barriers to self-care.	Respect individual and family preferences for degree of active engagement in care process. Acknowledge the many factors affecting self-management capability and seek to maximize skills, abilities, and resources. Recognize the individual and family's expectations influence outcomes in management of pain or suffering.	Marrero & Ackerman, 2007 Baumann & Dang, 2012 Cole, Smith, & Cupples, 2013 Schulman-Green, Jaser, Park, & Whittemore, 2016 Cronenwett et al., 2007
Integrate understanding of multiple dimensions of person-centered care: • Individual/family. • Community preferences, values. • Coordination and integration of care. • Information, communication, and education. • Physical comfort and emotional support. • Involvement of family and friends. • Transition and continuity.	Elicit individual and family values, preferences, and expressed needs as part of clinical interview. Communicate individual and family values, preferences, and expressed needs to other members of the health care team. Provide person-centered care with sensitivity and respect for the diversity of the human experience.	Value seeing health care situations "through [individual's] eyes." Respect and encourage individual expression of values, preferences, and needs. Value the individual's expertise with own health and symptoms. Willingly support [person]-centered care for individuals and groups whose values differ from own.	Cronenwett et al., 2007

continued on next page

**Table 6-1. (continued)
Support for Self-Management: Knowledge, Skills, and Attitudes for Competency**

Knowledge	Skills	Attitudes	Sources
Understand concepts of self-management and the individual's and family's central role in managing health.	Support individual and family development of the following self-management skills: 1. Goal-setting and self-monitoring. 2. Reflective thinking. 3. Decision-making. 4. Development of an action plan and implementation. 5. Self-evaluation and tailoring. 6. Management of physical, emotional, and cognitive responses related to the behavior change. Utilize appropriate engagement/activation skills such as motivational interviewing, 5 A's, health coaching, and positive psychology.	Recognize need for individuals and families to develop skills in these areas and include preventing illness as well as managing existing illness. View individual and family as full partners in care. Seek ways to promote independence. Value individual and family decisions and accept decisions not consistent with recommendations. Recognize and encourage successes. Value the use of engagement, activation skills, and shared decision-making. Recognize the importance of practice in becoming expert in the application of these skills.	Ryan & Swain, 2009 Grady & Gough, 2014 Battersby et al., 2010 Robert Wood Johnson, 2013 Olsen & Nesbitt, 2010
Understand the importance of performing a comprehensive self-management support assessment.	Employ effective interviewing techniques. Perform appropriate assessment activities, including use of standardized tools.	Appreciate that a comprehensive assessment becomes the foundation of the collaborative plan of care. View individuals as experts in their own lives.	Battersby et al., 2010 Grady & Gough, 2014
Synthesize critical information to develop a person-centered collaborative plan of care.	Utilize active listening principles. Utilize adult learning principles when working with adult individuals. Develop goals that are I-SMART (important, specific, measureable, achievable, realistic, and timely).	Value individual wishes and priorities for goal setting. Value contributions of interprofessional team, including community team members. Exercise creativity in plan development. Identify own biases and values related to health behaviors and goals. Respect and encourage individual/family expression of values, preferences, and needs. Value the individual's expertise with his/her own health and symptoms.	Battersby et al., 2010 Lenzen et al., 2017 Ryan & Swain, 2009 Grady & Gough, 2014 Tang, Funnell, Gillard, Nwankwo, & Heisler, 2011 Darnell & Dunn, 2013

continued on next page

**Table 6-1. (continued)
Support for Self-Management: Knowledge, Skills, and Attitudes for Competency**

Knowledge	Skills	Attitudes	Sources
Demonstrate the ability to identify, obtain, and coordinate resources needed (e.g., multiple health care providers, community, other caregivers) to provide integrated, comprehensive care.	Identify resources available to assist individual/family in meeting needs. Identify safety issues and follow up as appropriate.	Accept that barrier to care can be met in a variety of ways and through multiple agencies/groups. Honor individual's wishes regarding use of community support.	Battersby et al., 2010 Baumann & Dang, 2012 Lorig & Holman, 2003
Evaluate collaborative plan of care; progress toward goal achievement and effectiveness of planned interventions; modify as needed.	Elicit cooperation of individual/family and health care team in review and revision of plan of care as needed.	Value importance of person-centered interdisciplinary plan. Exercise creativity in meeting individual needs. Value keeping team informed of changes.	Lenzen et al., 2017

Self-Management Support Outcome Measure

Chronic Disease Self-Care Behavior	Measures	Validated Scale
Self-efficacy in the management of chronic conditions.	Self-efficacy measure at enrollment, 6 months and 1 year.	Stanford/Garfield Kaiser Chronic Disease Dissemination Study (Lorig et al., 2001). Self-Efficacy for Managing Chronic Disease 6-Item Scale (Daniali, Darani, Eslami, & Mazaheri, 2017).

Source: Adapted from Cronenwett et al. (2007). *Nursing Outlook, 55*(3), 122-131. Reprinted with permission from Elsevier.

Chapter 6

Case Study 6-1.
Diabetes Self-Management

Introduction

Mr. Jones is a 68-year-old Vietnam Veteran with a medical history including: uncontrolled type 2 diabetes mellitus, hypertension, hyperlipidemia, peripheral neuropathy, obesity, and post-traumatic stress disorder. He has been referred to see you today by his primary care provider following a recent visit to the emergency department for an infected wound on his left fifth toe. He has already been referred to see a podiatrist and has home health (skilled nursing) set up for dressing changes. He lives alone about 40 miles away from the clinic. His only next of kin is his daughter, Audrey, who lives 3 hours away but visits one weekend a month.

Clinical Interaction

You will be coordinating Mr. Jones's wound care and providing support for diabetes self-management. During the visit, Mr. Jones tells you that he accidentally kicked his bed frame over a month ago, resulting in the wound on his toe. Audrey was the one who had "forced" him to come into the emergency department for evaluation. Mr. Jones's wound is healing well and he reports 3 more days remain for course of oral antibiotics. He tells you that he does not check his home blood sugars and takes his insulins, "when I can remember to." His most recent A1c was 9.8%. His current diabetes medications are: insulin glargine 40 units QHS and insulin aspart® 12 units TID with meals.

Clinical Implications

As the CCTM® RN, you discuss with Mr. Jones that Audrey is a support person and the benefits of involving her in his plan of care. He agrees to have the RN call Audrey. Audrey agrees to accompany him to all of his visits to ensure that he does not miss any appointments. They are both provided education, using the teach-back method, on the pathophysiology of diabetes, treatment options for diabetes, and the long-term complications of chronic uncontrolled diabetes. You ask that the home health service provide a home safety evaluation and medication compliance check, in addition to wound care. You also refer them to a dietician and enroll Mr. Jones into a home telehealth program for daily blood sugar monitoring and medication reminder. Utilizing your motivational interviewing skills, you help Mr. Jones to develop I-SMART goals to better self-manage his diabetes.

Case Study 6-2.
Adolescent Weight Management

Introduction

Kelsey is a 15-year-old female who has been brought to the office by her mother on the recommendation from her school nurse due to frequent absenteeism. The pediatric nurse practitioner refers Kelsey to you for care coordination and, specifically, weight management. Her family is medically uninsured. Kelsey is otherwise healthy. Her height is 5'3" and her weight is 250 lbs. (BMI = 44.3). Her fasting lab work is normal. Her mom is also overweight.

Clinical Interaction

The family has already been referred to a social worker for assistance with applying for medical insurance. Your nursing assessment includes health literacy, depression screening, activity screening, diet history, family context, and school context. You identify that Kelsey does not want to go to school on the days her "favorite" clothes that fit her well are in the laundry and on days when she must change into a tight-fitting physical education uniform or bathing suit. You recognize the problem of a diet high in fast foods and carbohydrates and little to no exercise. With input from both Kelsey and her mom, you identify goals for self-management related to exercise and diet. Kelsey and mom both have smartphones and like the idea of using electronic apps for tracking progress. They choose to (1) Walk together for 10 minutes every evening regardless of the weather (Kelsey thinks walking in rain or snow will be a "fun adventure") and (2) Drink eight 8 oz glasses of water each day. You identify free apps for tracking activity and water intake: Fit and Gulp. Kelsey agrees to do her own laundry so that her favorite clothes are always clean. You offer to call the school RN to discuss solutions related to physical education class.

Clinical Implications

As the CCTM® RN, you follow-up with Kelsey and her mom monthly by phone to coach, monitor progress, and adjust goals. You meet with them anytime they are in the office. You tailor your nursing care to food and activity preferences, taking into consideration cost and neighborhood factors. Kelsey continues to desire the social support of her mom in diet and exercise so you refer her mom to an adult primary care practice to be sure her mom's health needs are also being met. You maintain excellent communication with both the school RN and the referring pediatric nurse practitioner.

Chapter 6

References

Agency for Healthcare Research and Quality (AHRQ). (2007). *Patient self-management support programs: An evaluation*. Retrieved from https://www.ahrq.gov/research/findings/final-reports/ptmgmt/index.html

Agency for Healthcare Research and Quality (AHRQ). (2013). *Outpatient case management for adults with medical illness and complex care needs*. Retrieved from https://effectivehealthcare.ahrq.gov/sites/default/files/pdf/case-management_research.pdf

Agency for Healthcare Research and Quality (AHRQ). (2016). *How to implement self-management support in your practice*. Retrieved from https://www.ahrq.gov/professionals/prevention-chronic-care/improve/self-mgmt/self/sms_how.html

American Academy of Ambulatory Care Nursing (AAACN). (2016). *Scope and standards of practice for registered nurses in care coordination and transition management*. Pitman, NJ: Author.

American Psychological Association (APA). (2018a). *Zarit Burden interview*. Retrieved from http://www.apa.org/pi/about/publications/caregivers/practice-settings/assessment/tools/zarit.aspx

American Psychological Association (APA). (2018b). *Caregiver reaction scale*. Retrieved from http://www.apa.org/pi/about/publications/caregivers/practice-settings/assessment/tools/caregiver-reaction.aspx

American Psychological Association (APA). (2018c). *Positive aspects of caregiving*. Retrieved from http://www.apa.org/pi/about/publications/caregivers/faq/positive-aspects.aspx

Baumann, L.C., & Dang, T.T. (2012). Helping patients with chronic conditions overcome barriers to self-care. *The Nurse Practitioner, 37*(3), 32-38. doi:10.1097/01.NPR.0000411104.12617.64

Beck, J., Greenwood, D.A., Blanton, L., Bollinger, S.T., Butcher, M.K., Condon, ... 2017 Standards Revision Task Force. (2017). 2017 national standards for diabetes self-management education and support. *Diabetes Care, 40*(10), 1409-1419. doi:10.2337/dci17-0025

Battersby, M., Von Korff, M., Schaefer, J., Davis, C., Ludman, E., Greene, S.M., ... Wagner, E.H. (2010). Twelve evidence-based principles for implementing self-management support in primary care. *The Joint Commission Journal on Quality and Patient Safety, 36*(12), 561-570.

Best, K.L., Miller, W.C., Eng, J.J., & Routhier, F. (2016). Systematic review and meta-analysis of peer-led self-management programs for increasing physical activity. *International Journal of Behavioral Medicine, 23*(5), 527-538. doi:10.1007/s12529-016-9540-4

Centers for Disease Control and Prevention (CDC). (2017). *Managing chronic obstructive pulmonary disease (COPD)*. Retrieved from https://www.cdc.gov/learnmorefeelbetter/programs/copd.htm

Centers for Disease Control and Prevention (CDC). (2018a). *What is self-management education?* Retrieved from https://www.cdc.gov/learnmorefeelbetter/sme/index.htm

Centers for Disease Control and Prevention (CDC). (2018b). *National center for chronic disease prevention and health promotion*. Retrieved from https://www.cdc.gov/chronicdisease/index.htm

Chao, A., Whittemore, R., Minges, K.E., Murphy, K.M., & Grey, M. (2014). Self-management in early adolescence and differences by age at diagnosis and duration of type 1 diabetes. *The Diabetes Educator, 40*(2), 167-177. doi:10.1177/0145721713520567

Cherniack, E.P., & Cherniack, A.R. (2014). The benefits of pets and animal-assisted therapy to the health of older individuals. *Current Gerontology and Geriatrics Research*. doi:10.1155/2014/623203

Cockayne, S., Pattenden, J., Worthy, G., Richardson, G., & Lewin, R. (2014). Nurse facilitated self-management support for people with heart failure and their family carers (SEMAPHFOR): A randomised controlled trial. *International Journal of Nursing Studies, 51*(9), 1207-1213. doi:10.1016/j.ijnurstu.2014.01.010

Cole, J.A., Smith, S.M., & Cupples, M.E. (2013). Do practitioners and friends support patients with coronary heart disease in lifestyle change? A qualitative study. *BMC Family Practice, 14*, 126. doi:10.1186/1471-2296-14-126

Cramm, J.M., & Nieboer, A.P. (2015). Chronically ill patients' self-management abilities to maintain overall well-being: What is needed to take the next step in the primary care setting? *BMC Family Practice, 16*, 123. doi:10.1186/s12875-015-0340-8

Cronenwett, L., Sherwood, G., Barnsteiner, J., Disch, J., Johnson, J., Mitchell, P., ... Warren, J. (2007). Quality and safety education for nurses. *Nursing Outlook, 55*(3), 122-131. doi:10.1016/j.outlook.2007.02.006

Cunningham, P. (2016). Patient perceptions of clinician self-management support for chronic conditions. *The American Journal of Managed Care, 22*(4), e125-e133.

Daniali, S.S., Darani, F.M., Eslami, A.A., & Mazaheri, M. (2017). Relationship between self-efficacy and physical activity, medication adherence in chronic disease patients. *Advanced Biomedical Research, 6*, 63. doi:10.4103/2277-9175.190997

Darnell, D., & Dunn, C. (2013). *Practicing MI skills with I-SMART goal-setting*. Retrieved from http://www.uihi.org/wp-content/uploads/2013/08/MI-Workshop-Goal-settings-Final-070313.pdf

Daoud, N., Hayek, S., Muhammad, A.S., Abu-Saad, K., Osman, A., Thrasher, J.F., & Kalter-Leibovici, O. (2015). Stages of change of the readiness to quit smoking among a random sample of minority Arab-male smokers in Israel. *BMC Public Health, 15*(672). doi:10.1186/s12889-015-1950-8.

Family Practice Notebook. (2018). *Geriatric medicine: Examination chapter*. Retrieved from https://fpnotebook.com/Geri/Exam/index.htm

Finney Rutten, L.J., Hesse, B.W., St. Sauver, J.L., Wilson, P., Chawla, N., Hartigan, D.B., ... Arora, N.K. (2016). Health self-efficacy among populations with multiple chronic conditions: The value of patient-centered communication. *Advances in Therapy, 33*(8), 1440-1451. doi:10.1007/s12325-016-0369-7

Fitzgerald, M., O'Tuathaigh, C., & Moran, J. (2015). Investigation of the relationship between patient empowerment and glycaemic control in patients with type 2 diabetes: A cross-sectional analysis. *BMJ Open, 5*(12). doi:10.1136/bmjopen-2015-008422.

Franklin, M., Lewis, S., Willis, K., Bourke-Taylor, H., & Smith, L. (2018). Patients' and healthcare professionals' perceptions of self-management support interactions: Systematic review and qualitative synthesis. *Chronic Illness, 14*(2), 79-103. doi:10.1177/1742395317710082

Funnell, M.M., Brown, T.L., Childs, B.P., Haas, L.B., Hosey, G.M., Jensen, B., ... Weiss, M.A. (2011). National standards for diabetes self-management education. *Diabetes Care, 34*(Suppl. 1), S89-S96. doi:10.2337/dc11-S089

Galdas, P., Fell, J., Bower, P., Kidd, L., Blickem, C., McPherson, K., ...Richardson, G. (2015). The effectiveness of self-management support interventions for men with long-term conditions: A systematic review and meta-analysis. *BMJ Open*. doi:10.1136/bmjopen-2014-006620

Glasgow, R.E., Davis, C.L., Funnell, M.M., & Beck, A. (2003). Implementing practical interventions to support chronic illness self-management. *Joint Commission Journal on Quality and Safety, 29*(11), 563-574.

Grady, P.A., & Gough, L.L. (2014). Self-management: A comprehensive approach to management of chronic conditions. *American Journal of Public Health, 104*(8): e25-e31.

Grey, M., Schulman-Green, D., Knafl, K., & Reynolds, N.R. (2015). A revised self- and family management framework. *Nursing Outlook, 63*(2), 162-170.

Hanlon, P., Daines, L., Campbell, C., McKinstry, B., Weller, D., & Pinnock, H. (2017). Telehealth interventions to support self-management of long-term conditions: A systematic metareview of diabetes, heart failure, asthma, chronic obstructive pulmonary disease, and cancer. *Journal of Medical Internet Research, 19*(5), e172. doi:10.2196/jmir.6688

Herre, A.J., Graue, M., Kolltveit, B.C., & Gjengedal, E. (2016). Experience of knowledge and skills that are essential in self-managing a chronic condition: A focus group study among people with type 2 diabetes. *Scandinavian Journal of Caring Sciences, 30*(2), 382-390. doi:10.1111/scs.12260

Hersh, L., & Salzman, B. (2013). Clinical management of urinary incontinence in women. *American Family Physician, 87*(9), 634-640.

Invisible Disabilities Association. (2018). *Service animals are working animals for many with invisible disabilities.* Retrieved from https://invisibledisabilities.org/ida-books-pamphlets/serviceanimals/service-animal/

Kemppainen, V., Tossavainen, K., & Turunen, H. (2013). Nurses' roles in health promotion practice: An integrative review. *Health Promotion International, 28*(4), 490-501.

Kos, D., van Eupen, I., Meirte, J., Van Cauwenbergh, D., Moorkens, G., Meeus, M., & Nijs, J. (2015). Activity pacing self-management in chronic fatigue syndrome: A randomized controlled trial. *American Journal of Occupational Therapy, 69*(5). doi:10.5014/ajot.2015.016287

Lee, H.Y., Stange, M.J., & Ahluwalia, J.S. (2015). Breast cancer screening behaviors among Korean American immigrant women: Findings from the health belief model. *Journal of Transcultural Nursing, 26*(5), 450-457. doi:10.1177/1043659614526457

Lee, J. (2015). Helping your patients set achievable goals. *AADE in Practice, 3*(5), 42-45. doi:10.1177/2325160315598289

Lenzen, S.A., Daniëls, R., van Bokhoven, M.A., van der Weijden, T., & Beurskens, A. (2017). Disentangling self-management goal setting and action planning: A scoping review. *PLoS One, 12*(11). doi:10.1371/journal.pone.0188822

Lenzen, S.A., van Dongen, J.J.J., Daniëls, R., van Bokhoven, M.A., van der Weijden, T., & Beurskens, A. (2016). What does it take to set goals for self-management in primary care? A qualitative study. *Family Practice, 33*(6), 698-703. doi:10.1093/fampra/cmw054.

Liddy, C., Johnston, S., Nash, K., Irving, H., & Davidson, R. (2016). Implementation and evolution of a regional chronic disease self-management program. *Canadian Journal of Public Health, 107*(2), E194-E201. doi:10.17269/cjph.107.5126.

Lorig, K.R. & Holman, H.R. (2003). Self-management education: History, definition, outcomes, and mechanisms. *Annals of Behavioral Medicine, 26*(1), 1-7.

Lorig, K., Holman, H., Sobel, D., Laurent, D., Gonzalez, V., & Minor, M. (2012). *Living a healthy life with chronic conditions* (4th ed.). Boulder, CO: Bull Publishing Company

Lorig, K.R., Sobel, D.S., Ritter, P.L., Laurent, D., & Hobbs, M. (2001). Effect of a self-management program for patients with chronic disease. *Effective Clinical Practice, 4,* 256-262.

Mann, E.G., Lefort, S., Vandenkerkhof, E.G. (2013). Self-management interventions for chronic pain. *Journal of Pain and Symptom Management, 3*(3), 211-22. doi:10.2217/pmt.13.9

Marrero, D.G., & Ackerman, R.T. (2007). Providing long-term support for lifestyle changes: A key to success in diabetes prevention. *Diabetes Spectrum, 20*(4), 205-209. doi:10.2337/diaspect.20.4.205

Moody, L., Turner, A., Osmond, J., Hooker, L., Kosmala-Anderson, J., & Batehup, L. (2015). Web-based self-management for young cancer survivors: Consideration of user requirements and barriers to implementation. *Journal of Cancer Survivorship, 9*(2), 188-200. doi:10.1007/s11764-014-0400-4

National Institute on Aging (NIA). (2018a). *Risks to cognitive health.* Retrieved from https://www.nia.nih.gov/health/risks-cognitive-health

National Institute on Aging (NIA). (2018b). *Assessing cognitive impairment in older patients.* Retrieved from https://www.nia.nih.gov/health/assessing-cognitive-impairment-older-patients

Olsen, J.M., & Nesbitt, B.J. (2010). Health coaching to improve healthy lifestyle behaviors: An integrative review. *American Journal of Health Promotion, 25*(1), e1-e11.

Palermo, T.M., Law, E.F., Bromberg, M., Fales, J., Eccleston, C., & Wilson, A.C. (2016). Problem-solving skills training for parents of children with chronic pain: A pilot randomized controlled trial. *Pain, 157*(6), 1213-1223. doi:10.1097/j.pain.0000000000000508

Pearson, M.L., Mattke, S., Shaw, R., Ridgely, M.S., & Wiseman, S.H. (2007). *Patient self-management support programs: An evaluation.* Publication #08-0011. Rockville, MD: Agency for Healthcare Research and Quality.

Pollack, A.H., Backonja, U., Miller, A.D., Mishra, S.R., Khelifi, M., Kendall, L., & Pratt, W. (2016). Closing the gap: Supporting patients' transition to self-management after hospitalization. *Proceedings of the 2016 CHI Conference on Human Factors in Computing Systems,* 5324-5336.

Ramar, K., & Olson, E.J. (2013). Management of common sleep disorders. *American Family Physician, 88*(4), 231-238.

Richardson, J., Loyola-Sanchez, A., Sinclair, S., Harris, J., Letts, L., MacIntyre, N.J., … Ginis, K.M. (2014). Self-management interventions for chronic disease: A systematic scoping review. *Clinical Rehabilitation, 28*(11), 1067-1077. doi:10.1177/0269215514532478

Ryan, P., & Sawin, K.J. (2009). The individual and family self-management theory: Background and perspectives on context, process and outcomes. *Nursing Outlook, 57*(4), 217-225. doi:10.1016/j.outlook.2008.10.004

Sahafi, L., Smith, D., Georgiou, K., Krishnan, J., & Battersby, M. (2016). Efficacy of the Flinders chronic condition management program in obese patients with hip or knee osteoarthritis: A study rationale and protocol. *Australasian Medical Journal, 9*(9), 297-307. doi:10.21767/AMJ.2016.2658

Schulman-Green, D., Jaser, S.S., Park, C., & Whittemore, R. (2016). A metasynthesis of factors affecting self-management of chronic illness. *Journal of Advanced Nursing, 72*(7), 1469-1489. doi:10.1111/jan.12902

Taylor, S.J.C., Pinnock, H., Epiphaniou, E., Pearce, G., Parke, H.L., Schwappach, A., … Sheikh, A. (2014). A rapid synthesis of the evidence on interventions supporting self-management for people with long-term conditions: PRISMS – Practical systematic review of self-management support for long-term conditions. *Health Services and Delivery Research, 2*(53), 1-622.

Tougas, M.E., Hayden, J.A., McGrath, P.J., Huguet, A., & Rozario, S. (2015). A systematic review exploring the social cognitive theory of self-regulation as a framework for chronic health condition interventions. *PloS One, 10*(8). doi:10.1371/journal.pone.0134977

Toukhsati, S.R., Driscoll, A., & Hare, D.L. (2015). Patient self-management in chronic heart failure – Establishing concordance between guidelines and practice. *Cardiac Failure Review, 1*(2), 128-131. doi: 10.15420/cfr.2015.1.2.128

Tu, H., Wen, C.P., Tsai, S.P., Chow, W.H., Wen C., Ye, Y., … Wu, X. (2018). Cancer risk associated with chronic diseases and disease markers: Prospective cohort study. *The BMJ, 360.* doi:10.1136/bmj.k134

van Hooft, S.M., Dwarswaard, J., Jedeloo, S., Bal, R., & van Staa, A. (2014). Four perspectives on self-management support by nurses for people with chronic conditions: A Q-methodological study. *International Journal of Nursing Studies, 52*(1), 157-166. doi:10.1016/j.ijnurstu.2014.07.004

van Dillen, S.M., Noordman, J., van Dulmen, S., & Hiddink, G.J. (2015). Quality of weight-loss counseling by Dutch practice nurses in primary care: An observational study. *European Journal of Clinical Nutrition, 69*(1), 73-78. doi:10.1038/ejcn.2014.129

Wildevuur, S.E., Thomese, F., Ferguson, J., & Klink, A. (2017). Information and communication technologies to support chronic disease self-management: Preconditions for enhancing the partnership in person-centered care. *Journal of Participatory Medicine, 6*(9).

Zahry, N.R., Cheng, Y., & Peng, W. (2016). Content analysis of diet-related mobile apps: A self-regulation perspective. *Health Communication, 31*(10), 1301-1310. doi:10.1080/10410236.2015.1072123

Tang, T.S., Funnell, M.M., Gillard, M., Nwankwo, R., & Heisler, M. (2011). Training peers to provide ongoing diabetes self-management support (DSMS): Results from a pilot study. *Patient Education and Counseling, 85*(2), 160-168. doi:10.1016/j.pec.2010.12.013

Chapter 7

Instructions for Continuing Nursing Education Contact Hours

Continuing nursing education credit can be earned for completing the learning activity associated with this chapter. Instructions can be found at aaacn.org/CCTMCoreCNE

Nursing Process

Jude Sell-Gutowski, MSN, BSN, RN-BC
Susan M. Paschke, MSN, RN-BC, NEA-BC
Kristine Meagher, MSN, RN, ACNS-BC, CCCTM®

Learning Outcome Statement

After completing this learning activity, the learner will be able to describe current thoughts related to the nursing process and enable readers to apply the nursing process in the context of Care Coordination and Transition Management (CCTM®).

Learning Objectives

After reading this chapter, the CCTM registered nurse (RN) will be able to:
- Describe the steps of the nursing process and how the steps promote critical thinking.
- Identify the knowledge and skills necessary for application of the nursing process in CCTM nursing (see Table 7-1 on page 146).
- Discuss potential actions to assess nursing care needs.
- Understand the rationale for using standard nursing nomenclature.
- Apply the nursing process in CCTM nursing.

AAACN Care Coordination and Transition Management Standards
Standard 1. Assessment
Standard 2. Nursing Diagnosis
Standard 3. Outcomes Identification
Standard 4. Planning
Standard 6. Evaluation

Source: AAACN, 2016.

Competency Definition
Possession of adequate knowledge and skill to follow the steps of the nursing process; including knowledge of nursing theory and the CCTM model, knowledge of wellness and disease processes including social determinants of health, ability to engage individuals and groups, critical thinking-skills, and use of accepted nursing nomenclature.

Nursing Process Definition
The *nursing process* is a person-centric, systematic, non-linear, scientific method for utilizing theoretical and scientific knowledge and nursing skills in determining health care needs; and implementing and evaluating personalized nursing interventions for individuals, families, and communities.

Source: Toney-Butler & Thayer, 2019.

For decades, the nursing process has been the essential core of nursing standards, legal definitions, and practice in western countries (Black, 2013). It is the common thread uniting professional nursing across the multiplicity of nursing practice settings and roles (Abdelkader & Othman, 2017; American Nurses Association [ANA], 2017). The CCTM RN uses the nursing process in many settings to improve the health of individuals, families, groups, communities, and populations (American Academy of Ambulatory Care Nursing [AAACN], 2017; Pérez Rivas et al., 2016). The nursing process requires the use of cognitive, interpersonal, and psychomotor skills. The nursing process is guided by a code of ethics and is applied within the context of the *Scope and Standards of Practice for Registered Nurses in Care Coordination and Transition Management* (AAACN, 2016) and state nursing practice acts.

I. Clinical Reasoning and Thinking

A. Clinical reasoning.
   1. Using data to come to a rational conclusion.
   2. Used at the point of care.
   3. Results in clinical judgment.
B. Critical thinking.
   1. Definitions proposed by many disciplines, both within and outside nursing literature.
      a. ". . . ability to apply higher-order cognitive skills (conceptualization,

analysis, evaluation) and the disposition to be deliberate about thinking (being open-minded or intellectually honest) that lead to action that is logical and appropriate" (Papp et al., 2014, p. 715).
    b. "Critical thinking is, in short, self-directed, self-disciplined, self-monitored and self-corrective thinking" (Paul & Elder, 2016, p. 4).
    c. Required to avoid the human tendency to think in an egocentric or social-centric manner, leading to biases.
    d. Acceptance of rigorous standards of excellence and thoughtful expertise (Foundation for Critical Thinking, 2017).
    e. Undergirded by professional standards and ethics.
    f. Requires asking questions related to assumptions about the person (Alfaro-LeFevre, 2017), how the circumstances may be regarded differently (Black, 2013), and what additional information is needed.
    g. Critically-thinking nurses scrutinize information and environment, consider all facets, understand and differentiate data, and link information together to synthesize appropriate choices or resolve problems (Chan, 2013).
    h. Includes clinical reasoning (Alfaro-LeFevre, 2017).
  C. Reflective thinking and practice.
    1. Process resulting in judgment related to self and others through viewing oneself and the environment critically (Burrell, 2014).
    2. Self-corrective, deliberate, after-the-fact analyzing reasoning.
    3. Continuous learning and adapting; connecting scientific knowledge to daily work.
    4. Examples: Journaling, chart review, and honest dialog (Alfaro-LeFevre, 2017).

II. **Person-Centered Care**

  A. In 2003, the Institute of Medicine (IOM) proposed five health care competencies, including person-centered care, that need to be addressed in the education of health professionals if the challenges of health care redesign are to be met. In response, the Quality and Safety Education for Nurses (QSEN) project (Cronenwett et al., 2007) defined person-centered care as recognizing "the patient or designee as the source of control and full partner in providing compassionate and coordinated care based on respect for patients' preferences, values and needs" (p. 123).
  B. All aspects of health care are guided by the individual's expressed values and preferences supporting realistic goals (American Geriatrics Society Expert Panel on Person-Centered Care, 2015). All persons important to the individual and all relevant providers must participate in the dynamic relationship.
  C. Person-centered care is associated with greater therapeutic alliance between person and provider, higher perception of provider support, and fewer beliefs about group disparities in care (different standards of care for different groups of people) (Hack, Muralidharan, Brown, Lucksted, & Patterson, 2017).
  D. Sidani and Fox (2014) describe three specific elements that define care as person-centered.
    1. Holistic.
    2. Collaborative.
    3. Responsive.
  E. Person-centeredness can also be described by its dimensions, principles, activities, and enablers (Scholl, Zill, Härter, & Dirmaier, 2014).
  F. The nursing process must be approached by the CCTM RN from an interprofessional and holistic perspective with the person and family at the center (AAACN, 2017; Hussey & Kennedy, 2016).

III. **The Nursing Process**

  A. Definition.
    1. Organizing framework for thinking through problems systematically and thoroughly.
    2. Universally accepted intellectual process by which problems are addressed (Agyeman-Yeboah, Korsah, & Okrah, 2017).
    3. Cyclic, dynamic, and flexible; not linear, fixed, static, or rigid (Kesner & Mayo, 2013).
    4. Deliberative, rational, and systematic method of critical thinking (Solbrekke, Englund, Karseth, & Beck, 2015).
    5. Person-centered, problem-oriented, and goal-directed.
    6. Holistic, interpersonal, and collaborative.
  B. Steps of nursing process (ANA, 2010; AAACN, 2017, 2018).
    1. Assessment.
    2. Nursing diagnosis.
    3. Identification of expected outcomes/goals.
    4. Planning.
    5. Implementation.

6. Evaluation.
C. Assessment: Systematic collection of "focused data relating to health needs and concerns of an individual, group, or population" (AAACN, 2017, p. 21). The nurse gathers or validates information about an individual's knowledge, psycho-socio-cultural, physiological, and spiritual status. Interviewing, observing, and examining are used deliberately to identify health problems and/or risk factors, as well as readiness and ability to realize health improvement, strengths, and resources (Alfaro-LeFevre, 2017). A holistic nursing assessment of the individual includes gathering data not only related to the individual's physical being, but also related to developmental goals, their lifestyle, available support systems, stressors, race and ethnicity, health beliefs, religious preference, sociocultural attributes, and any use of complementary health practices (Lilley, Rainforth Collins, & Snyder, 2017).
  1. Purpose of assessment is to ascertain the individual's responses to actual or potential problems and, if applicable, to treatment and intervention.
  2. Assessment occurs each time the individual interacts with the CCTM RN in person or through telehealth means.
  3. Data collection must be prioritized and occurs:
     a. Comprehensively, holistically (e.g., new individual with chronic illness encounter).
     b. Problem-focused (e.g., symptomatic visit, urgent care, health care setting transition, or telehealth encounter) (Ashton, 2017).
     c. Emergently (e.g., triage).
     d. Over time, a reassessment (e.g., chronic care management, responses to treatment or intervention).
  4. Types of data:
     a. Objective: Observed directly or indirectly through measurement or use of the senses (sight, touch, sound, and smell).
     b. Subjective: Stated, described, and/or verified by the individual, family, or caregivers through verbal and nonverbal communication. Subjective data include feelings, perceptions, and concerns.
  5. Interview of individual and/or family members and/or caregivers, when necessary.
     a. Complete investigation of symptoms is key to avoid missing a potentially life-threatening situation.
     b. The CCTM RN must know what cues to look for and questions to ask (AAACN, 2017).
     c. Complete investigation is especially important in telehealth nursing assessments prior to providing advice (Koehne, 2017).
  6. Physical assessment.
     a. Organized and systematic process, using general survey and techniques of inspection, palpation, percussion, and auscultation, typically in that order.
  7. Nursing assessment contributes to the overall interprofessional database of information about the individual.
  8. Documentation must be organized, comprehensible, and retrievable by other members of the health care team (AAACN, 2017).
  9. Hidayat and Kes (2015) recommend that nursing assessment be accomplished based on 11 functional health patterns to facilitate the accurate creation of nursing diagnoses.
     a. Health perception and management.
     b. Nutritional metabolic.
     c. Elimination.
     d. Activity exercise.
     e. Sleep; rest.
     f. Cognitive-perceptual.
     g. Self-perception/self-concept.
     h. Role relationship.
     i. Sexuality; reproductive.
     j. Coping-stress tolerance.
     k. Value-belief pattern.
  10. CCTM RNs must extrapolate from the data (Alfaro-LeFevre, 2017). The collected data must be critically analyzed, synthesized, and prioritized in preparation for the creation of one or more nursing diagnoses.
D. Nursing diagnosis: Clinical judgment based on the nursing assessment about individual, family, or community responses to actual or potential health problems/life developments stated in standardized terminology (AAACN, 2017). A nursing diagnosis has a label and clear definition. Nursing diagnoses document distinct nursing contributions to the individual's plan of care (Grant, 2017) and serve as clear, concise, and consistent interprofessional communication tools (Herdman & Kamitsuru, 2018).
Implementation of nursing diagnosis enhances every aspect of nursing practice, from garnering professional respect to assuring consistent documentation representing nurses'

professional clinical judgment, and accurate documentation to enable reimbursement. NANDA International exists to develop, refine and promote terminology that accurately reflects nurses' clinical judgments. (NANDA-I, 2018a, para. 3).
1. Responses to health problems/life processes are the "central concern" (Herdman & Kamitsuru, 2018, p. 35) of the delivery of nursing care. Nursing diagnoses address these responses.
2. Nursing diagnoses are formulated by analyzing the data collected.
   a. Distinguish relevant from irrelevant (Alfaro-LeFevre, 2017).
   b. Transform data into information.
   c. Apply clinical judgment to know what the collected data means (Grant, 2017).
3. Classify by grouping significant and related data to create a list of suspected problems that can be addressed with nursing interventions (Alfaro-LeFevre, 2017).
4. NANDA-I nursing diagnoses are the most evidence-based and comprehensive (Herdman & Kamitsuru, 2018).
   a. Exclude non-nursing diagnoses.
   b. Include environmental stressors.
   c. Include medication issues.
5. Nursing diagnoses may be problem-focused diagnoses, risk diagnoses, or health-promotion diagnoses (Herdman & Kamitsuru, 2018). A few syndrome diagnoses include chronic pain syndrome, disturbed sleep pattern, impaired physical mobility, fatigue, and social isolation.
   a. Problem-focused diagnosis example (three parts).
      (1) Constipation (condition) related to abdominal muscle weakness (cause), as evidenced by distended abdomen, abdominal pain, and rectal pressure.
   b. Risk diagnosis example (two parts).
      (1) Risk for acute confusion related to progression of Parkinson's disease and planned upcoming hospitalization.
      (2) Risk of strained caregiver role related to progression of individual's increasing self-care deficits.
   c. Health-promotion diagnosis example (two parts).
      (1) Readiness for enhanced coping as evidenced by expressing desire to enhance social supports.
6. Avoid common errors in application of nursing diagnoses.
   a. Naming a nursing diagnosis must be consistent with person-centered care and not be person-blaming. For example, a person who does not speak English should not be diagnosed with "altered verbal communication."
   b. Nursing diagnoses should lead to interventions (nursing or others) at the time (rather than later) that promote, protect, or restore health to the individual, family, or community (Lunney, 2011).
7. A nursing diagnosis provides the basis for selection of nursing interventions to achieve outcomes for which the nurse has accountability (NANDA-I, n.d.).

E. Outcomes/goals identification: A nursing-sensitive outcome can be defined as "an individual, family, or community state, behavior, or perception that is measured along a continuum in response to nursing intervention(s)" (Moorhead, Johnson, Maas, & Swanson, 2018, p. 3). Defining outcomes creates a continuous feedback loop that is essential to ensuring evidence-based care and the best possible outcomes, including improving the experience, improving population health, and reducing health care costs (Ballantyne, 2016).
1. Establish priorities of applicable nursing diagnoses first. Safety issues are always a high priority.
2. Derive outcomes from nursing diagnoses (AAACN, 2017).
3. Involve the individual and/or family in determining appropriate outcomes. Shared decision-making is required for authentic evidence-based practice (Hoffmann & Tooth, 2017).
4. Use the SMART acronym when writing outcome statements (Haughey, 2014):
   a. Specific – Concrete and well-defined terms.
   b. Measurable – Quantifiable with a specified source of measurement.
   c. Attainable/achievable – Possible for the given time frame and resources.
   d. Relevant/realistic – Related to the overarching goal.
   e. Time bound – Set deadlines.
5. Use of the Nursing Outcomes Classification (NOC) informs the nursing

Chapter 7

Figure 7-1.
Healthy Eating, Weight Control, Increased Physical Activity

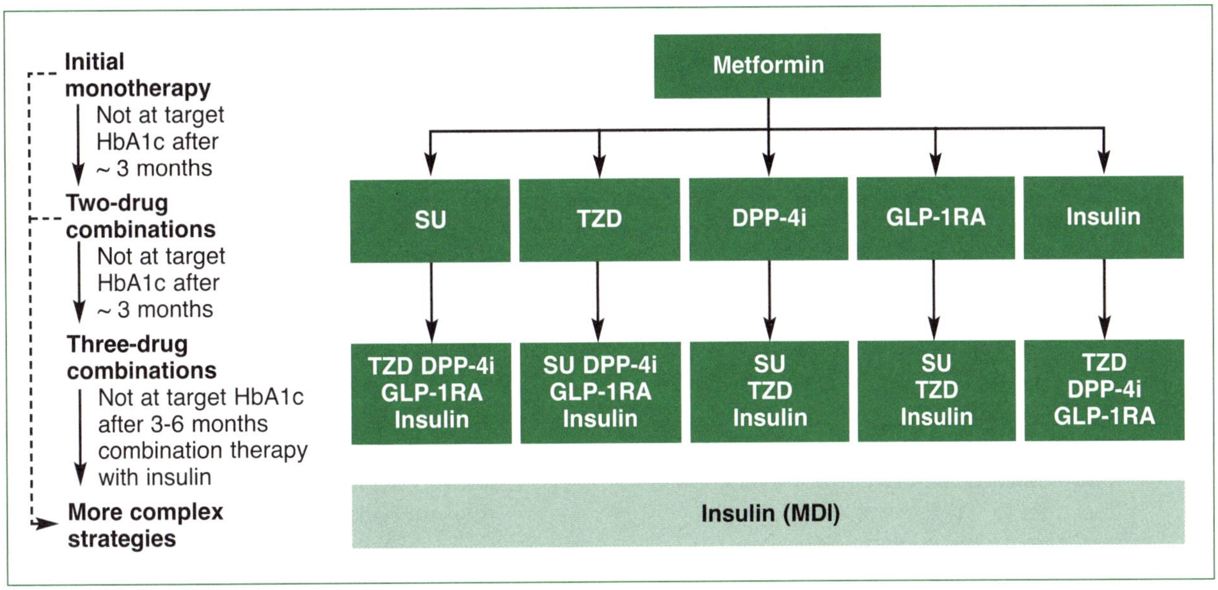

```
Initial
monotherapy                          Metformin
  Not at target
  HbA1c after
  ~ 3 months
                    ┌──────────┬──────────┼──────────┬──────────┐
Two-drug
combinations       SU         TZD       DPP-4i    GLP-1RA     Insulin
  Not at target
  HbA1c after
  ~ 3 months
                    ↓          ↓          ↓          ↓          ↓
Three-drug        TZD DPP-4i  SU DPP-4i    SU         SU       TZD
combinations      GLP-1RA     GLP-1RA     TZD        TZD      DPP-4i
  Not at target   Insulin     Insulin    Insulin    Insulin   GLP-1RA
  HbA1c after 3-6 months
  combination therapy
  with insulin                          Insulin (MDI)
More complex
strategies
```

Source: Wangou et al., 2014. Reprinted with permission from Wolters Kluwer Medknow Publications.

process and assists the nurse to document individual status before and after nursing interventions are deployed.
Example: Individual Engagement Behavior – 1638.
Definition: Personal action to actively participate in one's health care through shared decision-making with health professionals.
Domain: Health Knowledge & Behavior (IV); Class: Health Behavior (Q).
Rated from *never demonstrated to consistently demonstrated* indicator examples:
  a. Obtains reputable health information.
  b. Follows a healthy lifestyle.
  c. Monitors medication side effects.
  d. Chooses among treatment options (Moorhead et al., 2018).
6. Individualize measurement times (e.g., every clinic visit, every 6 months), with the minimum measurement interval at baseline and when nursing care is completed.
7. Use Likert-type scale (used with NOC outcomes).
  a. Five or seven-point scale used to allow individuals to express how much they agree or disagree with a particular statement (estimate of magnitude).
  b. Individuals can rate their own status.
  c. Marks incremental progress toward a goal.
  d. May increase individual motivation.
8. Treat-to-target: Therapeutic concept (titration of interventions).
  a. Employs well-defined, specific, and clinically relevant physiologic targets (quantitative measures such as weight, lab values, blood pressure) aimed at controlling pathophysiology (Wangnoo, Sethi, Sahay, John, & Sharma, 2014).
  b. Uses comprehensive, evidence-based, and generally accepted target values such as:
    (1) Has demonstrated effectiveness in treatment of cardiovascular disease (e.g., blood pressure, low-density lipoprotein cholesterol), rheumatoid arthritis (e.g., pain, swollen and tender joint counts, erythrocyte sedimentation rate, and C-reactive protein), and diabetes (e.g., hemoglobin A1c, fasting plasma glucose, and postprandial plasma glucose).
  c. Applies multifactorial approach, dependent on individual.
  d. Effective control of hypertension has been demonstrated when there is focused time with individuals, tools are provided to manage their condition, and follow up with stated goals has occurred (Frellick, n.d.).
  e. See Figure 7-1 for examples of treat-to-target for type 2 diabetes.
9. Mutual goal-setting with individuals and families, including the integration of symptom pattern recognition and triggers,

CHAPTER 7 – *Nursing Process*

Chapter 7

assists in the prioritization of desired outcomes (Ackley, Ladwig, & Flynn Makic, 2016).
   10. Expected outcomes must be modified based on re-evaluation of the situation or changes in health status (AAACN, 2016).
   11. Correlation between the standardized language systems of NANDA-I nursing diagnoses and NOC indicators has limitations that require further exploration (de Carvalho et al., 2018).
F. Planning: Prioritize nursing diagnoses and set time frames; obtain special equipment needed and gather any additional knowledge necessary for implementation (Lilley, Rainforth Collins, & Snyder, 2017).
   1. Identify person-centered, specific nursing (not medical management) interventions designed to "(1) prevent, manage, and eliminate problems and risk factors; (2) reduce the likelihood of undesired outcomes and increase the likelihood of desired outcomes; and (3) promote health and independence" (Alfaro-LeFevre, 2017, p. 174).
   2. Nursing diagnoses are prioritized by immediate needs from the perspective of individual, family, and health care team.
   3. Clinical judgment and knowledge of evidence-based nursing practices are required for selection of nursing interventions and activities for a particular individual considering: "(1) desired patient outcomes, (2) characteristics of the nursing diagnosis, (3) research base for intervention, (4) feasibility for performing the intervention, (5) acceptability to the patient, and (6) capability of the nurse" (Butcher, Bulechek, McCloskey Dochterman, & Wagner, 2018, p. 5).
   4. Consider cost effectiveness, integrating current trends, and available research (AAACN, 2017).
   5. Identify standardized Nursing Interventions Classification (NIC) interventions directed at etiology of nursing diagnoses.
   6. Individualize through selection of appropriate activities, realistic time frames, and individual and family inclusion in plan.
G. Implementation of the plan is the action component of the nursing process (Kesner & Mayo, 2013).
   1. Function may be independent, collaborative, or dependent functions.
   2. NIC is standardized classification of interventions nurses perform, physiological and psychological, and direct and indirect (e.g., supply management) (Butcher et al., 2018). Interventions included for:
      a. Illness treatment (e.g., hyperglycemia management).
      b. Illness prevention (e.g., fall prevention).
      c. Health promotion (e.g., exercise promotion).
   3. CCTM RN employs delegation and referral skills with thorough understanding of roles and scope.
   4. Activities occur during face-to-face clinical encounters or through telehealth activities.
   5. CCTM RN uses knowledge regarding educational methods and adult learning theory, as well as motivational interviewing skills to promote the desired behavior change.
   6. CCTM RN uses knowledge of evidence-based coaching and shared decision-making methods.
   7. CCTM RN includes CCTM activities (AAACN, 2017).
      a. CCTM RN practice has a strong emphasis on coordination of care in the implementation phase of the nursing process; particularly related to communication, teamwork, and collaboration with the individual and caregivers, and the interprofessional team across the continuum of care (AAACN, 2016).
   8. Involves health teaching and health promotion.
      a. Health teaching includes "healthy lifestyles, risk-reducing behaviors, disease management strategies, psychosocial needs, and self-care" (AAACN, 2016, p. 19). See Chapter 3, "Education and Engagement of Individuals, Families/Caregivers."
      b. Providing individual with skills to cope with chronic disease and overcome barriers.
   9. Requires consultation with appropriate stakeholders.
   10. Links individuals and caregivers to other members of the team and to other appropriate resources in the community.
   11. Requires documentation of interventions and individual responses.
H. Evaluation: Systematic, ongoing, and criteria-based activity that includes ongoing assessment – thus, the dynamic nature of the nursing process.
   1. Entire interprofessional care team helped by nurses' documentation of responses to interventions, whether nursing interventions

Chapter 7

   or other.
2. Assess progress toward the NOC goal and reassess usefulness and attainability of the goal.
3. Continual reflection supports timely changes and safer care (Alfaro-LeFevre, 2017).
4. May need to modify or set new outcome goals.
5. May need to redefine the problem if interventions are not working as expected.
6. May need to reassess the appropriateness of the selected intervention(s) (Alfaro-LeFevre, 2017).
7. CCTM RN is accountable for care variances.

IV. **Applying the Nursing Process to Family Care**

A. Terminology.
   1. Family: Two or more individuals coming from the same or different kinship groups who are involved in a continuous living arrangement, usually residing in the same household, experiencing common emotional bonds, and sharing certain obligations toward each other and toward others (Jejurkar, 2016, slide 3).
   2. Family health: "A condition including the promotion and maintenance of physical, mental, spiritual, and social health for the family unit and for individual family members" (Jejurkar, 2016, slide 3).
   3. Family process: "The ongoing interaction between family members through which they accomplish their instrumental and expressive tasks. The nursing process considers the family, not the individual as the unit of care" (Jejurkar, 2016, slide 3).
B. Approaches to family-centered nursing assessment. Thorough, accurate assessment is foundational.
   1. Family as the context: Primary focus is on the individual family member.
   2. Family as the client: Focus is on each individual as he or she affects the family as a whole.
   3. Family as a system.
      a. Family as client applied simultaneously with family as the context.
      b. Implies that when something happens to one, all are affected.
   4. Family as a social determinant of heath.
   5. Family as a component of society.
      a. As an institution, family interacts with other institutions, including health care, education, religious, and economic.
      b. Community nursing generally begins at the interface of family and other institutions.
   6. Areas of inquiry to consider:
      a. Family structure, characteristics and dynamics, such as family communication/interaction, decision-making patterns.
      b. Socio-economic and cultural characteristics, including educational attainment, occupation(s), significant others, role in community.
      c. Home and environment, including safety, sanitation, and available services.
      d. Health status of each family member.
      e. Values, health beliefs and practices, lifestyle, disease prevention, stress management, and immunization status.
C. Nursing diagnoses.
   1. Many NANDA-I nursing diagnoses can be applied or are specific to family care planning.
      a. Examples that can be applied to families: Risk for infection, impaired verbal communication, grieving, and imbalanced nutrition – less than body requirements.
      b. Examples specifically for families: Dysfunctional family processes, compromised family coping, and ineffective family health management.
D. Interventions.
   1. Many NIC interventions are for use with families (e.g., family integrity promotion) (Butcher et al., 2018).
E. Continue dynamic and cyclical nursing process through outcomes/goal setting and planning.

V. **The Nursing Process and Chronic Disease Management**

A. Chronic diseases are responsible for 7 of 10 deaths each year, and treating people with chronic diseases accounts for 86% of our nation's health care costs (Centers for Disease Control and Prevention, 2018).
B. According to the Institute for Healthcare Improvement, optimized team-based care and the chronic care model have had a positive impact on office visit cycle time, access to care, preventive screening, self-management goal setting and action planning, and medication

reconciliation (Hupke, 2014).
C. CCTM RN work is informed by Wagner's Chronic Care Model (Wagner, 1998) and the CCTM RN Model (see Chapter 1, "Introduction").
D. Interprofessional, team-based, across the span of care enhances chronic disease management.
E. CCTM RNs are ideally placed for chronic care interprofessional planning, care coordination, and evaluation of outcomes (Bodenheimer, Ghorob, Willard-Grace, & Grumbach, 2014; Harris et al., 2015).
F. For individuals with chronic conditions, interventions must include self-management support.
G. Professional CCTM RNs bring "unique and critical knowledge to both an individual with a new diagnosis, and individuals and families . . . as they integrate a chronic illness into their lives" (Rondinelli, Omery, Crawford, & Johnson, 2014, p. e113).

VI. **Plan of Care**

Care coordination and transition management is becoming increasingly important as health care systems assume more outcomes and quality-related financial responsibility. Focusing on hospital readmissions is no longer adequate.
A. Theoretically, an individual's plan of care should never be closed and should follow the individual across the continuum of care (Boston-Fleischhaure, Rose, & Hartwig, 2017).
B. Robust electronic tools for care coordination are still needed (Bates, 2015).
C. CCTM RNs have the knowledge to serve as the care coordinator in the interprofessional team necessary for individuals with complex medical needs. Social determinants of health can further complicate the navigation of health care in the fragmented system currently in place (AAACN, 2016).

VII. **Decision Support**

Clinical decision support systems (CDSS) aim to reduce variation and improve quality and safety of care by providing timely information to clinicians, individuals, and others to inform health care decision- making. Medicare and Medicaid electronic health records and incentive programs required CDSS to demonstrate "meaningful use." Clinical decision support systems are "intended to provide clinicians with intelligently filtered information at appropriate times to foster better processes, better individual patient care, and population health" (Singh & Wright, 2016, p. 111). Such systems have been demonstrated to improve individual care in medication ordering, chronic disease management, health screening, and vaccination (County Health Rankings & Roadmaps, 2018).
A. CDSS imbedded in electronic health records are being developed for inpatient nursing but are still in their infancy for CCTM care nursing, generally (Miranda et al., 2017).
B. Participants in one design study of a probability-based clinical decision support tool preferred elements that supported, rather than interrupted, nurses' cognitive processes (Jeffrey, Novak, Kennedy, Dietrich, & Mion, 2017).
C. Miranda and colleagues (2017) concluded that CDSS for all phases of the nursing process are needed and must be supported by a nursing theory foundation.
D. Developers of nursing clinical support systems need to be aware of "alert fatigue" phenomenon identified in medical CDSS (Robert Wood Johnson Foundation, 2015).
E. Efforts are underway to promote the inclusion of social and behavioral domains into electronic health records certified by the Office of the National Coordinator for Health Information Technology and the Centers for Medicare and Medicaid Services (IOM, 2015).
   1. Functional status and onset and progression of illness is contributed to by social and behavioral factors.
   2. The United States has an unfavorable balance between health care costs and health of the population relative to other developed countries.

VIII. **Expanding the CCTM RN Role and Nursing Process**

A. Nurses increased access to care in underserved areas almost 3 decades prior to development of nurse practitioner role (Keeling, 2015).
B. Role of clinical nurse specialist is expanding (Negley, Cordes, Evenson, & Schad, 2016) to support full scope practice, standardization, and safety.
C. Current call exists for expanded roles of RNs in primary care (Bauer & Bodenheimer, 2017), episodic and preventive care (Smolowitz et al., 2015), and in a variety of roles in accountable care organizations (Pittman & Forrest, 2015).
D. Functions that overlap with practice of medicine.
   1. Standing orders, protocols, standardized procedures, depending on the state, may permit the nurse to perform functions that overlap with the practice of medicine.

Figure 7-2.
Standardized Nursing Terminology

If nursing data is organized in a standardized way, it can be used to identify new opportunities for nursing research, improve practice, recognize trends, and for comparison. NANDA-I, Nursing Interventions Classification (NIC) and the Nursing Outcomes Classification (NOC) are recognized by the American Nurses Association (ANA) and are included in the National Library of Medicine's Metathesaurus for a Unified Medical Language and the Cumulative Index to Nursing Literature (CINAHL). They are mapped into the Systematized Nomenclature of Medicine (SNOMED) and registered in Health Level Seven International (HL7). NANDA-I, NOC and NIC are the terms used in this chapter to describe nursing judgments, treatments, and nursing-sensitive outcomes.

Source: Keenan, 2014.

2. Depending on state, advance practice nurses (e.g., nurse practitioners, certified nurse midwives) may or may not provide an advanced level of care (e.g., diagnosing, prescribing) without physician delegation via protocols or standardized procedures.
3. Debate continues regarding independent practice of nursing, supervising medical home, payment equal to physicians for same services, etc.

IX. Conclusion

The use of the nursing process, with individuals positioned centrally and considered holistically, in a collaborative interprofessional health care delivery system must be the nursing profession's strategy at an individual, institutional, and societal level. Conscientiously employing the nursing process has been demonstrated to have a positive effect on length of stay, perceived quality of nursing care and cost in the hospital environment (Johny, Moly, Sreedevi, & Nair, 2017), and improved control of chronic conditions with lower cost in the ambulatory care setting (Pérez Rivas et al., 2016). Health care provision is continually evolving, and not necessarily in a manner designed to facilitate health.

CCTM RNs' opportunities in the evolving health care transformation is supported by nursing's core values (such as empathy, ethics, and advocacy), in addition to expertise and clinical knowledge. Use of standardized terminology (see Figure 7-2) is essential for measuring, clarifying, and understanding nursing care and to evaluate care provided using nurse-sensitive outcomes that demonstrate value and characterize the unique care rendered by nurses (Törnvall & Janssen, 2017). CCTM RNs must join with other nurses in the development and advancement of nurse-sensitive indicators. Nursing must actively engage to ensure its contributions are understood at an interprofessional level across the span of care.

Table 7-1.
Nursing Process: Knowledge, Skills, and Attitudes for Competency

	Evidence-Based Practice (EBP)

Integrate best current evidence with clinical expertise and individual/family preferences and values for delivery of optimal health care (Cronenwett et al., 2007).

Knowledge	Skills	Attitudes	Sources
Demonstrate knowledge of basic scientific methods and processes. Describe evidence-based practice (EBP) to include the components of research evidence, clinical expertise, and individual/family values.	Participate effectively in appropriate data collection and other research activities. Adhere to institutional review board guidelines. Base individualized care plan on individual values, clinical expertise, and evidence.	Appreciate strengths and weaknesses of scientific bases for practice. Value the need for ethical conduct of research and quality improvement. Value the concept of EBP as integral to determining best clinical practice.	Cronenwett et al., 2007
Differentiate clinical opinion from research and evidence summaries. Describe reliable sources for locating evidence reports and clinical practice guidelines.	Read original research and evidence reports related to area of practice. Locate evidence reports related to clinical practice topics and guidelines.	Appreciate the importance of regularly reading relevant professional journals.	Cronenwett et al., 2007
Explain the role of evidence in determining best clinical practice. Describe how the strength and relevance of available evidence influences the choice of interventions in provision of person-centered care.	Participate in structuring the work environment to facilitate integration of new evidence into standards of practice. Question rationale for routine approaches to care that result in less-than-desired outcomes or adverse events.	Value the need for continuous improvement in clinical practice based on new knowledge.	Cronenwett et al., 2007
Discriminate between valid and invalid reasons for modifying evidence-based clinical practice based on clinical expertise or individual/family preferences.	Consult with clinical experts before deciding to deviate from evidence-based protocols.	Acknowledge own limitations in knowledge and clinical expertise before determining when to deviate from evidence-based best practices.	Cronenwett et al., 2007

	Quality Improvement

Use data to monitor the outcomes of care processes and use improvement methods to design and test changes to continuously improve the quality and safety of health care systems (Cronenwett et al., 2007).

Knowledge	Skills	Attitudes	Sources
Describe approaches for changing processes of care.	"Design a small test of change in daily work (using an experiential learning method (such as Plan-Do-Study-Act). Practice aligning the aims, measures, and changes involved in improving care. Use measures to evaluate the effect of change" (p. 127).	Value local change (in individual practice or team practice on a unit) and its role in creating joy in work. Appreciate the value of what individuals and teams can do to improve care.	Cronenwett et al., 2007

continued on next page

Chapter 7

Table 7-1. (continued)
Nursing Process: Knowledge, Skills, and Attitudes for Competency

Safety			
Minimize risk of harm to individuals and providers through both system effectiveness and individual performance (Cronenwett et al., 2007).			
Knowledge	**Skills**	**Attitudes**	**Sources**
Delineate general categories of errors and hazards in care. Describe factors that create a culture of safety (such as open communication strategies and organizational error-reporting systems).	Communicate observations or concerns related to hazards and errors to individuals, families, and health care team. Use organizational error-reporting systems for near-miss and error reporting.	Value own role in preventing errors.	Cronenwett et al., 2007
Describe processes used in understanding causes of error and allocation of responsibility and accountability (such as root cause analysis and failure mode effects analysis).	Actively participate in analyzing errors and designing system improvements. Engage in root cause analysis rather than blaming when errors or near misses occur.	Value vigilance and monitoring (even of own performance of care activities) by individuals, families, and other members of the health care team.	Cronenwett et al., 2007
Discuss potential and actual impact of national individual safety resources, initiatives, and regulations.	Use national individual safety resources for own professional development and to focus attention on safety in care settings.	Value relationship between national safety campaigns and implementation in local practices and practice settings.	Cronenwett et al., 2007

Person-Centered Care			
Recognize the individual or designee as the source of control and full partner in providing compassionate and coordinated care based on respect for individual's preferences, values, and needs (Cronenwett et al., 2007).			
Knowledge	**Skills**	**Attitudes**	**Sources**
Demonstrate comprehensive understanding of the concepts of pain and suffering, including physiologic models of pain and comfort.	Assess presence and extent of pain and suffering. Assess levels of physical and emotional comfort. Elicit expectations of individual and family for relief of pain, discomfort, or suffering. Initiate effective treatments to relieve pain and suffering in light of individual values, preferences, and expressed needs.	Recognize personally held values and beliefs about the management of pain or suffering. Appreciate the role of the nurse in relief of all types and sources of pain or suffering. Recognize individual expectations influence outcomes in management of pain or suffering.	Cronenwett et al., 2007

continued on next page

Table 7-1. (continued)
Nursing Process: Knowledge, Skills, and Attitudes for Competency

Person-Centered Care (continued)			
Knowledge	**Skills**	**Attitudes**	**Sources**
Integrate understanding of multiple dimensions of person-centered care: • Individual/family/community preferences, values • Coordination and integration of care • Information, communication, and education • Physical comfort and emotional support • Involvement of family and friends • Transition and continuity Describe how diverse cultural, ethnic, and social backgrounds function as sources of individual, family, and community values.	Elicit individual values, preferences, and expressed needs as part of clinical interview, implementation of care plan, and evaluation of care. Communicate individual values, preferences, and expressed needs to other members of health care team. Provide person-centered care with sensitivity and respect for the diversity of human experience.	Value seeing health care situations through individuals' eyes. Respect and encourage individual expression of individual values, preferences, and expressed needs. Value the individual's expertise with own health and symptoms. Seek learning opportunities with individuals who represent all aspects of human diversity. Recognize personally held attitudes about working with individuals from different ethnic, cultural, and social backgrounds. Willingly support person-centered care for individuals and groups whose values differ from own.	Cronenwett et al., 2007
Examine how the safety, quality, and cost effectiveness of health care can be improved through the active involvement of individuals and families. Examine common barriers to active involvement of individuals in their own health care processes. Describe strategies to empower individuals or families in all aspects of the health care process.	Remove barriers to presence of families and other designated surrogates based on individual preferences. Assess level of individual's decisional conflict and provide access to resources. Engage individuals or designated surrogates in active partnerships that promote health, safety and well-being, and self-care management.	Value active partnership with individuals or designated surrogates in planning, implementation, and evaluation of care. Respect individual's preferences for degree of active engagement in care process. Respect individual's right to access to personal health records.	Cronenwett et al., 2007

continued on next page

Table 7-1. (continued)
Nursing Process: Knowledge, Skills, and Attitudes for Competency

Nursing Process (continued)			
Knowledge	**Skills**	**Attitudes**	**Sources**
Know questions to ask and cues to look for regarding physical, psychological, and social readiness to learn. (Assessment) Identify questions to ask to holistically design an integrated care plan that encompasses a variety of care methods to provide individuals with complex care needs with the resources needed to maintain the highest level of function. (Assessment and Diagnosis) Have awareness of known risk factors that place a person at risk for rehospitalization or exacerbation and utilize knowledge and critical thinking to identify actions to mitigate risk. (Diagnosis and Plan)	Use techniques that invite/engage person and significant others in learning. Use techniques to assess learning such as "teach back." Identify full range of medical, functional, social, and emotional problems that increase individual's risk of adverse health events. Monitor for progress and early signs of problems. Utilize data collection and analysis to design interventions to improve outcomes.	Demonstrate creativity in planning appropriate learning experiences for individuals and significant others. Value the services available to individuals by delivering services that facilitate beneficial, efficient, safe, and high-quality experiences and improve health care outcomes.	Alfaro-Lefevre, 2017 Ashton, 2017 Lilley et al., 2017 Alfaru-LeFevre, 2019 Koehne, 2017
Understand the importance of instilling confidence in individuals and caregivers regarding their ability to manage future transitions. (Plan and Implementation)	Competence in medication review and reconciliation, experience in helping people communicate their needs to different health care professionals, and ability to shift from doing things for them to encouraging them to do as much as possible independently. Ability to impart skills to individuals and caregivers for effectively communicating care needs during subsequent encounters.	Value the importance of empowering people with knowledge and self-confidence to self-manage safely through care transitions.	AAACN, 2016 Anderson, 2017
Know the information and clinical skills needed to support and teach the person in the process of self-management. (Implementation)	Use evidence-based clinical guidelines to direct care.	Require flexibility, creativity, and an understanding everyone learns differently.	Butcher et al, 2018

continued on next page

Table 7-1. (continued)
Nursing Process: Knowledge, Skills, and Attitudes for Competency

Nursing Process (continued)			
Knowledge	**Skills**	**Attitudes**	**Sources**
Understand the themes of effective interpersonal interaction. (Implementation and Outcomes/Goals Identification)	Use effective communication within the context of a trusting, therapeutic relationship. Can assess the cognition/aptitude of a person and readiness to learn. Able to set clear expectations, goals, and boundaries from the beginning.	Require the ability to stick with a person over the "long haul," as this could be a relationship that needs to be in place for years.	O'Hagan et al., 2014
Understand illness and chronic care management of specific disease. (Diagnosis, Plan, Outcomes/Goals Identification and Implementation) Understanding of and ability to utilize community resources effectively. (Implementation)	Effective communication and leadership. Be able to provide individuals with skills to overcome barriers and cope with chronic illness.	Ability to be a confident and compassionate leader in a person's health care experience. Commitment and longevity.	Grant, 2017 Herdman & Kamitsuru, 2018 Parker & Fuller, 2016
Understand the goals of person-centered care and community resources that are available and appropriate. (Plan and Implementation)	Ability to link people with resources and other team members.	Holistic team approach is necessary.	Grumbach, Bodenheimer, & Grundy, 2009
Knowledge in use of nursing process in home setting. Understand sources of evidence-based nursing interventions. (Implementation)	Perform comprehensive nursing assessment including of the home environment. Create care plan.	Value EBP and lifelong learning.	American Home Health, n.d.
Demonstrate awareness of effective team communication methods and nursing role within team. (Implementation and Evaluation)	Utilize effective communication methods. Function competently within own scope of practice as a member of the health care team.	Value nurse role and scope of practice as part of interprofessional team.	AAACN, 2016
Demonstrate understanding of various electronic medical record features and use, including personal health records. (Assessment, Diagnosis, Outcomes/Goal Identification, Implementation and Evaluation)	Navigate the electronic health record and document and plan care in an electronic health record. Employ communication technologies to coordinate care and communicate.	Value technologies that support clinical decision-making, communication with individuals, and care coordination. Protect confidentiality of protected health information in electronic health records.	Morton et al., 2015

continued on next page

Table 7-1. (continued)
Nursing Process: Knowledge, Skills, and Attitudes for Competency

Nursing Process (continued)			
Knowledge	**Skills**	**Attitudes**	**Sources**
Know all aspects of the individual's disease, treatment, and support. (Assessment, Diagnosis, Plan, Implementation, Evaluation)	Critical thinking. Manages the care process. Development and communication of the care plan. Timely needs assessment. Assessment for symptoms and provision of interventions or other required management. Information provision. Ability to develop therapeutic relationships.	Belief it is the nurses' responsibility to navigate the health care system for the individual.	Nutt & Hungerford, 2010
Knowledge of chronic illness and needs of transitional care. Knowledge regarding education and adult learning theory (assessing individuals and teaching what individuals need; involving them in their plan of care). Knowledge of motivational interviewing skills to foster behavior change.	Ability to assess individuals and caregivers to determine learning needs; build upon strengths.	Open and accepting attitude toward individuals; coaching.	Coleman et al., 2007 Coleman & Berenson, 2004
Evidence-based, clinical guidelines of care for defined chronic conditions. Interdependence of clinical conditions. Medication indications, interactions, side effects, refill management, and safe administration. "Six domains of practice activity that are critical to the quality of care in a medical home: 1. organizational capacity, 2. chronic condition management, 3. care coordination, 4. community outreach, 5. data management, 6. quality improvement" (p. 783).	Advocate for individual and family needs. Communication, teaching. Use of survey instruments for data collection and data analysis.	Holistic, family-centered philosophy. Individual as partner. Adaptable to changing individual needs and complexity.	Berry et al., 2011

Source: Cronenwett et al. (2007). *Nursing Outlook, 55*(3), 122-131. Reprinted with permission from Elsevier.

Chapter 7

Case Study 7-1.
CCTM® Care Plan

Joan S.
DOB: 03/15/1947

The individual is a 71-year-old female with past medical history of chronic obstructive pulmonary disease and bipolar disorder who presents with shortness of breath.

The individual was initially doing well until she developed an upper-respiratory infection in late March. She was treated at this time with azithromycin. She was improving until about 1 week ago. Since that time, she has had increased dyspnea. However, she was having increased anxiety using her nebulizer (albuterol causes her to be shaky) so had been avoiding it. Her daughter-in-law reports she has periods of insomnia and irritability when she calls the patient to check up on her. Other times she reports increased sleepiness and feeling depressed. She is also noncompliant with bi-polar meds at times.

She presented to the emergency department 1 week later with continued symptoms. At that time, she was started on 40 mg of prednisone by mouth as well as doxycycline. She had difficulty tolerating the doxycycline due to gastrointestinal upset and continued to not take the albuterol secondary to feeling jittery.

She then returned to the emergency department for worsening symptoms.

In the emergency room, the individual was given an additional dose of 20 mg prednisone (60 mg total for the day) and started on azithromycin. She also was given three doses of ipratropium but declined albuterol nebulizers. She displayed shortness of breath and dyspnea on exertion. She can only walk about two blocks at this time, which is half of her usual. Additionally, she complained of a productive cough with green sputum. She denied any fevers/chills, nausea, or vomiting. With her cough, she has chest pain but no pain at rest or with exertion.

She was then admitted for further management. She lives alone, recently widowed. She is accompanied by her daughter-in-law who lives about an hour away.

- CT chest 2015 reviewed with individual: Extensive emphysema, two small nodules < 4mm.
- PE: GENERAL: She is oriented to person, place, and time. She appears well-developed and well-nourished. She does not appear distressed.
- HENT: Exam performed. Mouth/Throat: The oropharynx is clear and moist.
- NECK: No JVD present.
- CV: Normal rate, regular rhythm and normal heart sounds. No murmur. There is no peripheral edema. Exam reveals no gallop and no friction rub.
- PULM/CHEST: Effort normal. No respiratory distress. She has wheezes. Poor air movement.
- Diffuse expiratory wheezing throughout.
- ABD: The abdomen is soft. Bowel sounds are normal. She has no distension. There is no tenderness. There is no guarding.
- MUSC/SKEL: There is no peripheral edema.
- LYMPH: No cervical adenopathy.
- NEURO: She is alert and oriented to person, place, and time.
- SKIN: Skin is warm and dry. She is not diaphoretic.

Medications:
- Atorvastatin (Lipitor®) 20 mg tablet: Take one tablet (20mg total) by mouth daily.
- Doxycycline (Monodox®) 100 mg capsule: Take one capsule (100 mg total) by mouth two times a day for 7 days.
- Duloxetine (Cymbalta®) 60 mg capsule: Take 60 mg by mouth daily
- Fluticasone furoate (Arnuity Ellipta®) 200 mcg/actuation blister with device: Inhale one puff daily
- Ipratropium-albuterol (Duo-Neb®) 0.5-2.5 mg/3 mL nebulizer solution: Inhale 3 mL every 4 hours
- Levalbuterol (Xopenex® HFA) 45mcg/actuation inhaler: Inhale two puffs every 6 hours as needed for wheezing or shortness of breath
- Lithium 150 mg capsule: Take 300 mg by mouth three times a day with meals
- Lorazepam (Ativan®) 0.5 mg tablet: Take 0.5 mg by mouth every 8 hours as needed
- Multivitamin capsule - Take one capsule by mouth daily
- Olanzapine (Zyprexa®) 10 mg tablet: Take 10 mg by mouth nightly
- Prednisone (Deltasone®) 20 mg tablet: Take two tablets (40 mg total) daily x 5 days
- Promethazine-DM (Promethazine-DM®) 6.25-15 mg/5 mL syrup: Take 2.5 mL by mouth four times a day as needed for cough for up to 7 days

Assessment
- Record review
- Interview
- Review subjective and objective data
- Stratify at-risk individual as high, moderate, or low risk
- Document data in database to share with all team members

Diagnosis
Acute exacerbation of COPD

Problem List:
- COPD
- Bipolar disorder
- Osteoarthritis of knee
- Hyperlipidemia
- History of tobacco use
- Shortness of breath
- Influenza B
- Elevated troponin

Nursing Diagnoses:
- Impaired gas exchange
- Risk for infection

Outcomes/Goals:
- Improved symptom control
- Compliance with medication regimen
- Regular visits with PCP

continued on next page

Case Study 7-1. (continued)
CCTM® Care Plan

Plan

Care Coordination Problems:
- Frequent emergency department visits
- Compliance with medications
- Keep primary care appointments

Goal:
- Individual develops action plan when symptoms worsen
- Promote independence

Intervention:
- CCTM RN performs action plan teach back at each visit
- Coordinate with daughter-in-law to discuss increased assistance at home and transportation to PCP appointments
- Smoking cessation plan

Implementation

- CCTM RN communicates with primary care provider for medication compliance
- Use of motivational interviewing to promote individual independence
- Use OARS (Open-end questions, Affirm, Reflective listening, Summarize) to develop person-centered goals including compliance with all medications and follow-up appointments
- Develop therapeutic relationship with individual; discuss challenges faced to meet goals

Evaluation

Self-Management Goals:
- CCTM RN assesses individual's response to plan of care
- CCTM RN to utilize structure monitoring to measure individual and health care team performance
- Chronic care management

Chapter 7

Case Study 7-2.
Nursing Process

Introduction

Helen G. is a 74-year-old with a recent history of increased medical problems and complications. Liz, the CCTM RN in the primary care provider's office, knows Mrs. G well and is charged with management of Mrs. G's ongoing nursing care needs and subsequent follow-up appointments in multiple clinical areas.

Mrs. G has a history of hypertension, type 2 diabetes, hypercholesterolemia, essential tremors, and developed a low-grade right-sided astrocytoma near the basal ganglia 1 year ago. She underwent tumor ablation (97% successful), 6 weeks of daily radiation therapy, but failed a course of oral chemotherapy due to bone marrow suppression. She subsequently developed multiple deep vein thrombosis in the right leg and was started on enoxaparin and transitioned to warfarin over a 3-month period.

Normal pressure hydrocephalus was discovered inadvertently during the brain tumor workup. Symptoms included increasing gait disturbance, urinary incontinence, and mild dementia which exacerbated over time to complete inability to walk, limited ability to eat, total urinary incontinence, inability to dress and undress, and need for total care. A ventriculoperitoneal shunt was placed about 6 months later. After the shunt surgery, Mrs. G was placed in a nursing facility for rehab. Over the next 3 months, Mrs. G demonstrated significant improvement of symptoms. She is walking with a rollator and is able to perform most activities of daily living independently, but has developed increased short-term memory loss with poor decision-making thus safety is a major concern.

Since Mrs. G lives alone and all of her family members live in different states. Her friend Mary is her power of attorney for health care and the primary caregiver who assists Mrs. G in making health care decisions. Mrs. G wants to return home or to a local assisted living facility.

Clinical Interaction

Nursing process includes plan for:
- Follow up of diabetes, increased cholesterol, hypertension – primary care
- Follow up for DVT and warfarin therapy – vascular medicine
- Follow up for brain tumor – neuro-oncology
- Follow up for shunt care and maintenance – neurology
- Safety regarding warfarin, falls risk, cognitive disability
- Change in living arrangements
- No longer driving

Clinical Implications

- Multiple clinical assessments required on ongoing basis
- Prioritization of clinical needs
- Medication compliance
- Transition from home to assisted living – home has stairs to basement and second floor
- Coordination of appointments
- Transportation arrangements to multiple appointments
- Mrs. G attends mass regularly at the rehab facility – she is no longer able to drive and will require transportation and assistance to attend services
- Evaluation of outcomes and individual's satisfaction

How will the CCTM® RN utilize the nursing process in managing Mrs. G's ongoing care?

Assessment

What is Mrs. G's priority health care issue?
What types of assessments will need to be completed for Mrs. G initially and ongoing?
- Status of chronic illnesses – DM, DVT, HTN, shunt functioning
- Current physical condition – ADLs, mobility

Cognitive assessment – short and long-term memory, safety concerns, decision making
- Emotional assessment – decreasing independence, coping skills
- Psychosocial assessment – support, socialization, etc.

Diagnosis

What nursing diagnoses are applicable to Mrs. G? Consider:
- Altered health maintenance
- Anxiety
- Urinary incontinence
- Altered mobility
- Sleep pattern disturbance
- Self-care deficit (potential)
- Recreation deficit
- Thought alteration
- Social isolation
- Altered perception (new environment)
- Altered nutrition (new environment)

Identify the three most important nursing diagnoses for Mrs. G as she transitions to her new living arrangement.

Plan

What actions will the CCTM RN take to alleviate the issues identified in the assessment?

Identify potential short and long-term goals to be discussed and determined with Mrs. G.

Implementation

What actions will the CCTM-RN take to assist Mrs. G in accomplishing the identified goals?

What nursing interventions can the CCTM-RN perform independently?

What interventions will be performed in collaboration with providers or other care team members?

Evaluation

What outcomes will be measured to determine effectiveness of the plan of care?
- Related to health issues
- Related to existing conditions
- Related to safety
- Related to independence and self-functioning

How will effectiveness be measured?

Chapter 7

References

Abdelkader, F.A., & Othman, W.N.E. (2017). Factors affecting implementation of nursing process: Nurses' perspective. *IOSR Journal of Nursing and Health Science, 6*(3), 76-82. doi:10.9790/1959-0603017682

Ackley, B.J., Ladwig, G.B., & Flynn Makic, M.B. (2016). *Nursing diagnosis handbook: An evidence-based guide to planning care* (11th ed.). St. Louis, MO: Elsevier.

Agyeman-Yeboah, J., Korsah, K.A., & Okrah, J. (2017). Factors that influence the clinical utilization of the nursing process at a hospital in Accra, Ghana. *BMC Nursing, 16*(30). doi:10.1186/s12912-017-0228-0

Alfaro-LeFevre, R. (2017). *Critical thinking, clinical reasoning, and clinical judgment* (6th ed.). Philadelphia, PA: Elsevier.

American Academy of Ambulatory Care Nursing (AAACN). (2018). *Scope and standards of practice for professional telehealth nursing* (6th ed.). T. Anglea, C. Murray, M. Mastal, & S. Clelland (Eds.).Pitman, NJ: Author.

American Academy of Ambulatory Care Nursing (AAACN). (2016). *Scope and standards of practice for registered nurses in care coordination and transition management.* Pitman, NJ: Author.

American Academy of Ambulatory Care Nursing (AAACN). (2017). *Scope and standards of practice for professional ambulatory care nursing* (9th ed.). Pitman, NJ: Author.

American Geriatrics Society Expert Panel on Person-Centered Care. (2015). Person-centered care: A definition and essential elements. *Journal of the American Geriatrics Society, 64*(1), 15-18. doi:10.1111/jgs.13866

American Home Health. (n.d.). *Nursing process.* Retrieved from https://www.ahhc-1.com/educational-pieces-clients-article.php?id=6

American Nurses Association (ANA). (2010). *Nursing's social policy statement: The essence of the profession.* Silver Spring, MD: Author.

American Nurses Association (ANA). (2017). *The nursing process.* Retrieved from https://www.nursingworld.org/practice-policy/workforce/what-is-nursing/the-nursing-process/

Anderson, M.L. (2017). *Patient-administered self-care.* [Report]. Retrieved from http://www.ihi.org/resources/Pages/Publications/Patient-Administered-Self-Care.aspx

Ashton, L.M. (2017). *Urgent care: A growing healthcare landscape. Nursing, 4*(77), 21-24. doi:10.1097/01.NURSE.0000520503.98804.11

Ballantyne, H. (2016). Developing nursing care plans. *Nursing Standard, 30*(26), 51-57. doi:10.7748/ns.30.26.51.s48

Bates, D.W. (2015). Health information technology and care coordination: The next big opportunity for informatics? *Yearbook of Medical Informatics, 10*(1), 11-14. doi:10.15265/iy-2015-0020

Bauer, L., & Bodenheimer, T. (2017). Expanded roles of registered nurses in primary care delivery of the future. *Nursing Outlook, 65*(5), 624-632. doi:10.1016/j.outlook.2017.03.011

Berry, S., Soltau, E., Richmond, N.E., Kieltyka, R.L., Tran, T., & Wiliams, A. (2011). Care coordination in a medical home in post-Katrina New Orleans: Lessons learned. *Maternal and Child Health Journal, 15*(6), 782-793.

Black, B.P. (2013). Critical thinking, the nursing process, and clinical judgement. In Black, B.P. (Ed.), *Professional Nursing: Concepts & Challenges* (7th ed.) (pp. 171-192). St, Louis, MO: Saunders.

Bodenheimer, T., Ghorob, A., Willard-Grace, R., & Grumbach, K. (2014). The 10 building blocks of high-performing primary care. *Annals of Family Medicine, 12*(2), 166-171. doi:10.1370/afm.1616

Boston-Fleischhauer, C., Rose, R., & Hartwig, L. (2017). Cross-continuum care continuity. *The Journal of Nursing Administration, 47*(7-8), 399-403. doi:10.1097/NNA.0000000000000503

Burrell, L.A. (2014). Integrating critical thinking strategies into nursing curricula. *Teaching and Learning in Nursing, 9*(2), 53-58. doi:10.1016/j.teln.2013.12.005

Butcher, H.K., Bulechek, G.M., McCloskey Dochterman, J.M., & Wagner, C. (2018). *Nursing interventions classification (NIC)* (7th ed). St. Louis, MO: Mosby Elsevier.

Centers for Disease Control and Prevention. (2018). *Chronic disease prevention and health promotion.* Retrieved from https://www.cdc.gov/chronicdisease/index.htm

Chan, Z.C. (2013). A systematic review of critical thinking in nursing education. *Nurse Education Today, 33*(3), 236-240. doi:10.1016/j.nedt.2013.01.007

Coleman, E.A., & Berenson, R. (2004). Lost in transition: Challenges and opportunities for improving the quality of transitional care. *Annals of Internal Medicine, 141,* 533-536.

Coleman, E.A., Parry, C., Chalmers, S., Chugh, A., & Mahoney, E. (2007). The central role of performance improvement in improving the quality of transitional care. *Home Health Care Service Quarterly, 26*(4), 93-104.

County Health Rankings & Roadmaps. (2018). *Computerized clinical decision support systems (CDSS).* Retrieved from http://www.countyhealthrankings.org/policies/computerized-clinical-decision-support-systems-cdss

Cronenwett, L., Sherwood, G., Barnsteiner, J., Disch, J., Johnson, J., Mitchell, P., ... Warren, J. (2007). Quality and safety education for nurses. *Nursing Outlook, 55*(3), 122-131. doi:10.1016/j.outlook.2007.02.006

de Carvalho, E.C., Eduardo, A.H.A., Romanzini, A., Simão, T., Zamarioli, C.M., Garbuio, D.C., & Herdman, T.H. (2018). Correspondence between NANDA International nursing diagnoses and outcomes as proposed by the nursing outcomes classification. *International Journal of Nursing Knowledge, 29*(1), 66-78. doi:10.1111/2047-3095.12135

Frellick, M. (n.d.). *HHC nurses cheer on patients.* Retrieved from https://www.nurse.com/blog/2014/04/07/hhc-nurses-cheer-on-patients/

Foundation for Critical Thinking. (2017). *Our concept and definition of critical thinking.* Retrieved from http://www.criticalthinking.org/pages/our-concept-of-critical-thinking/411

Grant, V. (2017). What's your diagnosis? *ViewPoint, 39*(1), 9.

Grumbach, K., Bodenheimer, T., & Grundy, P. (2009). *The outcomes of implementing patient-centered medical home interventions: A review of the evidence on quality, access and costs from recent prospective evaluation studies.* San Francisco, CA: UCSF Center for Excellence in Primary Care. Retrieved from http://familymedicine.medschool.ucsf.edu/cepc/pdf/outcomes%20of%20pcmh%20for%20White%20House%20Aug%202009.pdf

Hack, S.M., Muralidharan, A., Brown, C.H., Lucksted, A.A., & Patterson, J. (2017). Provider behaviors or consumer participation: How should we measure person-centered care? *The International Journal of Person Centered Care, 7*(1), 14-20. doi:10.5750/ijpcm.v7i1.602

Harris, T., Kerry, S.M., Victor, C.R., Ekelund, U., Woodcock, A., Iliffe, S., ... Cook, D.G. (2015). A primary care nurse-delivered walking intervention in older adults: PACE (pedometer accelerometer consultation evaluation)-Lift cluster randomised controlled trial. *PLoS Med, 12*(2). doi:10.1371/journal.pmed.1001783

Haughey, D. (2014). *A brief history of smart goals.* Retrieved from https://www.projectsmart.co.uk/brief-history-of-smart-goals.php

Herdman, H.T., & Kamitsuru, S. (Eds.). (2018). *Nursing diagnoses: Definitions & classification 2018-2020* (11th ed). New York, NY: Thieme.

Hidayat, A.A.A., & Kes, M. (2015). Model documentation of assessment and nursing diagnosis in the practice of nursing care management for nursing students. *International Journal of Advanced Nursing Studies, 4*(2), 156-168. doi:10.14419/ijans.v4i2.5116

Hoffmann, T., & Tooth, L. (2017). Shared decision making. In Hoffmann, T., Bennett, S., & Del Mar, C., (Eds.), *Evidence-Based Practice Across the Health Professions* (2nd ed.). St. Louis, MO: Elsevier Mosby.

Hupke, C. (2014). *Team-based care: Optimizing primary care for patients and providers.* Retrieved from http://www.ihi.org/communities/blogs/team-based-care-optimizing-primary-care-for-patients-and-providers-

Hussey, P.A., & Kennedy, M.A. (2016). Instantiating informatics in nursing practice for integrated patient centered holistic models of care: A discussion paper. *Journal of Advanced Nursing, 72*(5), 1,030-1,041. doi:10.1111/jan.12927

Institute of Medicine (IOM). (2003). *Health professions education: A bridge to quality.* Washington, DC: The National Academies Press.

Institute of Medicine (IOM). (2015). *Capturing social and behavioral domains and measures in electronic health records: Phase 2.* Washington, DC: The National Academies Press.

Jeffrey, A.D., Novak, L.L., Kennedy, B., Dietrich, M.S., & Mion, L.C. (2017). Participatory design of probability-based decision support tools for in-hospital nurses. *Journal of the American Medical Informatics Association, 24*(6), 1,102-1,110. doi:10.1093/jamia/ocx060

Johny, S.A., Moly, K.T., Sreedevi. P.A., & Nair, R.R. (2017). Effectiveness of nursing process based clinical practice guideline on quality of nursing care among post CABG patients. *International Journal of Nursing Education, 9*(2), 120-126. doi:10.5958/0974-9357.2017.00048.4

Jejurkar, K. (2016). *A seminar on family health nursing.* [Presentation]. Retrieved from https://www.slideshare.net/kunal770909/family-health-nursing

Keeling, A.W. (2015). Historical perspectives on an expanded role for nursing. *Online Journal of Issues in Nursing, 20*(2). doi:10.3912/OJIN.Vol20No02Man02

Keenan, G.M. (2014). Big data in health care: An urgent mandate to change nursing EHRs! *Online Journal of Nursing Informatics, 18*(1). Retrieved from https://www.ncbi.nlm.nih.gov/pmc/articles/PMC4618496/pdf/nihms-592469.pdf

Kesner, K., & Mayo, W. (2013). Application of the nursing process in ambulatory care. In Laughlin, C.B. (Ed.), *Core Curriculum for Ambulatory Care Nursing* (3rd ed.). Pitman, NJ: American Academy of Ambulatory Care Nursing.

Koehne, K. (2017). Telehealth practice: Be inquisitive. *ViewPoint, 39*(4), 16-17.

Lilley, L.L., Rainforth Collins, S., & Snyder, J.S. (2017). *Pharmacology and the Nursing Process* (8th ed.). St. Louis, MO: Elsevier Mosby.

Lunney, M. (2011). *Avoiding errors in using NANDA International (I) diagnoses in clinical and educational settings.* [Abstract]. Retrieved from http://kb.nanda.org/article/AA-00961/0/Avoiding-Errors-in-Using-NANDA-International-I-Diagnoses-in-Clinical-and-Educational-Settings.html

Miranda, L.N., Farias, I.P., Almeida, T.G., Cizino da Trinadade, R.F., Freitas, D.A. & Vasconselos, E.L. (2017). Decision-making system for nursing: integrative review. *Journal of Nursing UFPE/Revista De Enfermagem UFPE, 11*(10), 4263-4272. doi: 10.5205/reuol.10712-95194-3-SM.1110sup201732

Moorhead, S., Johnson, M., Maas, M. L., & Swanson, E. (2018). *Nursing outcomes classification (NOC)* (6th Ed.). St. Louis: Elsevier Mosby.

Morton, K., Beauchamp, M., Prothero, A., Joyce, L., Saunders, L., Spencer-Bowdage, S., ... Pedlar, C. (2015). The effectiveness of motivational interviewing for health behaviour change in primary care settings: A systematic review. *Health Psychology Review, 9*(2), 205-223. doi:10.1080/17437199.2014.882006

NANDA International (NANDA-I). (2018a). *About us.* Retrieved from http://nanda.org/about-us/

NANDA International (NANDA-I). (n.d.). *Knowledge-based terminologies defining nursing.* Mountain, WI: Author.

Negley, K.D., Cordes, M.E., Evenson, L.K., & Schad, S.P. (2016). From hospital to ambulatory care: Realigning the practice of clinical nurse specialists. *Clinical Nurse Specialist (CNS), 30*(5), 271-276. doi:10.1097/NUR.0000000000000231

Nutt, M., & Hungerford, C. (2010). Nurse care coordinators: Definitions and scope of practice. *Contemporary Nurse, 36*(1-2), 71-81.

O'Hagan, S., Manias, E., Elder, C., Pill, J., Woodward-Kron, R., McNamara, T., ... McColl, G. (2014). What counts as effective communication in nursing? Evidence from nurse educators' and clinicians' feedback on nurse interactions with simulated patients. *Journal of Advanced Nursing, 70*(6), 1,344-1,355. doi:10.1111/jan.12296

Papp, K.K., Huang, G.C., Lauzon Clabo, L.M., Delva, D., Fischer, M., Konopasek, L., Schwartzstein, R.M., & Gusic, M. (2014). Milestones of critical thinking: A developmental model for medicine and nursing. *Academic Medicine, 89*(5), 715-720. doi:10.1097/ACM.0000000000000220

Parker, S., & Fuller, J. (2016). Are nurses well placed as care coordinators in primary care and what is needed to develop their role: A rapid review? *Health and Social Care in the Community, 24*(2), 113-122. doi: 0.1111/hsc.12194

Paul, R., & Elder, L. (2016). *The miniature guide to critical thinking: Concepts and tools* (7th ed.). Tomales Bay, CA: Foundation for Critical Thinking.

Pérez Rivas, F.J., Martin-Iglesias, S., Pacheco del Cerro, J.L., Minguet Arenas, C., Garcia López, M., & Beamud Lagos, M. (2016). Effectiveness of nursing process use in primary care. *International Journal of Nursing Knowledge, 27*(1), 43-48. doi:10.1111/2047-3095.12073

Pittman, P., & Forrest, E. (2015). The changing roles of registered nurses in Pioneer Accountable Care Organizations. *Nursing Outlook, 63*(5), 554-565. doi:10.1016/j.outlook.2015.05.008

Rondinelli, J.L., Omery, A.K., Crawford, C.L., & Johnson, J.A. (2014). Self-reported activities and outcomes of ambulatory care staff registered nurses: An exploration. *The Permanente Journal, 18*(1), e108-e115. doi:10.7812/TPP/13-135

Robert Wood Johnson Foundation. (2015). *Computerized clinical decision support systems (CDSS).* Retrieved from http://www.countyhealthrankings.org/take-action-to-improve-health/what-works-for-health/policies/computerized-clinical-decision-support-systems-cdss

Scholl, I., Zill, J.M., Härter, M., & Dirmaier, J. (2014). An integrative model of patient-centeredness – A systematic review and concept analysis. *PLoS One, 9*(9). doi:10.1371/journal.pone.0107828

Sidani, S., & Fox, M. (2014). Patient-centered care: Clarification of its specific elements to facilitate interprofessional care. *Journal of Interprofessional Care, 28*(2), 134-141. doi:10.3109/13561820.2013.862519

Singh, K., & Wright, A. (2016). Clinical decision support. In Finnell, J., Dixon, B. (Eds.), *Clinical Informatics Study Guide Text and Review.* Cham, Switzerland: Springer. doi:10.1007/978-3-319-22753-5

Smolowitz, J., Speakman, E., Wojnar, D., Whelan, E.M., Ulrich, S., Hayes, C., & Wood, L. (2015). Role of the registered nurse in primary health care: Meeting health care needs in the 21st century. *Nursing Outlook, 63*(2), 130-136. doi:10.1016/j.outlook.2014.08.004

Solbrekke, T.D., Englund, T., Karseth, B., & Beck, E.E. (2015). Educating for professional responsibility: From critical thinking to deliberative communication, or why critical thinking is not enough. In Trede, F. and McEwen, C. (Eds.), *Educating the Deliberate Professional: Preparing Practitioners for Future Practices.* New York, NY: Springer.

Toney-Butler, T.J., & Thayer, J.M. (2019). *Nursing process.* Treasure Island, FL: StatPearls Publishing.

Törnvall, E., & Janssen, I. (2017). Preliminary evidence for the usefulness of standardized nursing terminologies in different fields of application: A literature review. *International Journal of Nursing Knowledge, 28*(2), 109-119. doi:10.1111/2047-3095.12123

Wagner, E.H. (1998). Chronic disease management: What will it take to improve care for chronic illness? *Effective Clinical Practice, 1*(1), 2-4. Retrieved from https://ecp.acponline.org/augsep98/cdm.pdf

Wangnoo, S.K., Sethi, B., Sahay, R.K., John, M., & Sharma, S.K. (2014). Treat-to-target trials in diabetes. *Indian Journal of Endocrinology and Metabolism, 18*(2), 166-174. doi:10.4103/2230-8210.129106

Additional Readings

Dykes, P.C., Samal, L., Donahue, M., Greenberg, J.O., Hurley, A.C., Hasan, O., ... Bates, D.W. (2014). A patient-centered longitudinal care plan: Vision versus reality. *Journal of the American Medical Informatics Association, 21*(6), 1,082-1,090. doi:10.1136/amlajnl-2013-002454

Edwards, S.T., Dorr, D.A., & Landon, B.E. (2017). Can personalized care planning improve primary care? *Journal of* the American Medical Association, 318(1), 25-26. doi:10.1001/jama.2017.6953

Ferguson, D. (2015). *Most healthcare providers unprepared for longitudinal care.* [Report]. FierceHealthcare. Retrieved from http://www.fiercehealthcare.com/healthcare/most-healthcare-providers-unprepared-for-longitudinal-care

Guldin, M. (2017). *Care management in an evolving healthcare industry.* [Blog post]. Retrieved from http://www.chilmarkresearch.com/care-management-in-an-evolving-healthcare-industry/

Harmon, D. (2017). Legislative support to increase the role of the nurse in population health management. *ViewPoint 39*(4), 12-13.

Jutterström, L., Hörnsten, Å,. Sandström, H., Stenlund, H., & Isaksson, U. (2016). Nurse-led patient-centered self-management support improves HbA1c in patients with type 2 diabetes – A randomized study. *Patient Education and Counseling, 99*(11), 1,821-1,829. doi:10.1016/j.pec.2016.06.016

Massimi A., De Vito, C., Brufola, I., Corsaro, A., Marzuillo, C., Migliara, M., ... Damiani, G. (2017) Are community-based nurse-led self-management support interventions effective in chronic patients? Results of a systematic review and meta-analysis. *PLoS One, 12*(3). doi:10.1371/journal.pone.0173617

Moriyama, M., Takeshita, Y., Haruta, Y., Hattori, N., & Ezenwaka, C.E. (2015). Effects of a 6-month nurse-led self-management program on comprehensive pulmonary rehabilitation for patients with COPD receiving home oxygen therapy. *Rehabilitation Nursing, 40*(1), 40-51. doi:10.1002/rnj.119

Reeves, D., Hann, M., Rick, J., Rowe, K., Small, N., Burt, J., ... Bower, P. (2014). Care plans and care planning in the management of long-term conditions in the UK: A controlled prospective cohort study. *British Journal of General Practice, 64*(626), e568-e575. doi:10.3399/bjgp14X681385

Reynolds, R., Dennis, S., Hasan, I., Slewa, J., Chen, W., Tian, D., ... Zwar, N. (2018). A systematic review of chronic disease management interventions in primary care. *BMC Family Practice, 19*(11). doi:10.1186/s12875-017-0692-3

Silver Dunker, K., Manning, K., & Knowles, S. (2017). Utilizing a QSEN based clinical orientation checklist as a standard for orientation. *International Journal of Nursing & Care, 1*(7), 1-7.

Tastan, S., Linch, G.C., Keenan, G.M., Stifter, J., McKinney, D., Fahey, L., ... Wilkie, D.J. (2014). Evidence for the existing American Nurses Association-recognized standardized nursing terminologies: A systematic review. *International Journal of Nursing Studies, 51*(8), 1,160-1,170. doi:10.1016/j.ijnurstu.2013.12.004.

Thede, L.Q., & Schwirian, P.M. (2014). Informatics: The standardized nursing terminologies: A national survey of nurses' experience and attitudes – SURVEY II: Participants' perception of the helpfulness of standardized nursing terminologies in clinical care. *Online Journal of Issues in Nursing, 20*(1). doi:10.3912/OJIN.Vol20No01InfoCol01

Westra, B.L., Latimer, G.E., Matney, S.A., Park, J.I., Sensmeier, J., Simpson, R.L., ... Delaney, C.W. (2015). A national action plan for sharable and comparable nursing data to support practice and translational research for transforming health care. *Journal of the American Medical Informatics Association, 22*(3), 600-607. doi:10.1093/jamia/ocu011

Zimmermann, T., Puschmann, E., van den Bussche, H., Wiese, B., Ernst, A., Porzelt, S., ... Scherer, M. (2016). Collaborative nurse-led self-management support for primary care patients with anxiety, depressive or somatic symptoms: Cluster-randomised controlled trial (findings of the SMADS study). *International Journal of Nursing Studies, 63*, 101-111. doi:10.1016/j.ijnurstu.2016.08.007

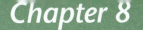

Teamwork and Collaboration

Maribeth Kelly, MSN, RN, PCCN, CCCTM®
Frances R. Vlasses, PhD, RN, ANEF, FAAN
Lisa Wus, DNP, RN, FNP-BC, PCCN-CMC, CCCTM®

Instructions for Continuing Nursing Education Contact Hours

Continuing nursing education credit can be earned for completing the learning activity associated with this chapter. Instructions can be found at aaacn.org/CCTMCoreCNE

Learning Outcome Statement

After completing this learning activity, the learner will be able to apply effective teamwork and collaboration knowledge and skills and overcome barriers to produce quality and effective person-centered outcomes when performing in the role of the Care Coordination and Transition Management registered nurse (CCTM® RN) across all care settings.

Learning Objectives

After reading this chapter, the CCTM RN will be able to:
- Define teamwork and collaboration.
- Identify integration of the relevant standards within the *Scope and Standards for Registered Nurses in Care Coordination and Transition Management* in the CCTM RN role.
- Identify the importance of teamwork and collaboration, and the effects on person-centered care processes and outcomes.
- Describe evidence-based strategies that support teamwork, including overcoming common barriers.
- Describe the role of the CCTM RN within a team.
- Demonstrate how the CCTM RN practices the knowledge, skills, and attitudes required for teamwork and collaboration (see Table 8-1 on page 168).
- Describe the interprofessional approach to partnering with individuals and families in shared decision-making.
- Describe the development of a care plan using guiding principles.

AAACN Care Coordination and Transition Management Standards

Standard 5a.	Coordination of Care
Standard 5c.	Consultation
Standard 6.	Evaluation
Standard 7.	Ethics
Standard 11.	Communication
Standard 13.	Collaboration
Standard 16.	Environment of Care

Source: AAACN, 2016.

Competency Definition

In the Quality and Safety Education for Nurses (QSEN) project, the teamwork and collaboration competency is defined as functioning "effectively within nursing and interprofessional teams, fostering open communication, mutual respect, and shared decision-making to achieve quality patient care" (American Association of Colleges of Nursing [AACN] QSEN, 2012, p. 4).

The Institute of Medicine (IOM) (2000, 2001) noted the American health care system is not yet adequately equipped to deliver chronic care with consistently positive effect, in part because there has been a focus on acute illness. Effective care of those with chronic conditions and diseases, the IOM notes, requires careful attention not only to what care is delivered, but also to how it is delivered. Moreover, it is necessary to appreciate that care is not given to just the individual, but also to caregivers and families. To make the necessary changes, the IOM says professionals need to use skills that build relationships with individuals and their peers. Although teamwork and collaboration share similarities and are often used interchangeably, different definitions have been used to describe teamwork and collaboration within interprofessional work. McEwan, Ruissen, Eys,

Chapter 8

Zumbo, and Beauchamp (2017) maintain that teamwork refers to team members who interact and convert team inputs into outcomes through interdependent behavioral processes. The American Nurses Association (2016) defines collaboration as individuals across professions working together through combining knowledge, skills, and values and attitudes with other health care workers, including individuals, families, and communities, when applicable, to improve health outcomes.

Gaglioti, Barlow, Thoma, and Bergus (2017) provide evidence that positive outcomes are attained when coordination and transition management are carried out within strong interprofessional teams. The Interprofessional Education Collaborative [IPEC] (2016) emphasized that interprofessional collaboration "is the key to safe, high-quality, accessible, patient-centered care desired by all" (p. 4). While there is a general need to deploy effective teams to serve those with chronic conditions and diseases, legislation has added to the urgency with which professionals in ambulatory and other settings across the care continuum must acquire the knowledge, skills, and values associated with highly effective teams.

Both the American Recovery and Reinvestment Act of 2009 and the Patient Protection and Affordable Care Act of 2010 began the stimulation of team-based approaches to providing care. The current stimulus for teamwork and collaboration, where communication is essential, addresses the concerns regarding pay for performance, cost of health care in the United States, health care quality, and denial of reimbursement for never events and readmissions within 30 days of discharge from the acute care setting (Salmond & Echevarria, 2017). Never events are defined as clear and measurable events that result in serious injury or death and are usually preventable (Agency for Healthcare Research and Quality [AHRQ], 2018).

The Medical Home model is just one example that relies on interprofessional teamwork and team-based care. Furthermore, federal legislation is pressuring the reconsideration of the concept of health and the relationship of primary care to that concept. The centrality of community is a theme across nearly all major health care reform laws that have emerged in recent years. Accountability in primary care for population health management of chronic disease goes beyond individuals and extends to the health care community in its entirety. There is a sharing of roles and responsibilities between health care delivery professionals and public health professionals across several domains, including health promotion, primary prevention care, and behavioral change. Members of these groups must work in a coordinated manner on behalf of individuals, families, and communities. Responsibilities of such teams extend to maintaining healthy environments and responding to public health emergencies, not just to the provision of primary care. Health care reform requires health care professionals connect within the community to work for the good of individuals, families, and communities as responsible members of interprofessional teams (IPEC, 2016).

Responding to the emerging changes in the structure of health care in the context of community, the IOM (2010), in its report *The Future of Nursing*, emphasized nurses must play a key role not just as members of interprofessional teams, but also as leaders within those teams. "Nurses have both the clinical and management knowledge and skill set needed to assume key coordination roles" (Salmond & Echevarria, 2017, p. 22). The role of collaboration and coordination of care across a variety of settings is part of the role of nurses and is needed to prepare nurses for coordination and collaboration (IOM, 2010). The knowledge, skills, and attitudes (KSAs) needed for nurses to undertake and participate in their role on interprofessional teams are described in Table 8-1. The KSAs are dependent upon one's own competence as a nurse and the ability to work with others, realizing team members all have differing levels of competencies. Team members who exhibit qualities of open and honest communication create an environment of mutual respect that supports shared decision-making which can result in quality care.

Seminal work by Mitchell and colleagues (2012) described basic principles and values to guide and accelerate team-based care effectiveness. As part of a Best Practices Innovation Collaborative, Mitchell and associates (2012) synthesized previous work, developed team-based principles and values, and then conducted interviews of team-based health care practices to further develop and validate efforts. This set of principles of team-based care is one product of their work. Additionally, five personal values identifying and characterizing the most effective members of well-functioning teams included honesty, discipline, creativity, humility, and curiosity (Mitchell et al., 2012). Among examples were putting a high value on effective communication and transparency, carrying out duties even when inconvenient, excitement in tackling problems creatively, reliance on others to help recognize and avoid failures regardless of hierarchy, and dedication to using insights for continuous improvement (Mitchell et al., 2012).

I. Collaboration, Teamwork and Professional Practice Standards

The discussion in the *Scope and Standards of Practice for Registered Nurses in Care Coordination and Transition Management* (American Academy of Ambulatory Care Nursing [AAACN], 2016) includes collaboration as a main characteristic. "The RN practicing CCTM interacts with the patient, family members, caregivers, and health care professionals to foster professional relationships that improve population health" (AAACN, 2016, p. 28). The components of teamwork and collaboration can be seen throughout the individual standards themselves.

A. Application of professional standards to the CCTM RN dimension of Teamwork and Collaboration Standard 13: Collaboration (AAACN, 2016, p. 28).
  1. Apply critical-thinking skills and use appropriate clinical judgments when implementing population health interventions or planning effective care for groups or individuals and their families.
  2. Partner with interprofessional team members in diverse settings regarding the promotion, prevention, and restoration of health in populations.
  3. Recognize that populations are composed of individuals.
  4. Provide outreach to individuals and their caregivers to identify health or psychosocial issues used in the development of an appropriate plan of care.
  5. Coordinate with local and community resources to improve the health of populations or individuals.
  6. Communicate recommended intervention(s) and plan(s) of care with expected outcomes with individuals or caregivers and applicable members of the interprofessional team.
  7. Interface with peers using shared decision-making to implement practice(s) to improve population health and CCTM performance and standards.
B. Application of Standard 11: Communication (AAACN, 2016, p. 26).
  1. Promote active communication using a method or manner that enhances learning and the sharing of information.
  2. Evaluate personal skills and styles of communication to identify areas needing improvement and/or education.
  3. Share best practices with peers, requesting feedback and evaluation.
  4. Maintain professional communication(s) with members of the health care team, families, and stakeholders to promote effective interactions.
  5. Create a positive environment that fosters an attitude of information sharing and learning.
  6. Share with the health care team hazards or barriers that could have a negative effect on individuals and/or caregivers.
  7. Seek opportunities to create positive mentoring relationships in regard to CCTM, as well as individual and departmental practices.
  8. Share and communicate knowledge and skills obtained from professional conferences and seminars to CCTM colleagues and staff.
  9. Exemplify an engaged attitude and professional nursing practice that fosters a sense of excellence and enthusiasm among peers and colleagues.
C. Application of Standard 5a: Coordination of Care (AAACN, 2016, p. 18).
  1. Demonstrate accountability across care settings in maintaining continuity of care.
  2. Facilitate individual and/or population progress toward positive person-centered clinical outcomes.
  3. Utilize an interprofessional approach to engage the individual, caregiver, and providers in the implementation of the plan of care across care settings.
  4. Facilitate the transition of individual/population to the appropriate level of care.
  5. Educate and activate the individual and/or caregiver for optimal disease management by promoting healthy lifestyle changes in the prevention of illness across population(s).
  6. Prevent disease progression by reducing risk factors.
  7. Recognize and maximize opportunities to increase the quality of care.
  8. Manage high-risk individuals and/or population(s) with the aim of preventing or delaying adverse outcomes.
  9. Communicate relevant information to the individual, caregiver, and interprofessional health care team across the care continuum.
  10. Apply effective teamwork and collaboration skills to overcome identified barriers to produce quality and effective individual outcomes.

D. Application of Standard 5c: Consultation (AAACN, 2016, p. 20).
   1. Synthesize clinical data and evidence when providing consultation across the care continuum.
   2. Communicate consultation recommendations to appropriate stakeholders.
E. Application of Standard 7: Ethics (AAACN, 2016, p. 22).
   1. Participate without recrimination in the identification of ethical concerns using the mechanisms provided by the applicable organization(s).
   2. Contribute input and/or serve on individuals' rights and ethics committees.
   3. Maintain awareness of emerging ethical trends that affect individual rights.
   4. Deliver nursing care that reflects the cultural, spiritual, intellectual, educational, and psychosocial differences among individuals, families, or communities, and that preserves individual autonomy, dignity, and rights.
   5. Advocate and support informed decisions by the individual or legally designated representative.
   6. Facilitate individual rights to voice opinions regarding care and services received without recrimination, as well as their rights to have issues addressed.
   7. Incorporate appropriate measures to deliver safe care in cases where individuals are not able to act in their own best interests or do not understand the consequences of their decisions.
   8. Promote access to quality health services that encompasses equality, confidentiality of information, and continuity of care.
F. Application of Standard 16: Environment (AAACN, 2016, p. 31).
   1. Participate in orientation and education programs that identify and evaluate current processes and best practices that enhance the creation and maintenance of a safe, hazard-free, confidential, ergonomically correct, and comfortable work/individual care setting.
   2. Monitor and identify the status and the quality of the environment of care.
   3. Make recommendations to ensure the environment is accessible, safe, and functional for individuals, staff, and visitors.
   4. Utilize preventive and screening programs and appropriate interventions if untoward occupational exposure occurs and/or if risk to occupational exposure is reasonably anticipated.
   5. Maintain confidentiality of employee exposure to untoward exposure, treatment, and follow-up.
   6. Comply with organizational policies, protocols, guidelines, and evidence-based practices addressing the prevention of infection, allergic reactions, disposal of biohazardous waste, and maintenance of a safe and comfortable environment.
   7. Maintain the physical space and professional practices that ensure individuals have access to care, ensuring privacy, security, and confidentiality of personal information.
   8. Utilize up-to-date medications, equipment, supplies, and technology in the practice environment.
   9. Ensure the care environment accommodates the delivery of CCTM practices and addresses age-specific, disability-specific, and diverse population needs.
G. Application of Standard 6: Evaluation (AAACN, 2016, p. 21)
   1. Conduct systematic, ongoing, and criterion-based evaluation of the outcomes of care coordination plans in relation to facilitating clinical management across transitions of care.
   2. Collaborate with the interprofessional team, individual, and/or family, and community resources involved in the transitional management of care in the evaluation process.
   3. Integrate current, evidence-based methods and tools in the evaluation process.
   4. Use ongoing assessment strategies to revise and adapt to changes in transition management of care.
   5. Assimilate and document results of the evaluative process in easily understood language for communication to the individual and/or family, interprofessional team, and community resources.
   6. Participate in a collaborative process with stakeholders to assess and assure appropriate use of interventions to facilitate care coordination and/or transition management, minimizing unnecessary treatment and individual safety risks.
   7. Evaluate the effectiveness of care coordination plans in facilitating care across transition points.

II. Interprofessional Approach

For the CCTM RN to be effective, he or she

must be adept at interprofessional collaboration. D'Amour and Oandason (2005) define interprofessionality as "the process by which professionals reflect on and develop ways of practicing that provides an integrated and cohesive answer to the needs of the client/family/population" (IPEC, 2011, p. 9). This represents a shift in the usual siloed approach to care delivery and requires information sharing and group problem solving with the individual at the center of the team.

In 2016, universal standards for interprofessional collaboration were refined outlining interprofessional competencies required for all health professionals. These include interprofessional knowledge of values and ethics, roles and responsibilities, and communication and teamwork (IPEC, 2016). These competencies include an orientation in community and population health in addition to person centeredness.

Research demonstrates that individuals want to be partners in their own health care (Bernabeo & Holmboe, 2013). A critical aspect of partnering with individuals and families is shared decision-making. In this model, the clinician and the person or family make health-related decisions collaboratively, based on both the best available evidence and the person's values, beliefs, and preferences (Bernabeo & Holmboe, 2013). Shared decision-making in addition to other practices, such as bedside shift report, shared medical records, teach-back, care partner programs, and collaborative goal setting, promote person and family partnering, especially if they are utilized at key individual touch points – before, during, and after a care episode (Frampton et al., 2017) and are instrumental to the effectiveness of the interprofessional team.

A. Interprofessional team members communicate regularly to discuss care focusing on the unique needs and desires of the individual. This communication may take place as rounds, regular huddles, or formal care conferences.
B. Interprofessional collaboration skills can be developed through training programs like TeamSTEPPS®. Such training provides skills needed to build strong teams, including specific communication and leadership tactics. Pillars of the program include leadership, communication, situational awareness, and mutual support. TeamSTEPPS is an evidence-based teamwork system aimed at optimizing individual outcomes through improving communication and teamwork skills among team members across the health care delivery system. It was developed by the Department of Defense's Patient Safety Program in collaboration with AHRQ (2014). It is available for free online at https://www.ahrq.gov/teamstepps/index.html
C. The development of an interprofessional care plan ideally includes the individual's stated goals with defined interventions from each contributing discipline. The following guiding principles are offered by Jones, Jamerson, and Pike (2012):
   1. Patient problems linked to mutual goals.
   2. Goals with outlined expectations.
   3. Outcomes (indicators) that document individual progress toward the goal.
   4. Evidence-based interventions that align with assessment and treatments.
   5. Education to prepare the individual and family for transitions in care.
D. Documenting interprofessional care plans continues to be challenging because most current documentation systems do not allow for the integration of data across disciplines. Therefore, teams must develop alternative communication processes to ensure all members continue to work on the same plan.

III. **Key Elements for Effective Teamwork and Evidence-Based Strategies that Support it, Including Methods to Overcome Common Barriers**

A. Characteristics of high-performing teams.
   1. Clear roles and responsibilities (AHRQ, 2014; Mitchell et al., 2012).
      a. Individual as key member of team.
      b. "There are clear expectations for each team member's functions, responsibilities, and accountabilities which optimize the team's efficiency and often make it possible for the team to take advantage of division of labor, thereby accomplish more than the sum of its parts" (Mitchell et al., 2012, p. 9).
         (1) Members of different backgrounds.
         (2) Discipline-specific knowledge and skills.
         (3) Influenced by cultural and organizational norms.
      c. Best utilization of resources, staff skills, and interests.
         (1) Interdependent actions needed, including coordination of steps and hand-offs (Edmonson, 2012).
         (2) Decrease unnecessary redundancy.
         (3) Consider assignments (e.g., assigning all physician's patients to same care coordinator, attributed to physician willingness to work

with care coordinators) (Brown, Peikes, Peterson, Schore, & Razafindrakoto, 2013).
   d. Focus all practice personnel to work at their highest education, potential, and scope of practice (Salmond & Echevarria, 2017). Performing duties permitted by the license and/or education and allowing other team members to concentrate or delegate other duties.
2. Clear, valued, and shared vision (AHRQ, 2014; Mitchell et al., 2012).
   a. Common purpose.
   b. High-functioning teams work to establish shared goals that reflect individual, family, and caregiver priorities that can be understood and supported by all team members (Mitchell et al., 2012).
3. Shared mental models (AHRQ, 2014; Westli, Johnson, Eid, Rasten, & Brattebo, 2010).
   a. Provide information (e.g., provide information before being asked).
   b. Provide support (e.g., provide assistance before being asked).
   c. Team initiative (e.g., provide guidance or makes suggestions to team members).
   d. Communicate situational awareness (e.g., provide situation updates)
4. Shared training among team members (McEwan et al., 2017; Mitchell et al., 2012).
   a. Substantial, positive effects can be obtained when team members actively participate in learning and practice activities, such as workshops, simulation training, and review-type activities (McEwan et al., 2017).
   b. Organizations should provide opportunities for interprofessional education and training to practice skills and enhance values of teamwork (Mitchell et al., 2012).
5. Mutual trust and confidence (AHRQ, 2014; Kumar, Deshmukh, & Adhish, 2014; Mitchell et al., 2012).
   a. Manage conflict.
   b. Strong team orientation.
   c. Team's collective ability to succeed.
   d. Team member's psychological safety and willingness to take interpersonal risks (Edmonson, 2012).
6. Strong team leadership (AHRQ, 2014; Mitchell et al., 2012).
   a. Two types of leaders (AHRQ, 2014).
      (1) Designated: The person assigned to lead and organize a designated core team, establish clear goals, and facilitate open communication and teamwork among team members.
      (2) Situational: Any team member who has the skills to manage the situation at hand.
         (a) Recognize when team communication is not functioning well and act as facilitator (Mitchell et al., 2012).
   b. Behaviors of effective team leaders (AHRQ, 2014).
      (1) Organize the team.
      (2) Articulate clear goals.
      (3) Empower members to speak up and challenge, when appropriate.
      (4) Actively promote and facilitate good teamwork.
      (5) Skillful at conflict resolution.
      (6) Project positive role model behaviors.
      (7) Motivating team members (Kumar et al., 2014).
   c. Effective communication, and timely, regular feedback (AHRQ, 2014; Mitchell et al., 2012).
      (1) Set high standard for consistent, clear, professional communication.
      (2) Communicate often and at right time.
      (3) Team members are empowered to speak up, and communication should include asking questions, seeking feedback, talking about errors, asking for help, offering suggestions, sharing ideas, and discussing problems and concerns.
   d. Training on skills for effective communication (AHRQ 2014; Mitchell et al., 2012).
      (1) Conflict resolution.
      (2) Use active listening and closed-loop communication.
   e. Continually strive to learn.
   f. Multiple methods for team communication and coordination.
      (1) Huddles, briefings, and team meetings.
         (a) Routine and ad hoc.
         (b) Happens on a consistent basis, whether daily, weekly, or other project-specific timing (Edmonson, 2012).

(c) Reflection that includes use of explicit observations, questions, and discussions of processes and outcomes (Edmonson, 2012).
(2) Weekly caseload reviews to assess new cases and individual progress (RN care manager with caseload consultant physicians) (McGregor, Lin, & Katon, 2011).
(3) Remote teams: Virtual communication methods.
(4) Electronic medical record standards.
(5) Individual portals for CCTM RN and individual communication.
(6) Enlisting individual assistance with information transfer (O'Malley, Tynan, Cohen, Kemper, & Davis, 2009).
g. Optimize resources available to the team and individuals. Listing, maintaining, and accessing resources available at all times and considering:
(1) Community-based, state, national, and institutional resources.
(2) Access, dependent on location and cost.
h. Measurable processes and outcomes (Mitchell et al., 2012).
(1) Lack of communication and resources places a barrier in the process and in producing positive outcomes.
7. Barriers and methods to overcome.
a. Unclear or blurred roles and responsibilities of team, variation in communication styles and practices, different levels of experience and training, multiple team members, and duplication of services (inefficiency) (AHRQ, 2014; Mitchell et al., 2012).
b. Role transitions, both self-identity and group identity (Cadmus, Reis, & Turner, 2013).
(1) Documentation of team roles at each transition setting and member responsibilities; clarify new roles upfront.
(2) Create new interprofessional workflows.
(3) Conduct orientation for team members.
(4) Develop orientation materials; conduct training and document attendance.
(5) Establish forums and methods for ongoing communication and follow up.
(6) Develop buddy system for new team members.
c. Team development processes are forming, storming, norming, performing, adjourning (Kumar et al., 2014).
(1) Team forming can include participants of different expertise, cultures, and ethics, complementing and supporting each other's skills, and defining and establishing roles and objectives.
(2) Storming occurs when members are establishing their position within the team, which can cause conflict and the need for clarification.
(3) The norming stage is where a clear agreement as to the roles and goals of the team, and collaboration and group interaction are more apparent.
(4) A performing team shares the vision, team members identify areas for continued refinement, and goals are achieved. This process allows for:
(a) Set clear objectives for team.
(b) Establish process and structure.
(c) Build good relationships among team members.
(d) Develop conflict resolution skills.
(e) Celebrate successes.
(5) The adjourning phase occurs at the end of team tasks; there is a sense of closure and bonding between members.
d. Communication challenges between team members or across care sites.
(1) Lack of information, coordination, sharing, and follow up (AHRQ, 2014).
(a) Act as facilitator to resolve.
(b) Act as coach for individuals and families not accustomed to or comfortable with active team membership and communication (Mitchell et al., 2012).
(c) Establish cross-site meetings or collaborative trainings to improve mutual understanding (Hesselink et al., 2013).

(2) Establish standardized methods of sharing information that best allows team members to participate (AHRQ, 2014).
  (a) Huddles.
  (b) Briefs and debriefs.
  (c) Case conferencing: Telephone, other virtual method, or in-person face to face.
  (d) Webinars.
e. Resources change or are not available.
  (1) Team members change, inconsistency of members.
    (a) Nurses can perform many roles of other health care team members "in the event that these team members are not available, such as nutrition education, medication education, psychosocial support, and clerical duties" (Paschke, 2018, p. 48).
    (b) Change management and adaptability of the members to interact with multiple roles, disciplines, incoming, and outgoing members are required to maintain an ongoing productive flow of work being done by the team.
    (c) Maintaining a log, minutes, examples, and communications that have occurred will provide an overview to assist new members joining at any time in the process.
  (2) Community resources change.
f. Unclear processes (AHRQ, 2014).
  (1) Establish guidelines, time frames, and deadlines to provide clear guidance.
  (2) Utilize tools such as guidelines, protocols, workflow documents, or checklists.
  (3) If unavailable, initiate/develop a guideline/workflow to provide clear direction, especially in tasks that are complex.
g. Collaborative behaviors required when working in teams create tensions and conflict.
  (1) Leaders should identify the nature of the conflict, model good communications, identify shared goals, and encourage difficult conversations (Edmonson, 2012).
  (2) Give timely and constructive feedback, providing examples as applicable (AHRQ, 2014; Kumar et al., 2014; Mitchell et al., 2012).
  (3) May be instances of "productive conflict," while must be moderated, may encourage climate of discussion and innovation (Edmonson, 2012).
h. Team member fear of being seen as ignorant, incompetent, negative, or disruptive.
  (1) Methods to create climate of psychological safety among team members (Edmonson, 2012).
    (a) Develop trust and respect; if a mistake is made or someone asks for help, others will not penalize.
    (b) Emphasize group tasks and what is needed to perform well.
    (c) Team leaders should be accessible and approachable, invite participation, use direct language, acknowledge limits of current knowledge, be willing to display fallibility, set boundaries and hold people accountable, and highlight failures as learning opportunities.
  (2) Benefits of psychological safety: Encourages speaking up, enables clarity of thought, supports productive conflict, promotes innovation, and increases accountability (Edmonson, 2012).

IV. **How the CCTM RN Participates as a Member or Leader of a Team**

A. Articulates CCTM RN role responsibilities to team members modeling person-focused care: population health management, nursing process, person-centered care planning, education and engagement of individual and family, coaching and counseling of individuals and families, support for self-management, advocacy, and care-setting communication and transitions (Haas, Swan, & Haynes, 2013).
B. Understands roles and contributions of each team member to person-focused care.
C. Builds collaborative relationships needed for teamwork, followership, and situational leadership.

D. Understands that team leadership is fluid and associated with individual priority. For example, if priority need is nutritional, dietitian needs to provide leadership. Ensures that leadership is appropriate to individual need.
E. Assumes leadership role when patient needs are related to CCTM RN role and individual transitions (Hesselink et al., 2013; Kelly & Penney, 2011).
F. Facilitates role transitions by participating and communicating new interprofessional workflows for team (Cadmus et al., 2013).
G. Facilitates communication and trust between team members by using professional feedback and situational monitoring, and offering mutual support.
H. Joins with team in debriefings to monitor accountability of all team members (Registered Nurses' Association of Ontario, 2006).

Chapter 8

Table 8-1.
Teamwork and Collaboration: Knowledge, Skills, and Attitudes for Competency

Knowledge	Skills	Attitudes	Sources
Team Development			
"Describe the process of team development and the roles and practices of effective teams" (p. 14).	"Communicate consistently the importance of teamwork in patient-centered and population health programs and policies" (p. 13). "Apply leadership practices that support collaborative practice and team effectiveness" (p. 14) "Develop consensus on the ethical principles to guide all aspects of teamwork" (p. 14). "Demonstrate high standards of ethical conduct and quality care in contributions to team-based care" (p. 11). "Act with honesty and integrity in relationships with patients, families, and other communities" (p. 11).		IPEC, 2016
Describe own strengths, limitations, and values in functioning as a member of a team.	Demonstrate awareness of own strengths and limitations as a team member. Initiate plan for self-development as a team member. Act with integrity, consistency, and respect for differing views.	Acknowledge own potential to contribute to effective team functioning. Appreciate importance of intra- and interprofessional collaboration.	Cronenwett et al., 2007
"Describe the impact of team based practice" (p. 9).		"Value the team approach to providing high quality care" (p. 9.) "Commit to being an effective team member" (p. 9). "Commit to interprofessional and intraprofessional collaboration" (p. 10). "Respect the boundaries of therapeutic relationships" (p. 12).	AACN QSEN Education Consortium, 2012
Describe ethics as a standard for professional CCTM RN nursing practice.			AAACN, 2016

continued on next page

Table 8-1. (continued)
Teamwork and Collaboration: Knowledge, Skills, and Attitudes for Competency

Knowledge	Skills	Attitudes	Sources
Team Roles			
Describe scopes of practice and roles of health care team members. Describe strategies for identifying and managing overlaps in team member roles and accountabilities. Recognize contributions of other individuals and groups in helping individual/family achieve health goals.	Function competently within own scope of practice as a member of the health care team. Assume role of team member or leader based on situation. Initiate requests for help when appropriate to situation. Clarify roles and accountabilities under conditions of potential overlap in team member functioning. Integrate the contributions to others who play a role in helping individual/family achieve health goals.	Value the perspectives and expertise of all health team members. Respect the unique attributes that members bring to a team, including variations in professional orientations and accountability. Respect the centrality of the individual/family as core members of any health care team.	Cronenwett et al., 2007
	"Engage diverse professionals who complement one's own professional expertise, as well as associated resources to develop strategies to meet specific care situation in shared patient-centered problem solving" (p. 12). "Communicate one's role and responsibility clearly to patients, families, community members, and other professionals" (p. 12). "Explain the roles and responsibilities of other care providers and how the team works together to provide care, promote health, and prevent disease" (p. 12).	"Share accountability with other professions, patients, and communities for outcomes relevant to prevention and health care" (p. 14).	IPEC, 2016
	"Partners effectively with key stakeholders and groups in care delivery to individuals, families, and groups" (p. 531).		Swider, Krothe, Reyes, & Cravetz, 2013
"Describe strategies to integrate patients/families as primary members of the health team" (p. 10).	"Use patient engagement strategies to involve patients/families in the healthcare team" (p. 10). "Work with team members to identify goals for individual patients and populations" (p. 9). "Ensure inclusion of patients and family members as part of the team based on their preferences to be included" (p. 9).	"Value patients/families as the source of control for their health" (p. 10).	AACN QSEN Education Consortium, 2012

continued on next page

Table 8-1. (continued)
Teamwork and Collaboration: Knowledge, Skills, and Attitudes for Competency

Knowledge	Skills	Attitudes	Sources
Communication			
Analyze differences in communication style preferences among individuals and families, nurses, and other members of the health team. Describe impact of own communication style on others. Discuss effective strategies for communicating and resolving conflict.	Communicate with team members, adapting own style of communicating to needs of the team and situation. Demonstrate commitment to team goals. Solicit input from other team members to improve individual and team performance.	Value teamwork and the relationships upon which it is based. Value different styles of communication used by individuals, families, and health care providers.	Cronenwett et al., 2007
		"Support the development of a safe team environment where issues can be addressed between team members and conflict can be resolved" (p. 9).	AACN QSEN Education Consortium, 2012
	"Give timely, sensitive, and instructive feedback to others about their performance on the team, responding respectfully as a team member to feedback from others" (p. 13). "Listen actively, and encourage ideas and opinions of other team members" (p. 13). Use "effective communication tools and techniques, including information systems and communication technologies, to facilitate discussions and interactions that enhance team function" (p. 13). "Use respectful language appropriate for a given difficult situation, crucial conversation, or conflict" (p. 13). Initiate actions to resolve conflict. Contribute to resolution of conflict and disagreement.	"Value conflict resolution as a means to improve team functioning" (p. 13).	IPEC, 2016 Cronenwett et al., 2007

continued on next page

Table 8-1 (continued)
Teamwork and Collaboration: Knowledge, Skills, and Attitudes for Competency

Knowledge	Skills	Attitudes	Sources
Impact of Team on Safety and Quality of Care			
Describe examples of the impact of team functioning on safety and quality of care. Explain how authority gradients influence team work and individual safety. Describe "the risks associated with handoffs among providers and across transitions of care" (p. 10).	Follow communication practices that minimize risks associated with handoffs among providers and across transitions in care. Assert own position/perspective in discussions about individual care. Choose communication styles that diminish the risks associated with authority gradients among team members. "Use process improvement strategies to increase effectiveness of the interprofessional teamwork and team based services, programs, and policies" (p. 14).	Appreciate the risks associated with handoffs among providers and across transitions in care.	Cronenwett et al., 2007 AACN QSEN Education Consortium, 2012 IPEC, 2016
Impact of Team on Systems			
Identify system barriers and facilitators of effective team functioning. Examine strategies for improving systems to support team functioning.	Lead or participate in the design and implementation of systems that support effective teamwork. Engage in state and national policy initiatives aimed at improving teamwork and collaboration.	Value the influence of system solutions in achieving team functioning.	Cronenwett et al., 2007

Source: Cronenwett et al. (2007). *Nursing Outlook,* 55(3), 122-131. Reprinted with permission from Elsevier.

Chapter 8

Case Study 8-1.
Huddles in Transitions of Care

Introduction

W.L., a 33-year-old Cantonese-speaking female, came in to the emergency department (ED) for complaint of sore throat. W.L. had difficulty swallowing for the past 5-6 days and vomiting over the past 3 days. W.L. is married and has two small children at home. W.L. has had no unusual travel, does not smoke, and does not consume alcohol. There is no pertinent family history.

In the ED, W.L. was assessed. She was awake, alert, oriented x4, well appearing, no acute distress. Review of systems were within normal limits, except oropharynx showing significant tonsillar enlargement. Initial complete blood count (CBC), basic metabolic panel, electrocardiogram, urinalysis and rapid strep were done. Initial CBC revealed white blood cell of 45 and platelet 22,000.

Computed tomography scans and bone marrow biopsy were done. W.L. was diagnosed with acute myeloid leukemia (AML) and received initial chemotherapy during her hospitalization.

W.L. has a history of hepatitis B, infectious viral hepatitis (diagnosed at age 18), C-section times two (last one 3 months ago), and tubal ligation. She is uninsured and does not speak any English. At home she was on docusate (Colace®), tenofovir (Viread®), ibuprophen, and oxycodone.

Daily huddles were convened to ascertain an assessment of care needs, and create an interprofessional plan of care and transitions of care. Included in the huddles were the CCTM® RN, MD, social worker, case manager, pharmacist, physical therapist, and admission/discharge coordinator.

Clinical Interaction

Teamwork and collaboration plan includes:
- Continued education of disease processes (AML, hepatitis B).
- Identification of barriers for successful care transition, including lack of insurance, transportation, culture, and language.
- Coordination of follow-up appointments (oncology, liver, obstetrics).
- Plan for management and adherence of medications post-discharge.
- Safety regarding falls risk, and signs and symptoms of infection related to chemotherapy.

Clinical Implications

- Multiple clinical assessments required on an ongoing basis.
- Prioritization of clinical needs.
- Medication compliance.
- Transition from acute care to specialty care (see Chapter 11, "Care Coordination and Transition Management Between Acute Care and Ambulatory Care").
- Transportation arrangements to multiple appointments.
- Utilization of wrap around services (Chinese Health Information Center, Leukemia/Lymphoma Society, Cancer Support Services).
- Evaluation of outcomes and individual satisfaction.

Chapter 8

Case Study 8-2.
Managing Complex Cases in Transitions of Care

Introduction

P.S., a 70-year-old married male who resides in Ohio, was staying with his wife in a senior living apartment in Pennsylvania recently to be closer to his daughter for needed assistance while his wife was recovering from knee surgery. Over the last 2 weeks, P.S. was noted to have some cognitive changes and confusion, as well as noted gait instability, so he was taken to the emergency room. Upon assessment in the hospital, he was noted to have diminished right eye visual acuity and subjective blurriness.

P.S. has a past medical history of coronary artery disease with stent placement in 2003, depression, delirium, type 2 diabetes mellitus, right-sided ocular lymphoma diagnosed 2014 and treated with intraocular methotrexate. He had a relapse in June 2017, and at that time, was treated bilaterally with radiation therapy.

Through multiple discussions with ocular oncology, neurology, neurosurgery, and ophthalmology, P.S. had a computed tomography (CT) scan and magnetic resonance imaging of his brain that showed a supracellular-enhancing mass, as well as left lateral third ventricular-enhancing mass, suggesting lymphoma. He then had a lumbar puncture CT of chest/abdomen/pelvis and an endoscopic transventricular biopsy. P.S was diagnosed with secondary central nervous system lymphoma.

P.S. received high-dose methotrexate and steroids during his hospital stay. His hospitalization was complicated by a witnessed fall and a rapid response to be called for vasovagal syncope due to dehydration. P.S. also developed primary adrenal insufficiency likely secondary to recent steroid use.

An occupational therapist (OT) and physical therapist (PT) followed the individual during his hospital stay. OT noted deficits in his overall occupational performance due to decreased balance, decreased coordination, decreased strength, decreased activity tolerance, and impaired cognition. PT noted poor safety and environmental awareness, and P.S. was recommended for sub-acute rehabilitation. Through case management and P.S.'s daughter and wife, who were at his bedside daily, P.S. was able to go to a rehab facility close to the daughter's home at discharge.

Clinical Interaction

Teamwork and collaboration plan will include:
- Continued education of disease processes (lymphoma).
- Identification of barriers for successful care transition, including current immobility of spouse, living arrangements, and transportation.
- Coordination of follow-up appointments (oncology, endocrinology).
- Plan for management and adherence of medications post discharge.
- Safety regarding falls risk, and signs and symptoms of infection related to chemotherapy.

Clinical Implications

- Multiple clinical assessments required on an ongoing basis.
- Prioritization of clinical needs.
- Medication compliance.
- Transition from acute care to specialty care (see Chapter 11, "Care Coordination and Transition Management Between Acute Care and Ambulatory Care").
- Coordination of appointments and next chemotherapy regimen.
- Transportation arrangements to multiple appointments.
- Utilization of wrap around services (Leukemia/Lymphoma Society, Cancer Support Services).
- Evaluation of outcomes and individual satisfaction.

References

Agency for Healthcare Research and Quality (AHRQ). (2014). *TeamSTEPPS®*. Retrieved from https://www.ahrq.gov/teamstepps/index.html

Agency for Healthcare Research and Quality (AHRQ). (2018). *Never events*. Retrieved from https://psnet.ahrq.gov/primers/primer/3/never-events

American Academy of Ambulatory Care Nursing (AAACN). (2016). *Scope and standards of practice for registered nurses in care coordination and transition management*. Pitman, NJ: Author.

American Association of Colleges of Nursing (AACN), QSEN Education Consortium. (2012). *Graduate-level QSEN competencies, knowledge, skills and attitudes*. Retrieved from http://www.aacnnursing.org/Portals/42/AcademicNursing/CurriculumGuidelines/Graduate-QSEN-Competencies.pdf

American Nurses Association (ANA). (2016). *Collaborative health care: How nurses work in team based settings*. Retrieved from https://www.nursingworld.org/education-events/career-center/nursing-career-resources/

American Recovery and Reinvestment Act of 2009. (2009). Retrieved from https://www.gpo.gov/fdsys/pkg/BILLS-111hr1enr/pdf/BILLS-111hr1enr.pdf

Bernabeo, E., & Holmboe, E.S. (2013). Patients, providers and systems need to acquire a specific set of competencies to achieve truly patient-centered care. *Health Affairs, 32*(2), 250-258.

Brown, R.S., Peikes, D., & Peterson, G., Schore, J., & Razafindrakoto, C.M. (2013). Six features of Medicare coordinated care demonstration programs that cut hospital admissions of high-risk patients. *Health Affairs, 31*(6), 1156-1166.

Cadmus, E., Reis, L., & Turner, B. (2013). Ever-evolving: Population care coordinators. *Nursing Management, 44*(12), 9-11.

Cronenwett, L., Sherwood, G., Barnsteiner, J., Disch, J., Johnson, J., Mitchell, P., … Warren, J. (2007). Quality and safety education for nurses. *Nursing Outlook, 55*(3), 122-131.

D'Amour, D., & Oandasan, I. (2005). Interprofessionality as the field of interprofessional practice and interprofessional education: An emerging concept. *Journal of Interprofessional Care, 19*(Suppl. 1), 8-20.

Edmonson, A. (2012). *Teaming: How organizations learn, innovate, and compete in the knowledge economy*. San Francisco, CA: Jossey-Bass.

Frampton, S.B., Guastello, S., Hoy, L., Naylor, M., Sheridan, S., & Johnson-Fleece, M. (2017). *Harnessing evidence and experience to change culture: A guiding framework for patient and family engaged care*. Retrieved from https://nam.edu/harnessing-evidence-and-experience-to-change-culture-a-guiding-framework-for-patient-and-family-engaged-care/

Gaglioti, A.H., Barlow, P., Thoma, K.D., & Bergus, G.R. (2017). Integrated care coordination by an interprofessional team reduces emergency department visits and hospitalizations at an academic health centre. *Journal of Interprofessional Care, 31*(5), 557-565.

Haas, S., Swan, B.A., & Haynes, T. (2013). Developing ambulatory care registered nurse competencies for care coordination and transition management. *Nursing Economic$, 31*(1), 44-49, 43.

Hesselink, G., Vernooig-Dassen, M., Pijnenborg, L., Barach, P., Gademan, P., Dudzik-Urbaniak, E., … Wollersheim, H. (2013). Organizational culture an important context for addressing and improving hospital to community patient discharge. *Medical Care, 51*(1), 90-98.

Institute of Medicine (IOM). (2000). *To err is human: Building a safer health system*. Washington, DC: National Academies Press.

Institute of Medicine (IOM). (2001). *Crossing the quality chasm*. Washington, DC: National Academies Press.

Institute of Medicine (IOM). (2003). *Health professions education*. Washington, DC: National Academies Press.

Institute of Medicine (IOM). (2010). *The future of nursing: Leading change, advancing health*. Washington, DC: National Academies Press.

Interprofessional Education Collaborative (IPEC). (2011). *Core competencies for interprofessional collaborative practice*. Retrieved from https://www.aacom.org/docs/default-source/insideome/ccrpt05-10-11.pdf?sfvrsn=77937f97_2

Interprofessional Education Collaborative (IPEC). (2016). *Core competencies for interprofessional collaborative practice*. Retrieved from https://hsc.unm.edu/ipe/resources/ipec-2016-core-competencies.pdf

Jones, K.L., Jamerson, C., & Pike, S. (2012). The journey to electronic interdisciplinary care plans. *Nursing Management, 43*(12), 9-12.

Kelly, N.M., & Penney, E.D. (2011). Collaboration of hospital case manaagers and home care liaisons when transitioning patients. *Professional Case Management, 16*(3), 128-136.

Kumar, S., Deshmukh, V., & Adhish, V.S. (2014). Building and leading teams. *Indian Journal of Community Medicine, 39*(4), 208-213.

McEwan, D., Ruissen, G.R., Eys, M.A., Zumbo, B.D., & Beauchamp, M.R. (2017). The effectiveness of teamwork training on teamwork behaviors and team performance: A systematic review and meta-analysis of controlled interventions. *PLOS ONE, 12*(1), e0169604.

McGregor, M., Lin, E.H., & Katon, W.J. (2011). TEAMcare: An integrated multicondition collaborative care program for chronic illnesses and depression. *Journal of Ambulatory Care Management, 34*(2), 152-162.

Mitchell, P., Wynia, M., Golden, R., McNellis, B., Okun, S., Webb, C.E., … Von Kohorn, I. (2012). *Core principles and values of effective team-based health care*. Retrieved from https://nam.edu/wp-content/uploads/2015/06/VSRT-Team-Based-Care-Principles-Values.pdf

O'Malley, O., Tynan, A., Cohen, G., Kemper, N., & Davis, M. (2009). Coordination of care by primary care physicians: Strategies, lessons and implications. *Research Brief, 12*, 1-16.

Patient Protection and Affordable Care Act, 42 U.S.C. § 18001. (2010). Retrieved from https://www.hhs.gov/sites/default/files/ppacacon.pdf

Paschke, S.M. (2018). Ambulatory care operations. In C.B. Laughlin (Ed.), *Core curriculum for ambulatory care nursing* (4th ed., pp. 47-55). Pitman, NJ: American Academy of Ambulatory Care Nursing.

Registered Nurses' Association of Ontario. (2006). *Collaborative practice among nursing teams*. Toronto, Canada: Author.

Salmond, S.W., & Echevarria, M. (2017). Healthcare transformation and changing roles for nursing. *Orthopaedic Nursing, 36*(1), 12-25.

Swider, S.M., Krothe, K., Reyes, D., & Cravetz, M. (2013). The Quad Council practice for competencies for public health nursing. *Public Health Nursing, 30*(6), 519-536.

Westli, H.K., Johnsen, B.H., Eid, J., Rasten, I., & Brattebo, G. (2010). Teamwork skills, shared mental models, and performance in simulated trauma teams: An independent group design. *Scandinavian Journal of Trauma, Resuscitation and Emergency Medicine, 18*, 47.

Additional Readings

Bodenheimer, T., & Laing, B.Y. (2007). The teamlet model of primary care. *Annals of Family Medicine, 5*(5), 457-461.

Manderson, B., McMurray, J., Piraino, E., & Stolee, P. (2011). Navigation roles support chronically ill older adults through healthcare transition: A systematic review of the literature. *Health and Social Care in the Community, 20*(2), 113-127.

Scholtes, P., Joiner, B., & Streibel, B. (2003). *The team handbook*. Madison, WI: Oriel.

Schottenfeld, L., Petersen, D., Peikes, D., Ricciardi, R., Burak, H., McNellis, R., & Genevro, J. (2016). *Creating patient-centered team based primary care* [White Paper]. Agency for Healthcare Research and Quality (AHRQ). Rockville, MD.

World Health Organization. (2010). *Framework for action on interprofessional education & collaborative practice*. Retrieved from http://www.who.int/hrh/resources/framework_action/en/

Chapter 9

Instructions for Continuing Nursing Education Contact Hours

Continuing nursing education credit can be earned for completing the learning activity associated with this chapter. Instructions can be found at aaacn.org/CCTMCoreCNE

Cross Setting Communications and Care Transitions

Tina Truong, MS, RN, CCCTM®
Stefanie Coffey, DNP, MBA, MN, FNP-BC, RN-BC
Jayme M. Speight, MSN, RN-BC
Cynthia R. Niesen, DNP, MA, RN, NEA-BC

Learning Outcome Statement

After completing this learning activity, the learner will be able to demonstrate the knowledge, skills, and attitudes required for effective cross-setting communication and transitions in care.

Learning Objectives

After reading this chapter, the Care Coordination and Transition Management registered nurse (CCTM® RN) will be able to:
- Explain the concept of care transitions.
- Identify common barriers to effective communication.
- Explain the communication deficiencies that commonly occur with care transitions.
- Define the role of the CCTM RN in cross-setting communication and care transition.
- Identify key characteristics of effective communication for care transitions.
- Design and implement processes to provide sufficient, timely, and useful information necessary to achieve successful care transitions.
- Analyze processes and identify improvement opportunities in cross-setting communication.
- Evaluate evidence and do small tests of change to improve cross-setting communication during care transitions.
- Demonstrate the knowledge, skills, and attitudes required for cross-setting communication and transitions in care (see Table 9-1 on page 185).

AAACN Care Coordination and Transition Management Standards
Standard 1.	Assessment
Standard 2.	Diagnoses
Standard 3.	Outcomes Identification
Standard 4.	Planning
Standard 5.	Implementation
Standard 5a.	Coordination of Care
Standard 5c.	Consultation
Standard 6.	Evaluation
Standard 11.	Communication
Standard 13.	Collaboration
Standard 15.	Resource Utilization
Standard 16.	Environment

Source: AAACN, 2016.

Competency Definition
Effective utilization of communication skills to gain and transmit information, encourage team participation, leverage electronic medical record and other standard communication tools, and design and implement processes to provide sufficient, timely, and useful information necessary to achieve successful patient care transitions (Cronenwett et al., 2007).

There has been an explosion of information regarding care coordination and the components needed to ensure a smooth process for care transitions since the Institute of Medicine (IOM) published its first quality chasm report in 2001. Several subsequent statements by the IOM further defined the problems found within the U.S. health care system that contributed to countless numbers of injury, illness, and death. Since 2001, federal, public, and private partnerships have focused on improving care coordination by enhancing communication and collaboration across multiple settings to improve care transitions. Lamb (2014) states "care coordination occurs at the intersection of patients, providers, and health care settings and relies on integrative activities including communication" (p. 3). The Agency for Healthcare Research and Quality (AHRQ) (2016) also recognizes that "care coordination involves deliberately organizing patient care activities and sharing information among all of the participants concerned with a patient's care to achieve safer and more effective care" (para. 1).

The concept of care coordination is expansive; thus, it would stand to reason that several of the vital concept components involved in this process, namely care transitions and communication, would be equally as complex. There is a difference when defining care transitions and transitional care.

Care transition refers to "the movement patients make between health care practitioners and settings as their condition and care needs change during a chronic or acute illness. For example, in the course of an acute exacerbation of an illness, an individual might receive care from a primary care physician or specialist in an outpatient setting, then transition to a hospital physician before moving on to yet another care team at a skilled nursing facility. Finally, the individual might return home, where he or she would receive care from a visiting nurse. Each of these shifts from care providers and settings is defined as a care transition" (Coleman & Boult, 2003, p. 556). This process is largely achieved through communication (Wenger & Young, 2007).

"*Transitional care* is defined as a broad range of time-limited services designed to ensure health care continuity, avoid preventable poor outcomes among at-risk populations, and promote the safe and timely transfer of individuals from one level of care to another or from one type of setting to another" (Kim & Flanders, 2013, p. ITC3-1).

Hallmarks of transitional care are the focus on highly vulnerable, chronically ill patients throughout critical transitions in health and health care, and the emphasis on educating individuals and family caregivers to address causes of poor outcomes and the avoidance of preventable rehospitalizations (Coleman & Boult, 2003).

I. **Transitions of Care**

There may be multiple transitions of care in the process of an individual's journey from and returning to his or her home setting or final destination. Each one of these transitions requires the efficient transfer of information between environments; thus, they are highly dependent on adequate communication for success (Cibulskis, Giardino, & Moyer, 2011).

A. The transition of care is driven by many factors, including health or illness acuity, resources, and individual preferences. The following example will assist in "visualizing" many care transitions an individual will have during an acute critical admission.
   1. Individual and caregiver present to the primary care clinic with complaints of dyspnea, cough, fever, and weakness.
   2. Primary care provider suspects pneumonia with sepsis and calls an ambulance.
   3. Emergency medical team transports individual to the nearest emergency department (ED).
   4. ED staff assess, treat, and admit the individual to the hospital.
   5. Hospitalist admits the individual to the intensive care unit and receives interprofessional care that promotes recovery of the illness. The care is comprehensive and includes members from different specialties, such as intensivist providers, nursing (RN, licensed practical nurse [LPN], and certified nursing assistant), respiratory, radiology, dietary, laboratory, pastoral services, social work, physical therapy, environmental services, utilization review, and hospital management.
   6. Hospitalist transfers the individual to a hospital telemetry unit for continued less-acute care by an interprofessional staff member until discharge criteria are met.
   7. Hospitalist discharges individual to a skilled nursing rehabilitation center to gain strength.
   8. Individual spends 3 weeks at a skilled nursing facility and works with an interprofessional team consisting of RN, physical therapist, occupational therapist, and providers in preparation to discharge home.
   9. Individual is discharged home with caregiver and home health nurse and/or aid.
   10. Individual is seen at primary clinic for the first time since her admission to the hospital.
   11. Individual is referred to specialty providers as needed for follow up of pneumonia, sepsis, and outpatient therapies.
   12. Individual completes visits with each specialty provider across different health systems.

B. As noted from the above example, there is an opportunity for fragmentation of care that could result in one or more negative consequences that contribute to poor outcomes and quality of care. Common factors that contribute to care transition mishaps or gaps include poor communication, incomplete transfer of information, inadequate education of older adults and their family caregivers, limited access to essential services, and the absence of a single point person to ensure continuity of care (Lim, Foust, & Van Cleave, 2016). Communication has been described as a complicated process of transfer and exchange of information affecting multiple aspects of individual care, including assessment, decision-making, goal planning, problem identification and prioritization, and care planning (Allen, Ottmann, & Roberts, 2013). This exchange of information occurs informally and formally between members of the health care team who say communication is critical in health care (Lancaster, Kolakowsky-Hayner, Kovacich, & Greer-Williams, 2015). Effective care transition communication is an expectation of quality individual care, yet adverse events and risk exposures occur due to ineffective or poor communication during transitions of care.
   1. Poor communication among health care providers and the lack of shared information about individuals are common causes of under-treatment, suboptimal therapy, adverse drug events, and hospital admissions or readmissions (IOM, 2013).
   2. The Joint Commission identified miscommunication as the main cause of serious, unexpected injuries, and was the second common cause of sentinel events reported during the first 6 months of 2013 (Ellison, 2015).
   3. The potential for medical errors increases when more than one health care provider or site of care is involved in providing services to an individual (Clancy, 2008). Up to 49% of individuals experience at least one medical error after discharge, and one in five individuals discharged from the hospital suffers an adverse event. Improved communication among providers could prevent up to half or more of these events (Society of Hospital Medicine [SHM], 2013).
   4. The average Medicare individual has seven providers across four care settings involved in his or her care – five specialty providers and two primary care providers (IOM, 2013).
   5. Communication is a vital component of the post-hospital discharge. Kripalani and colleagues (2007) conducted a systematic review of the literature and found that direct communication between hospital physicians and primary care physicians only occurs 3% to 20% of the time, and written communication in the form of the discharge summary is only available 12% to 34% of the time.
   6. One in five Medicare patients discharged from hospitals are readmitted within 30 days, and 34% within 90 days (Brown, 2018; Robert Wood Johnson Foundation [RWFJ], 2013a, b).
   7. Four out of five individuals are discharged from hospitals without direct communication with a primary care provider (RWFJ, 2013a, b).
   8. Within 30 days of discharge from the hospital, 60% of individuals on Medicare make one transfer in care settings, 18% have two transfers, 9% have three transfers, and 4% have four or more transfers in care settings. Each movement increasing the opportunity for communication failure (Brown, 2018; IOM, 2013).
C. Given the potential for adverse events and possible rehospitalization, cross-setting communication, using standardized tools to clearly communicate, becomes a critical intervention to improve care quality, decrease cost, and prevent harm (Arnold & Underman Boggs, 2016; Cibulskis et al., 2011). Effective cross-setting communication is further compounded by patient acuity, co-morbidities, reduced lengths of stay, and increasing financial pressures (IOM, 2013). In 2015, Dusek, Pearce, Harripaul, and Lloyd published a systematic review of 127 studies highlighting best care transition practices. These referenced documents provided the basis for the authors' guideline for evidence-based recommendations associated with promoting safe and effective care transitions. The authors cited that much of the literature focused on coordination and communication of critical aspects of client care that, if not managed well by the interprofessional health care team, resulted in adverse outcomes, such as sentinel events and readmission to the hospital. During different transitions, communication with accurate information is essential. Their review of numerous bodies of knowledge emphasized the importance of the nurse's role in care transitions and the need for nurses to actively serve as crucial communicators and collaborators in the coordination of an individual's care.

Chapter 9

II. **Communication and Care Coordination**
   A. Definitions.
      1. Communication: "Sharing knowledge among participants in a patient's care...*interpersonal communication* is distinguished from information transfer by a two-way exchange of knowledge through personal interactions, while *information transfer* is characterized by the transfer of data – whether orally, in writing, or electronically – and does not necessarily involve direct interaction between sender and receiver" (McDonald et al., 2014, p. 23).
         a. TeamSTEPP (Team Strategies and Tools to Enhance Performance and Patient Safety): Components of monitoring utilized to improve communication and collaboration among teams while preventing error and injury (AHRQ, 2018).
            (1) **S**tatus of individual.
            (2) **T**eam members.
            (3) **E**nvironment.
            (4) **P**rogress toward goal.
   B. Cross-setting communication challenges. The Center for Transforming Healthcare and others have identified numerous risk factors related to inadequate communication.
      1. Differing expectations between senders and receivers of information (Vermeir et al., 2015).
      2. Lack of teamwork and respect.
      3. Inadequate amount of time devoted to the hand-off process.
      4. Lack of standardized process or procedure for successful hand-off communication, such as the Situation, Background, Assessment, and Recommendation (SBAR) tool (The Joint Commission, 2013).
      5. Direct involvement of primary care physicians during hospitalization has become less common, and the involvement of multiple specialist providers is more common (Cibulskis et al., 2011).
      6. Failure to produce a timely discharge summary or transition document.
      7. Lack of integrated or accessible electronic medical records (EMRs) (Bonner, Schneider, & Weissman, 2010).
      8. Lack of longitudinal responsibility across settings (Bonner et al., 2010).
      9. Failure to complete diagnostic testing, specialty visits, therapy (Kim & Flanders, 2013).
      10. Lack of a team-based approach to care across settings (Bonner et al., 2010).
      11. Failure to re-engage primary care through a post-discharge office visit (Kim & Flanders, 2013).
      12. Failure to provide accurate information (Dusek et al., 2015).
      13. Missing information or lacking quality information (Vermeir et al., 2015).
   C. Pediatric considerations.
      1. Communication with the individual's school nurse.
         a. Many schools without nurses (RN or LPN).
         b. Many school districts have one nurse who covers multiple schools.
      2. Lack of pediatric community services.
      3. Failure to treat pediatric individuals in an individual-family centered model of care (Cady & Belew, 2017; Council on Children with Disabilities and Medical Home Implementation Project Advisory Committee, 2014).
      4. Failure to consider pediatric developmental stages and milestones that may affect communication (Council on Children with Disabilities and Medical Home Implementation Project Advisory Committee, 2014).

III. **Communication and Continuity of Care**

The term *continuity of care* was first described by Haggerty and colleagues (2003) as a complex longitudinal construct in health care that is focused on coordination. *Informational continuity* outlines the use of individual data available in current time and includes individualized plans of care shared from one provider to another across locations (Haggerty et al., 2008). A vital role of the ambulatory care CCTM RN is cross-setting communication for safe transitions of care (Brady & Ricciardi, 2016).

Designed to improve communication among health care professionals and improve safety for individuals, electronic health records (EHRs) and computerized provider order entries are part of the 2009 Health Information Technology for Economic and Clinical Health (HITECH) Act (HealthIT.gov, 2014; U.S Department of Health & Human Services, 2017). The addition of EHRs and computerized systems has improved team communications among health care providers (Kennedy, 2014; Pilcher & Bradley, 2013). Informational continuity often involves electronic information, team meetings or messaging, huddles, progress reports, handoffs, discharge plans, referral contact information, and individual care summaries

(Arnold & Underman Boggs, 2016). Collaboration allows a variety of health care professionals to work together with shared goals that focus on the individual.
A. As stated by AAACN's former CEO Cynthia Nowicki Hnatiuk, EdD, RN, CAE, FAAN, "Care coordination is a role that synchronizes all aspects of patient care, from admission to discharge home or to another care setting, and follow-up with other care providers" (Filipek, 2015). Care coordination transitions occur within organized activities and processes (Radwin, Castonguay, Keenan, & Hermann, 2016).
 1. Communicate care information among clinicians and with the individual and family.
 2. Designate and enforce accountability for each team member's responsibilities.
 3. Facilitate care transition with clear communication of information and emphasize accountability.
 4. Link individuals to necessary resources.
B. Early and ongoing individual assessment across the continuum of care is essential in transition planning (Arnold & Underman Boggs, 2016; Dusek et al., 2015).
C. Needed care is uninterrupted, and success is dependent on the relatedness between the care transition sequences (Wenger & Young, 2007).

IV. **Cross-Setting Communication Methods**
A. Care transition interventions involving self-management education, dismissal planning, and follow-up coordination have resulted in significantly improved outcomes over time and contribute to lowered mortality, emergency department visits, and hospital readmissions for chronically ill older adults (Le Berre, Maimon, Sourial, Guériton, & Vedel, 2017).
B. A study conducted by Jackson and colleagues (2016) found successful hand-off communication involves active listening, complete and accurate documentation, and detailed verbal communication between providers.
 1. Communicating in real time allows for the participants to ask clarifying questions regarding the plan of care and other details.
    a. Include face-to-face communication, teleconferencing, or phone conversation (recorded messages are ineffective).
    b. Identify a time agreed upon by all individuals involved in the hand-off communication.
    c. Minimize interruptions during communication with a designated area free of disruptions.
    d. Conduct a verbal communication report involving key personnel (e.g., RN to RN, RN to other interprofessional members) who have in-depth knowledge of the individual's care.
    e. Use ISBAR format (Marshall, Harrison, & Flanagan, 2009).
       (1) **I**dentification of self and individual information.
       (2) **S**ituation: State the purpose.
       (3) **B**ackground: Tell the story of the current problem.
       (4) **A**ssessment: Describe what you think is happening.
       (5) **R**ecommendation: State what you are requesting.
    f. Use BOOST Universal Discharge Checklist and General Assessment and Preparedness (GAP) tool to summarize individual and family information at discharge (SHM, 2013).
C. Provide hand-off communication at all levels of transition.
 1. Consider individual needs when choosing the transition site.
 2. Include individual and families in all transitions to establish contact information and understanding of the plan of care and individual goals.
D. Use a plan that outlines care details as a communication tool.
E. Include a written list of appointments to the individual, family, and transition site.
F. Begin dismissal and admission planning at each point of admission to a new site.
G. Electronic health record (American Academy of Family Physicians, 2014).
 1. Pros.
    a. Customizable and able to achieve standard format and content.
    b. Individual information easily shared across the continuum of care if access available.
    c. Up-to-date medication and allergy lists.
    d. Order entry available on-site or remotely.
    e. Standardized order sets.
    f. Ability to develop and share individual's plan of care and individual's goals.
    g. Ability to identify team members and contact information.
    h. Ability to trend data for individual monitoring and population management.

i. Create individual-specific problem lists.
2. Cons.
   a. Lack of universal design and access within and across systems.
   b. Content can be overwhelming, decreasing usefulness.
   c. Cost.
   d. Time required for training.
H. MyChart® is a tool that provides individuals with secure access to their medical record in an online and app format. It allows individuals to manage and receive the following information (University of Virginia Health System, 2018):
   1. Communicate with providers.
   2. View test results.
   3. Request prescriptions.
   4. Review visit information.
   5. Track health records.

V. **Principles of Communication with Individuals and Caregiver**

A. Results of a 12-month Communication Catalyst program identified 12 curriculum topics for the AAACN *CCTM Core Curriculum* (Swan & McGinley, 2016). This education for all nurses supports the improvement of nurse-patient communication, care transitions, and positive outcomes for individuals and families.
B. The curriculum enhanced the knowledge and skills required for care transitions for individuals and staff. The curriculum dimensions of CCTM include (Swan & McGinley, 2016):
   1. Advocacy.
   2. Education and engagement of individuals and families.
   3. Coaching and counseling of individuals and families.
   4. Person-centered care planning.
   5. Support for self-management.
   6. Nursing process.
   7. Teamwork and collaboration.
   8. Cross-setting communication and care transitions.
   9. Population health management.
   10. Care coordination and transition management between acute care and ambulatory care.
   11. Informatics nursing practice.
   12. Telehealth nursing practice.
C. Ensure clear communication with health care team members and individuals and families. Use strategies that enhance communication and transition planning (Dusek et al., 2015).
   1. Assess early for comprehensive planning.
   2. Determine individual readiness for transition.
   3. Actively involve the individual in planning and setting goals for transition.
   4. Discuss pros and cons of transition changes with the individual and family.
   5. Provide self-management education.
D. Begin transition of care from one setting to another planning early and before discharge (Arnold & Underman Boggs, 2016).
   1. Perform a needs assessment of medical and functional status, cognition, psychosocial support needs, and the current level of support available for individuals.
   2. Promote an adequate next care transition setting.
   3. Identify and confirm financial/insurance coverage.
   4. Gather the dismissal summary information, problem list, and plan for ongoing care.
   5. Provide a dismissal and episode of care medication list.
   6. Provide a list of follow-up visits that includes names, time/location, dates, and telephone numbers.
E. Ensure the individual's instructions and plan of care are congruent among multiple team members, individuals, and families at points of transition (Lees, 2013).
   1. Utilize resources and design health information using the three A's (Accurate, Accessible, and Actionable) (Centers for Disease Control and Prevention, 2016) to accommodate the individual and family's health care literacy and improve comprehension.
      a. Accurate: Use health literacy practices to ensure information can be understood and is accurate.
      b. Accessible: Ensure individuals can see information created.
         (1) Place where people will see it.
         (2) Consider placement of information to reach those not actively seeking the education.
         (3) Highlight the main message.
         (4) Consider an easy-to-skim presentation with bullets, large font, and plenty of spacing.
         (5) Use captions and images.
         (6) Use multiple formats and channels of communication.
      c. Actionable: Start, stop, or do more or less of something.
         (1) Provide a brief background of information.
         (2) Make actionable recommendations.

2. Print information to support verbal instructions. Adapt teaching materials and methods to benefit literacy and learning styles (The Joint Commission, 2010).
   a. Create education materials written at a reading level of 5th grade or lower.
   b. Use the "teach-back" method to ensure information is understood.
   c. Consider use of The Joint Commission's checklist for advancing effective communication, cultural competence, and person- and family-centered care (The Joint Commission, 2010).
F. Pediatric considerations.
   1. Pediatric developmental stage (Council on Children with Disabilities and Medical Home Implementation Project Advisory Committee, 2014).
   2. School and education setting of the child (Baker, Anderson, & Johnson, 2017; Duff & Poole, 2016).
   3. Community resources or lack thereof (Bentti Vockell, Wimberg, Britto, & Nye, 2018).
   4. In pediatrics, should consider including school health nurses and daycare providers as needed (Baker et al., 2017).

VI. Communication Failures

A communication breakdown occurs when information impacting an individual or individual's care is not shared or shared inappropriately among interprofessional team members, the individual, their care team, community, and across care settings. Communication breakdowns could be related to human or systematic errors that lead to delay in transfer of necessary information. Fragmented care within complex health care systems, miscommunication during handoffs, punitive work climates leading to under-reported errors, and work-related fatigue have been identified as barriers to safe, effective communication in health care (Arnold & Underman Boggs, 2016).

A. Effective communication can be negatively influenced by individual factors, such as cultural differences, hierarchies, time constraints, workload, fatigue, and distraction. In addition, professional and organizational barriers can include professional jargon, organizational structure, and hierarchies (Ellison, 2015).
B. A prospective cohort study published in 2003 found 19% of individuals discharged from a single U.S. academic medical center had an adverse event within 2 weeks of hospital discharge; one-third could have been prevented and another third minimized (Kim & Flanders, 2013).
C. Ineffective communication in transitions of care can lead to adverse outcomes and risk for individuals, as well as higher hospital readmission rates and cost (Arnold & Underman Boggs, 2016; Vermeir et al., 2015).
D. Complications.
   1. Medication errors.
   2. Procedure-related complications.
   3. Falls.
   4. Readmissions.
      a. Most undesired by the individual, family, and hospital.
         (1) Frustration.
         (2) Increased cost.
         (3) Increased mortality and morbidity.
         (4) Loss of potential earnings.
   5. Sentinel events.
   6. Delay in diagnosis, treatment, procedures, and results (IOM, 2013; Vermeir et al., 2015).
   7. Trauma to individuals related to repeating their stories and information to providers.
      a. Typical surgery individual can see up to 27 providers while in the hospital (IOM, 2013).
   8. Increased length of stay.
   9. Increased cost and waste.
E. Contributing factors.
   1. Medication injuries most prevalent.
      a. Polypharmacy.
      b. Unfamiliar provider admits individual to hospital but does not provide post-hospital care.
      c. Inaccurate medication reconciliations.
         (1) Individual and family are unsure of medications.
         (2) Incomplete or inaccurate records from outside facilities/providers.
         (3) Isolated/lack of interface of EHRs.
      d. Medication discrepancies occur in 87% of discharge and follow-up lists, with 26% related to dosing changes (Albert, 2016).
      e. Medication non-adherence.
         (1) Misunderstanding of instructions.
         (2) Cognitive impairments.
         (3) Lack of follow-up care.
         (4) Language barriers.
         (5) Low health literacy.
         (6) Access to medications.
         (7) Fear of medications or associated side effects.
         (8) Psychosocial and mental health factors.

2. Health literacy.
   a. Lack of assessment of the individual's ability to understand and comprehend verbal and written material presented.
   b. 50% of adults have the skills to use written material accurately and consistently (Nouri & Rudd, 2015).
   c. Information not presented at or below a 5th grade level.
   d. Information only presented in a single format.
   e. Individual health factors not considered in material comprehension.
3. Access to information.
   a. Individual is not provided with enough information to understand or follow up during transitions.
   b. Individual provided with too much information to comprehend or retain.
   c. Delay in completion of discharge summaries.
      (1) 11% of summaries never get to the primary care provider (Vermeir et al., 2015).
   d. Health care protected information through Health Insurance Portability and Accountability Act (HIPAA) without proper release can cause delays, particularly accessing mental health or substance use information.
   e. Varying EHR systems incapable of sharing with other systems.
4. Unclear role definitions and responsibilities.
   a. Each interprofessional team member should understand his or her role in care coordination and communication (Dusek et al., 2015).
   b. Clear rule definitions prevent missed communications and duplication.
5. Time.
   a. Not enough time dedicated to assuring information is communicated accurately, efficiently, and timely.
6. Lack of continuity.
   a. Communication is continual.
   b. Communication needs to occur before, during, and after a transition (Dusek et al., 2015).
F. Pediatric considerations.
   1. Disagreements between the nurse and parent(s) regarding ideas about the prioritization of goals for the child and family (Bentti et al., 2018).
   2. Misunderstanding about the parent perspective by nurses and other providers (Bentti et al., 2018).

VII. Interventions

Methods to prevent communication breakdown and failure should target the timeliness of communication, clarity, and consistency, and promote standardization in communication across settings (Albert, 2016; Vermeir et al., 2015).
A. Assess current care transition process.
   1. Comprehensive assessment of an individual's health goals and preferences; physical, emotional, cognitive, and functional capacities and needs; and social and environmental considerations (Naylor & Sochalski, 2010).
B. Evaluate existing evidence-based programs for adoption and implement evidence-based plan of transitional care (Naylor & Sochalski, 2010).
C. Identify current members involved in individual's care.
D. Build a coordinated acute care enterprise from admission to discharge to home or transfer to a post-acute facility to post-discharge follow up (The Advisory Board Company, 2013).
   1. Interprofessional communication and collaboration from admission through discharge or transition.
E. Involvement of a consistent care team member who oversees all care transitions.
F. Structured hand-off reports with consistent content.
   1. Discharge checklist (RWJF, 2013a, b).
   2. Engagement of all team members, including individual and family (Naylor & Sochalski, 2010).
G. Improved access to EMR systems or products.
   1. Standardized documentation.
   2. Simple, HIPAA-compliant process for obtaining appropriate access.
H. Notification of primary care provider when the individual experiences a care transition.
   1. Admission and discharge.
   2. Early and consistent primary care involvement.
I. Explicit assignment of longitudinal responsibility for follow-up care and testing; shared accountability along the continuum of care.
J. Building a culture of communication and team-based approach to individual care across disciplines.
K. Building capacity and process to achieve timely primary care re-engagement post-discharge.
L. Pediatric considerations.
   1. Provide family support and address parent and family needs in addition to the child (Looman, Hullsiek, Pryor, Mathiason, & Finkelstein, 2018).

Chapter 9

VIII. Care Transition Models

Transitional care is defined as a set of actions taken by a trained individual to coordinate and ensure continuity of health care for individuals they transfer between care settings, change in health status, and health care providers (Brown, 2018; Dusek et al., 2015). Models for transitional care each have specific target populations, but all have the fundamentals of communication, follow up, hand off, care coordination, ongoing assessment, individual involvement, and proactive planning.

A. Care Transitions Intervention (Coleman, Parry, Chalmers, & Min, 2006).
   1. Developed by Eric Coleman, MD, MPH.
   2. Designed to promote effective and practical care transitions for vulnerable adults.
   3. Forged partnerships between hospitals and community-based organizations to facilitate seamless discharges.
   4. Provided individuals with transition coaches who taught individuals how to manage their complex medical conditions, including medication management, maintenance of personal health records, the importance of seeing their primary care provider post-discharge, and knowledge regarding red flags related to their conditions.

B. Better Outcomes for Older Adults through Safe Transitions (Project BOOST) (SHM, 2013).
   1. Developed by the Society of Hospital Medicine.
   2. Utilizes interprofessional mentors to work with individuals and care providers as they transition from hospital to home.
   3. Identifies essential elements of the discharge process, communication with primary care provider before discharge, telephone contact within 72 hours post-discharge, assess individuals for discharge plan comprehension and adherence ("teach back") citation.
   4. BOOST tool incorporates the 8 P's that are evidence-based predictors of unsuccessful transitions used as a guide for information sharing in the transition process. The 8 P's include:
      a. Problem medications (e.g., anticoagulants, insulin).
      b. Psychological concerns (e.g., depression).
      c. Principal diagnosis (e.g., cancer, stroke, diabetes).
      d. Polypharmacy (five or more routine medications).
      e. Individual support (absence of caregiver to assist post discharge).
      f. Inadequate health literacy (inability to demonstrate "teach back").
      g. Prior hospitalization (nonelective) within last 6 months.
      h. Palliative care (would you be surprised if the individual died within the next year?).

C. The Bridge Model (Altfeld, Pavle, Rosenberg, & Shure, 2013).
   1. Developed and refined by Rush University Medical Center Older Adult Programs and Aging Care Connections.
   2. Utilizes masters-prepared social workers.
   3. Provides transitional care through intensive care coordination that starts in the hospital and continues after discharge.
   4. Bridge model consists of three intervention phases.
      a. Pre-discharge: An in-hospital assessment to identify unmet needs and to set up community-based services (including medical provider linkages) before discharge.
      b. Post-discharge: Secondary assessment made via a phone call 2 days after discharge to identify and intervene on additional identified needs.
      c. Follow-up: Conducted 30 days post-discharge to track participant's progress, address any emerging needs, and provide a stable connection to services.

D. Guided Care (Boult, Karm, & Groves, 2008).
   1. Developed at the Johns Hopkins Bloomberg School of Public Health.
   2. Focuses on coordinated, interprofessional, person-centered, and cost-effective teams.
   3. Includes in-home nursing assessments, care planning, individual self-management, smooth transitions, and access to community resources.

E. Geriatric Resources for Assessment and Care of Elders (GRACE) (Counsell, Callahan, Buttar, Clark, & Frank, 2006).
   1. Includes a certified RN practitioner and social worker to address health care needs of low-income seniors.
   2. Develops individualized care plan, including GRACE-based protocols for care of the elderly.
   3. Utilizes EMR and ongoing tracking system to monitor longitudinal progress.

F. Re-Engineered Discharge (Project RED) (AHRQ, 2013).
   1. Developed by Dr. Brian Jack of Boston University Medical Center and funded by AHRQ.

2. A person-centered, standardized approach to discharge planning.
3. Developed strategies to improve the hospital discharge process to promote individual safety and decrease readmission rates.
4. Identified 12 discrete interventions or practices that reduce readmissions.

G. State Action on Avoidable Rehospitalizations (Institute for Healthcare Improvement, 2013).
1. Identified key changes in the ideal transition to clinical office practice.
   a. Provide timely access to care following hospitalization.
   b. Develop standardized processes outlining the expected content of communication, format, preferred method of communication, responsibility.
   c. Review anticipated discharges on a daily basis. Risk-stratify hospitalized individuals into high-risk, moderate, low-risk categories.
   d. Adjust post-discharge care based upon risk.
   e. Complete post-discharge phone calls, focusing on medication management, self-care, worsening symptoms, and action plan, date, and time for a follow-up appointment.
   f. Schedule regular follow up with hospitalist and primary care provider.
   g. Develop a standardized process for communication between hospitalist and primary care provider.
   h. Prepare individual and clinical team before the post-hospital visit.
      (1) Assure access to post-hospital appointments (carve-outs, group visits for medium or low-risk individuals).
      (2) Place a reminder call to the individual before the post-hospital visit to remind him or her of the future appointment, need to bring medications, individual knowledge of available resources.
      (3) Communicate with home-care providers and case managers as appropriate prior to visit.
         (a) Assess individual and review or revise the plan of care.
      (4) Ask individual about health-related goals, medication reconciliation, instruct individual in self-management, explain warning signs, and how to contact help; hospitalist to compare admission medications to discharge medications.
      (5) Discuss end-of-life wishes as applicable.
      (6) Instruct individual in self-care management using "teach back."
   i. At the conclusion of the visit, communicate and coordinate an ongoing plan of care.
      (1) Print the reconciled, dated, medication list and provide a copy to individual and caregiver.
      (2) Ensure next visit is scheduled.

H. Pediatric to adult care transition.
1. Preparing children and families for the transition to adult care.
   a. Assess for readiness of both child and caregiver(s) (McManus et al., 2015).
   b. Begin to solidify child self-care management skills through education about disease management and regular prevention strategies (Abernethy, 2018).
   c. Transition activities for children should include a co-management transition plan (Cooley & Sagerman, 2011).
2. Planning for the pediatric transition to adult care (McManus et al., 2015).
   a. Identifying individual and caregiver(s) preferences for adult follow up and transitions.
   b. Start making children and families aware of transition policies as young as age 12 years (White, 2015).
   c. Some practices may start the planning phase as early as age 14 years.
   d. Informing adult providers of plans to transition children to their level of care at adulthood.
   e. Utilizing EHRs to begin the transition of care.
   f. Begin transition to adult approach to care at age 18 (White, 2015).
3. Transfer of care for pediatric practice to adult practice, age 18 to 22 years (McManus et al., 2015, White, 2015).
   a. Determine practice age limitations.
   b. Provide information and education about navigating adult practices (provider lists, how to schedule appointments, etc.).
   c. Advise adult practices of any special needs or accommodations.

Chapter 9

Table 9-1.
Cross Setting Communications and Transitions: Knowledge, Skills, and Attitudes for Competency

Communication			
"Understand and utilize communication skills with patients, team members, and across care transition settings to communicate effectively and build consensus" (Cronenwett et al., 2009, p. 341).			
Knowledge	**Skills**	**Attitudes**	**Sources**
Analyze own communication style. Describe impact of own communication style on others. Analyze differences in communication style preferences among individuals and families, advanced practice nurses, and other members of the health care team.	Reflect, solicit feedback, and utilize assessment tools to gain insight into personal communication skills, areas for improvement, and techniques to bridge communication styles. Initiate actions to resolve conflict. Communicate respect for team member competence in communication. Assess for health literacy of care team members and individuals.	Appreciate your impact on communication success. Value different styles of communication.	Cronenwett et al., 2009 The Joint Commission, 2010
Discuss principles of effective communication. Describe the basic principles of consensus building and conflict resolution. Examine nursing roles in assuring coordination, integration, and continuity of care.	Assess own level of communication skill in encounters with individuals and families through reflection and feedback. Participate in building consensus or resolving conflict in the context of individual care. Communicate care needed and provided at each transition in care.	Value continuous improvement of own communication and conflict resolution skills.	Cronenwett et al., 2007 Marshall et al., 2009 Jackson et al., 2016
Define communication styles. Describe differences in communication approaches in care coordination. Examine role of nurses in different communication styles.	Utilize multimodal communication techniques to assure complete transfer and retrieval of information from all individual and care team members. Participate in discussions in individual care and assess for appropriate involvement of individual and team members at each transition in care.	Value the input, suggestions, and ideas of all members. Acknowledge and reflect on the importance of each communication style.	McDonald et al., 2014

continued on next page

Table 9-1. (continued)
Cross Setting Communications and Transitions: Knowledge, Skills, and Attitudes for Competency

Team Building and Collaboration			
"Build, support, and participate effectively within nursing and inter-professional teams, fostering open communication, mutual respect, and shared decision-making to achieve quality patient care during care transitions" (Cronenwett et al., 2007, p. 125).			
Knowledge	**Skills**	**Attitudes**	**Sources**
Describe examples of the impact of team functioning on safety and quality of care. Analyze authority gradients and their influence on teamwork and individual safety.	Follow communication practices that minimize risks associated with handoffs among providers and across transitions in care. Choose communication styles that diminish risks associated with authority gradients among team members. Assert own position/perspective and supporting evidence in discussions about individual care.	Appreciate risks associated with handoffs among providers and across transitions in care.	Cronenwett et al., 2007
	Communicate regularly with the individual, support teams, and providers to discuss the plan of care. Demonstrate awareness of the complex individual with multi-specialty involvement. Identify relationships and systems to provide an organized communication pathway between team members, Patient-Centered Medical Home (PCMH), individual, and caregivers. Establish regular gathering of stakeholders to evaluate processes and design improvements.	Value the solutions obtained through systematic, interprofessional collaborative efforts.	Cronenwett et al., 2009 Dusek et al., 2015
Analyze own strengths, limitations, and values as a member of a team. Describe scopes of practice and roles of all health care team members.	Demonstrate awareness of own strengths and limitations as a team member. Continuously plan for improvement in the use of self in effective team development and functioning. Act with integrity, consistency, and respect for differing views. Function competently within own scope of practice as a member of the health care team. Assume the role of team member or leader based on the situation.	Acknowledge own contributions to effective or ineffective team functioning. Respect the unique attributes that members bring to a team, including variation in professional orientations, competencies, and accountabilities. Respect the centrality of the individual/family as core members of any health care team.	Cronenwett et al., 2007

continued on next page

Chapter 9

Table 9-1. (continued)
Cross Setting Communications and Transitions: Knowledge, Skills, and Attitudes for Competency

Team Building and Collaboration (continued)			
Knowledge	**Skills**	**Attitudes**	**Sources**
Analyze strategies for identifying and managing overlaps in team member roles and accountabilities.	Function as the primary point of contact for care coordination for the individual and the team, PCMH stakeholders, and other team leaders. Guide the team in managing areas of overlap in team member functioning. Solicit input from other team members to improve individual as well as team performance. Facilitate interprofessional team meetings for care coordination and transitions of care. Empower contributions of others who play a role in helping patients/families achieve health goals.	Value individual and team contributions toward achieving individual goals. Respect unique roles and perspectives of each team member.	Cronenwett et al., 2009
Identify system barriers and facilitators of effective team functioning. Examine strategies for improving systems to support team functioning. Analyze strategies that influence the ability to initiate and sustain effective partnerships with members of nursing and interprofessional teams. Analyze the impact of cultural diversity on team functioning.	Initiate and sustain effective health care teams. Communicate with team members, adapting own style of communicating to needs of the team and situation. Lead or participate in the design and implementation of systems that support effective teamwork. Engage in state and national policy initiatives aimed at improving teamwork and collaboration.	Value the influence of system solutions in achieving team functioning. Appreciate importance of interprofessional collaboration. Value collaboration with nurses and other members of the nursing team.	Cronenwett et al., 2007 Cronenwett et al., 2009

continued on next page

Table 9-1. (continued)
Cross Setting Communications and Transitions: Knowledge, Skills, and Attitudes for Competency

Quality Improvement Using Evidence-Based Practice			
"Evaluate practice evidence and research, and use data to monitor the outcomes of care processes and improvement methods to design and test changes to continuously improve the quality and safety of health care systems" (Cronenwett et al., 2007, p. 126).			
Knowledge	**Skills**	**Attitudes**	**Sources**
Differentiate clinical opinion from research and evidence summaries. Describe reliable sources for locating evidence reports and clinical practice guidelines. Identify principles that compose the critical appraisal of research evidence. Summarize current evidence regarding major diagnostic and treatment actions within the practice specialty. Determine evidence gaps within the practice specialty. Describe strategies for learning about the outcomes of care in the setting in which one is engaged in clinical practice.	Read original research and evidence reports related to area of practice. Locate evidence reports related to clinical practice topics and guidelines. Critically appraise original research and evidence summaries related to area of practice. Exhibit contemporary knowledge of best evidence related to practice specialty. Promote research agenda for evidence needed in practice specialty. Initiate changes in approaches to care when new evidence warrants evaluation of other options for improving outcomes or decreasing adverse events. Seek information about outcomes of care for populations served in care setting. Seek information about quality improvement projects in the care setting.	Appreciate the importance of regularly reading relevant professional journals. Value knowing the evidence base for practice specialty. Value public policies that support evidence-based practice. Appreciate that continuous quality improvement is an essential part of the daily work of all health professionals.	Cronenwett et al., 2007 Cronenwett et al., 2009
Describe the benefits and limitations of quality improvement data sources, and measurement and data analysis strategies.	Design and use databases as sources of information for improving individual care. Select and use relevant benchmarks.	Appreciate the importance of data that allows one to estimate the quality of local care.	Cronenwett et al., 2009
Describe processes used in understanding causes of error and allocation of responsibility and accountability (such as root cause analysis and failure mode effects analysis).	Participate appropriately in analyzing errors and designing system improvements. Engage in root cause analysis rather than blame when errors or near misses occur.	Value vigilance and monitoring (even of own performance of care activities) by individuals, families, and other members of the health care team.	Cronenwett et al., 2007

continued on next page

Table 9-1. (continued)
Cross Setting Communications and Transitions: Knowledge, Skills, and Attitudes for Competency

Quality Improvement Using Evidence-Based Practice (continued)			
Knowledge	**Skills**	**Attitudes**	**Sources**
"Analyze the differences between micro-system and macro-system change" (p. 344). "Understand principles of change management" (p. 344). "Analyze the strengths and limitations of common quality improvement methods" (p. 344). "Analyze potential and actual impact of national patient safety resources, initiatives, and regulations on care transitions" (p. 346).	"Use principles of change management to implement and evaluate care processes at the micro-system level" (p. 344). "Design, implement, and evaluate tests of change in daily work (using an experiential learning method such as Plan-Do-Study-Act)" (p. 344). "Align the aims, measures and changes involved in improving care" (p. 344). Use measures to evaluate the effect of change. Use national patient safety resources to design and implement improvements in care.	"Appreciate the value of what individuals and teams can do to improve care" (p. 344). "Value local systems improvement (in individual practice, team practice on a unit, or in the macro-system) and its role in professional job satisfaction" (p. 344). "Appreciate that all improvement is change but not all change is improvement" (p. 344). "Value relationship between national patient safety campaigns and implementation in local practice and practice settings" (p. 346).	Cronenwett et al., 2009

Informatics			
"Use and support the use of information and technology to communicate, manage knowledge, mitigate error, and support decision-making" (Cronenwett et al., 2007, p. 129).			
Knowledge	**Skills**	**Attitudes**	**Sources**
Contrast benefits and limitations of common information technology strategies used in the delivery of individual care. Evaluate the strengths and weaknesses of information systems used in individual care.	Participate in the selection, design, implementation, and evaluation of information systems. Communicate the integral role of information technology in nurses' work. Model behaviors that support implementation and appropriate use of electronic health records. Assist team members to adopt information technology by piloting and evaluating proposed technologies.	Value the use of information and communication technologies in individual care.	Cronenwett et al., 2009

continued on next page

Table 9-1. (continued)
Cross Setting Communications and Transitions: Knowledge, Skills, and Attitudes for Competency

Informatics (continued)			
Knowledge	**Skills**	**Attitudes**	**Sources**
Formulate essential information that must be available in a common database to support individual care in the practice specialty. Evaluate benefits and limitations of different communication technologies and their impact on safety and quality.	Promote access to individual care information for all professionals who provide care to individuals. Serve as a resource for how to document nursing care at basic and advanced levels. Develop and utilize standard communication tools for care transitions based on evidence and available technology. Develop safeguards for protected health information. Champion communication technologies that support clinical decision-making, error prevention, care coordination, and protection of individual privacy. Develop order sets, alerts and tools to aid in care transitions. Advocate for a central documentation location, format, and exchange process to improve care transitions.	Appreciate the need for consensus and collaboration in developing systems to manage information for individual care. Value the confidentiality and security of all individual records.	Cronenwett et al., 2009
Describe and critique taxonomic and terminology systems used in national efforts to enhance interoperability of information systems and knowledge management systems.	Access and evaluate high-quality electronic sources of health care information. Participate in the design of clinical decision-making supports and alerts. Search, retrieve, and manage data to make decisions using information and knowledge management systems. Anticipate unintended consequences of new systems.	Value the importance of standardized terminologies in conducting searches for individual information. Appreciate the contribution of technological alert systems. Appreciate the time, effort, and skill required for computers, databases and other technologies to become reliable and effective tools for individual care.	Cronenwett et al., 2009

Sources: Cronenwett et al. (2007). *Nursing Outlook, 55*(3), 122-131. Reprinted with permission from Elsevier. Cronenwett et al. (2019). *Nursing Outlook, 57*(6), 338-348. Reprinted with permission from Elsevier and the author.

Chapter 9

Case Study 9-1.
Chronic Care

Introduction

Jenny has been admitted to the hospital for 5 days for an exacerbation of her congestive heart failure (CHF). This is her second admission in 3 months, and she will be discharged tomorrow. You are her CCTM® nurse; here is what you know about Jenny's situation.

Jenny is a 67-year-old female living alone on the third floor of an apartment complex and works full time at the postal office. Aside from CHF, Jenny is also diagnosed with pre-diabetes, hypercholesterolemia, hypertension, fibromyalgia, and chronic obstructive pulmonary disease. Jenny presented to the emergency department after a week of progressive shortness of breath to the point where she was unable to get dressed without taking breaks.

Clinical Interaction

Per the chart notes, Jenny told the bedside nurse that since her last admission, she has been taking her medications as directed; however, has not followed up with a doctor due to "not having the time or energy." Jenny also reports she is unable to miss additional time from work for any appointments. Her assigned primary care provider, through her insurance company, is located at a health clinic 8 miles from her home. The electronic health record notes are unclear as to whether or not Jenny has a local cardiologist. The doctors have told you they are concerned about the individual's adherence to the prescribed medication regimen and diet restrictions. The team has requested that you meet with Jenny to offer her and perhaps her family support after her hospitalization.

Clinical Implications

1. Jenny's complex diagnoses can be better managed through the involvement of multiple health care professionals located at different settings: cardiologist, primary care physician, social services, diabetes nurse, case manager within her insurance health maintenance organization, and others. Care coordination would help facilitate the necessary communication between the multiple professionals involved in her care. She has been hospitalized and readmitted in a short timeframe with an exacerbation of her CHF in the presence of multiple co-morbidities. A social worker may be able to help her receive community service assistance in transporting her to and from clinic appointments or other needs. A diabetes nurse and case manager could help with her trouble in self-managing medication administration and adhering to diet restrictions. There may be opportunities to better involve her family to help support her at home. Jenny's care involves members at home, in the community, primary care, specialty clinics, and hospital settings, which is critical for CCTM cross-setting communication support.
2. When meeting Jenny, a CCTM RN would want to ask Jenny the following questions:
   a. Who is supporting her at home? Who does she turn to when she needs help?
   b. Does she currently have any providers that she is working with outside of the hospital (primary care provider, cardiologist, endocrinologist, pulmonologist, naturopath, pain management provider, etc.)?
   c. What does Jenny know about her multiple medical conditions; review each one separately.
   d. What does she know about her medications?
   e. What resources does Jenny have access to? Transportation, phone, income, and insurance?
   f. What are Jenny's plans after the hospitalization?
3. Risk factors for communication failure and breakdown include:
   a. Multiple care team members.
   b. Multiple care environments.
   c. Multiple episodes of care.
   d. Inconsistency in care team members through duration of admission.
   e. Health literacy of individual and family for understanding the plan of care and fulfilling the self-management interventions and goals.
4. Opportunities for improved communication:
   a. Individual – Most interactions and assessments were completed through chart notes and review of the electronic health record; it would be helpful for the CCTM RN to assess the individual directly and include any family members as appropriate.
   b. Providers – Additional information is needed from providers regarding their concerns and assessments. What is the background? What are the recommendations regarding Jenny's care moving forward?
   c. Interprofessional care team – Team members could introduce themselves to one another and then introduce each other to the individual seeking care for continuity. Using multi-modal communication methods, oral, and written notes to assure complete handoffs.
   d. Community services – Identifying primary care and specialty providers working with Jenny to provide hand-off communication after hospitalization. Talking with community service professionals and family support currently involved in the individual's care. Assuring a connection to community services prior to discharge, calling on community services and cross-setting providers helps to support the individual in meeting the plan of care goals.
5. ISBAR tool or TeamSTEPP communication tool could be used to transition an individual into community or home setting after discharge. The CCTM RN would identify current health status, pending test and labs, and need for follow up. The CCTM RN would reach out to the appropriate provider and care team to provide pertinent hand-off information. Whether that communication occurs with a primary care provider or specialist, the individual's information should be communicated in person, writing, or through the electronic health record ensuring confidentiality is maintained. If possible, a discussion with Jenny and her family would occur regarding her health information and plan of care. This discussion ensures the individual and families are involved and can voice concerns and preferences regarding transitional care needs. The CCTM RN should present these concerns and preferences to the next provider and/or caregiver.

Case Study 9-2.
Emergency Care

Introduction

Mr. D.P. is a 68-year-old homeless Veteran transported to a community hospital emergency department (ED) via ambulance with an altered level of consciousness and unstable vital signs. He was emergently intubated and placed on a ventilator. He has identification on his person, although the next of kin is not listed. He has not previously received care at the community hospital and is unable to provide any information. The emergency medical team brought his belongings, which include several adequately identified medication bottles with pertinent information, including his Veterans Healthcare Administration (VA) provider's name and phone number. The medications include diabetic and blood pressure pills and pulmonary inhalers.

The ED care team (provider, RNs, technicians) arrived in the room and received the hand-off report. The paramedic states, "He's been living in the woods with people who said that he's been sick with fever, shortness of breath, and a cough. When checking on him in his tent, we found him delirious. We grabbed anything we could that might be helpful with his care. The people in the woods said he's only been in this area a few weeks, and he smokes cigarettes and some pot, but doesn't do any other drugs. His blood glucose is 88 mg/dl, tympanic temperature is 102.7° F, heart rate is 122 beats per minute, respiratory rate is 24 breaths per minute, blood pressure is 96/54, and SaO_2 is 84% on room air. We put a non-rebreather mask on him and started a peripheral intravenous (IV) line. We also gave a total of 0.8 mg of naloxone (Narcan®) IV with no response."

Clinical Interaction

The ED CCTM® RN contacted the VA hospital listed on the medication bottles and spoke with Medical Records personnel to explain the emergent situation. They requested a faxed copy of the Veteran's identification card so they could release medical information for continuity of care. The CCTM RN obtained an emergency contact name and phone number, and called the D.P.'s sister who said, "He doesn't like to take his medication for his schizophrenia, and he will often disappear for periods of time. He has had pneumonia several times and had a recent hospitalization for his high blood sugars. I am his health care surrogate and power of attorney, and will bring the paperwork with me to the hospital. We will leave now and can be there in about 2 hours. Let me give you my cell phone number to call if you need."

The CCTM RN forecasted the need for medical records from the VA hospital and the need to contact family or friends. This communication was vital to coordinate care within the ED and for his care transition to the intensive care unit (ICU), and possibly subsequent care transitions. This coordination also facilitated VA notification and future care transition back into the VA health care system.

Clinical Implications

1. Identify the points of communication that need to occur at each transition.
   a. Emergency medical services (EMS) to ED.
   b. ED to ICU.
   c. Possible other transitions within the hospital among care units and procedural areas.
   d. Possible transition to another facility (rehabilitation, skilled nursing facility, morgue, community/home health, etc.).
2. Key points of communication that need to occur at each point of transition:
   a. Person-centered hand-off communication (e.g., health care professional).
      (1) Background for admission.
      (2) Synopsis of unit stay with current individual assessment.
      (3) Social/family information.
      (4) Plan of care.
   b. Organizational (e.g., unit to unit).
      (1) Same information hand-off communication as above (1.a).
      (2) More detail focused on anticipated needs (medical, nursing, social/family, etc.).
   c. Cross-setting.
      (1) A brief synopsis of above information with focus on current needs (medications, therapy, treatments, progress toward goals, etc.).
      (2) Involvement and contact information of family.
3. The CCTM RN adapts to utilizing a different communication style depending on to whom the information exchange is occurring between and how the information is being shared.
   a. Initially, the communication style that occurred between the EMS and ED contact would be brief (situation, assessment findings, treatments administered), and then, questions/requests for additional treatments from the ED provider could be requested by the EMS team, if needed. This communication is succinct when radioing information while en route to the hospital. The EMS team communicates with the ED team, providing details of their assessment, individual response to medical treatments, and any other information that was not appropriate to communicate over the radio. This in-depth communication changes as the ED provider delivers verbal orders to the ED staff in a clear, direct, and succinct manner.
   b. The communication style becomes more formal and focused, using a pre-approved reporting style, when the individual is transferred from one hospital unit to another. For example, a provider speaking with another provider will probably share more medical information, whereas nursing communication

continued on next page

Case Study 9-2. (continued)
Emergency Care

will focus on the nursing care, treatments, and social aspects involving the individual. Nursing staff would include only the pertinent information when communicating with a specialty health care team member; for example, a respiratory therapist. At this stage, communication is two-way and becomes interpersonal.

    c. Communication between a health care team member and the individual's sister would be entirely different than dialogue among health care professionals and should contain less medical jargon. It is important to convey empathy and concern, and offer support for family member(s) (e.g., chaplain, social services, etc.).

4. List the ISBAR components involved in the above transition of care.
    a. **I**dentify/Introduce yourself and the individual; state your full name, title, and work location and provide the individual's name and demographics.
    b. **S**ituation: The purpose for admission during an ED to hospital ICU transfer is to provide a higher level of care.
    c. **B**ackground: Provide the background information from the EMS transfer communication and initial physical assessment information.
    d. **A**ssessment: Provide current physical assessment information, treatments (respiratory support equipment, IV lines, etc.) tests/procedures, medications or blood products administered and effect.
    e. **R**ecommendation: Coordinate time of transfer, equipment, personnel needed, and care needs during transfer.

5. Consider and anticipate the probable transition from a higher-level of care unit to a lower-care unit and, eventually, discharge.
    a. Pre-hospital to EMS.
    b. EMS to ED.
    c. ED to ICU (also any tests or procedures transfers while admitted to the ICU; e.g., radiology scans, surgery, etc.).
    d. ICU to unit (floor).
    e. Unit to home, rehabilitation facility, skilled nursing facility.

6. Communication tools, other than ISBAR that could be used to transfer information for this individual as he moves between care settings.
    a. Internal and external electronic health record.
    b. BOOST Universal Patient Discharge Checklist.
    c. GAP (General Assessment and Preparedness) tool to summarize the presence of any issues an individual may be experiencing regarding a transition to home.
    d. A written list of follow-up appointments.
    e. MyChart®: A tool that provides individuals with secure access to their medical record.

Chapter 9

References

Abernethy, S.H. (2018). Neonatal diabetes: Nurse navigator role. *Journal of Pediatric Nursing, 38*, 145-146.

Agency for Healthcare Research & Quality (AHRQ). (2013). *Re-Engineered Discharge (RED) Toolkit.* Retrieved from https://www.ahrq.gov/professionals/systems/hospital/red/toolkit/index.html

Agency for Healthcare Research and Quality (AHRQ). (2016). *Care coordination.* Rockville, MD: Author. Retrieved from http://www.ahrq.gov/professionals/prevention-chronic-care/improve/coordination/index.html

Agency for Healthcare Research and Quality (AHRQ). (2018). *TeamSTEPPS 2.0.* Rockville, MD: Author. Retrieved from http://www.ahrq.gov/teamstepps/instructor/index.html

American Academy of Ambulatory Care Nursing (AAACN). (2016). *Scope and standards of practice for registered nurses in care coordination and transition management.* Pitman, NJ: Author.

American Academy of Family Physicians. (2014). *Understanding features & functions of an EHR.* Retrieved from http://www.aafp.org/practice-management/health-it/product/features-functions.html

Albert, N.M., (2016). A systematic review of transitional-care strategies to reduce rehospitalization in patients with heart failure. *Heart and Lung 45*(2), 100-113.

Allen, J., Ottmann, G., & Roberts, G. (2013). Multi-professional communication for older people in transitional care: A review of the literature. *International Journal of Older People Nursing, 8*(4), 253-269. doi:10.1111/j.1748-3743.2012.00314.x

Altfeld, A., Pavle, K., Rosenberg, W., & Shure, I. (2013). Integrating care across settings: The Illinois transitional care consortium's bridge model. *The Journal of American Society on Aging.* Retrieved from http://www.asaging.org/blog/integrating-care-across-settings-illinois-transitional-care-consortium%E2%80%99s-bridge-model

Arnold, E.C., & Underman Boggs, K. (2016). *Interpersonal relationships: Professional communication skills for nurses.* St. Louis, MO: Elsevier.

Baker, D., Anderson, L., & Johnson, J. (2017). Building student and family-centered care coordination through ongoing delivery system design. *NASN School Nurse, 32*(1), 42-49.

Bentti Vockell, A.L., Wimberg, J., Britto, M., & Nye, A. (2018). Using a parent coordinator to support the role of the pediatric nurse practitioner in care coordination. *Journal of Pediatric Health Care, 32*(1), 36-42.

Brady, J., & Ricciardi, R. (2016). *Making care transitions safer: The pivotal role of nurses.* Rockville, MD. Agency for Healthcare Research and Quality (AHRQ). Retrieved from https://www.ahrq.gov/news/blog/ahrqviews/pivotal-role-nurses.html

Brown, M.M. (2018). Transitions of care. In T.P. Dalleman & M.R. Helton (Eds.), *Chronic Illness Care* (pp. 369-373). Chapel Hill, NC: Springer International Publishing.

Bonner, A., Schneider, C.D., & Weissman, J.S. (2010). *Massachusetts strategic plan for care transitions.* Boston, MA: Massachusetts Executive Office of Health and Human Services.

Boult, C., Karm, L., & Groves, C. (2008). Improving chronic care: The "guided care" model. *Permanente Journal, 12*(1), 50-54.

Cady, R.G., & Belew, J.L. (2017). Parent perspective on care coordination services for their child with medical complexity. *Children, 4*(6), 45-59.

Centers for Disease Control and Prevention. (2016). *Health literacy.* Retrieved from https://www.cdc.gov/healthliteracy/developmaterials/index.html

Cibulskis, C.C., Giardino, A.P., & Moyer, V.A. (2011). Care transitions from inpatient to outpatient settings: Ongoing challenges and emerging best practices. *Hospital Practice, 39*(3), 128-139.

Clancy, C.M. (2008). Improving the safety and quality of care transitions. *AORN Journal, 88*(1), 111-113.

Coleman, E., & Boult, C. (2003). Improving the quality of transitional care for persons with complex care needs. *Journal of the American Geriatrics Society. 51*(4), 556-557.

Coleman, E.A., Parry, C., Chalmers, S., & Min, S.J. (2006). The care transitions intervention. *Archives of Internal Medicine, 166*(1), 1822-1828.

Cooley, W., & Sagerman, P. (2011). Supporting the health care transition from adolescence to adulthood in the medical home. *Pediatrics, 128*(1), 198-200.

Council on Children with Disabilities and Medical Home Implementation Project Advisory Committee. (2014). Patient- and family-centered care coordination: A framework for integrating care for children and youth across multiple systems. *Pediatrics, 133*(5), 1451-1460.

Counsell, S.R., Callahan, C.M. Buttar, A.B., Clark, D.O., & Frank, K.I. (2006). Geriatric Resources for Assessment and Care of Elders (GRACE): A new model of primary care for low income seniors. *Journal of American Geriatrics Society, 54*(7), 1136-1141.

Cronenwett, L., Sherwood, G., Barnsteiner, J., Disch, J., Johnson, J., Mitchell, P., ... Warren, J. (2007). Quality and safety education for nurses. *Nursing Outlook, 55*(3), 122-131.

Cronenwett, L., Sherwood, G., Pohl, J., Barnsteiner, J., Moore, S., Sullivan, D., ... Warren, J. (2009). Quality and safety education for advanced nursing practice. *Nursing Outlook, 57*(6), 338-348.

Duff, C.L., & Poole, C.R. (2016). School nurses: Coordinating care through a community/school health partnership. *NASN School Nurse, 31*(6), 342-346.

Dusek, B., Pearce, N., Harripaul, A. & Lloyd, M. (2015). Care transitions: A systematic review of best practices. *Journal of Nursing Care Quality, 30*(3), 233-239.

Ellison, D. (2015). Communication skills. *Nursing Clinics of North America, 50*(1), 45-57. doi:10.1016/j.cnur.2014.10.004

Filipek, D. (2015). *AAACN and AONE offer joint leadership in care coordination.* Retrieved from https://www.nurse.com/blog/2015/11/18/aaacn-and-aone-offer-joint-leadership-in-care-coordination-2/

Haggerty, J.L., Reid, R.J., Freeman, G.K., Starfield, B.H., Adair, C.E., & McKendry, R. (2003). Continuity of care: A multidisciplinary review. *British Medical Journal, 327*(7425), 1219-1221. doi:10.1136/bmj.327.7425.1219

Haggerty, J.L., Pineault, R., Beaulieu, M.D., Brunelle, Y., Gauthier. J., Goulet, F., & Rodrigue, J. (2008). Practice features associated with patient-reported accessibility, continuity, and coordination of primary health care. *Annals of Family Medicine, 6*(2), 116-123. doi:10.1370/afm.802

HealthIT.gov. (2014). *Meaningful use: Meaningful use and the shift to merit-based incentive payment systems.* Retrieved from https://www.healthit.gov/providers-professionals/ehr-implementation-steps/step-5-achieve-meaningful-use

Institute for Healthcare Improvement. (2013). *How-to guide: Improving transitions from the hospital to community settings to reduce avoidable rehospitalizations.* Cambridge, MA: Author.

Institute of Medicine (IOM). (2001). *Crossing the quality chasm: A new health system for the 21st century.* Washington, DC: National Academies Press.

Institute of Medicine (IOM). (2013). *Best care at lower cost: The path to continuously learning healthcare in America.* Washington, DC: The National Academies Press.

Jackson, P.D., Biggins, M.S., Cowan, L., French, B., Hopkins, S.L., & Uphold, C.R. (2016). Evidence summary and recommendations for improved communication during care transitions. *Rehabilitation Nursing, 41*(3), 135-148.

The Advisory Board Company. (2013). *Building the coordinated acute care enterprise: Critical transition points in the continuum of care.* Washington, DC: Author.

Kennedy, A. (2014). Looking back and moving forward: The journey to consumer-driven healthcare continues. *Journal of AHIMA, 85*(1), 10.

Kim, C.S., & Flanders, S.A. (2013). Transitions of care. *Annals of Internal Medicine, 158*(5, Part 1), ITC3-1.

Kripalani, S., LeFevre, F., Phillips, C.O., Williams, M.V., Basaviah, P., & Baker, D.W. (2007). Deficits in communication and information transfer between hospital-based and primary care physicians: Implications for patient safety and continuity of care. *JAMA, 297*(8), 831-841.

Lamb, G. (2014). *Care coordination: The game changer.* Silver Spring, MD: American Nurses Association.

Lancaster, G., Kolakowsky-Hayner, S., Kovacich, J., & Greer-Williams, N. (2015). Interdisciplinary communication and collaboration among physicians, nurses, and unlicensed assistive personnel. *Journal of Nursing Scholarship, 47*(3), 275-284. doi:10.1111/jnu.12130

Le Berre, M., Maimon, G., Sourial, N., Guériton, M., & Vedel, I. (2017). Impact of transitional care services for chronically ill older patients: A systematic evidence review. *Journal of the American Geriatrics Society, 65*(7), 1597-1608. doi:10.1111/jgs.14828

Lees, L. (2013). Key principles of effective discharge planning. *Nursing Times, 109*(3), 18-19.

Lim, F., Foust, J., & Van Cleave, J. (2016). Transitional care. In M. Boltz, E. Capezuti, T. Fulmer, D. Zwicker, & A. O'Meara (Eds.), *Evidence-based geriatric nursing protocols for best practice* (5th ed., pp. 633-668). New York, NY: Springer

Looman, W.S., Hullsiek, R.L., Pryor, L., Mathiason, M.A., & Finkelstein, S.M. (2018). Health-related quality of life outcomes of a telehealth care coordination intervention for children with medical complexity: A randomized controlled trial. *Journal of Pediatric Health Care, 32*(1), 63-75.

Marshall, S., Harrison, J., & Flanagan, B. (2009). The teaching of a structured tool improves the clarity and content of interprofessional clinical communication. *Quality & Safety in Healthcare, 18*(2), 137-140. doi:10.1136/qshc.2007.025247

McDonald, K.M., Schultz, E. Albin, L., Pineda, N., Lonhart, J., Sundaram, V., ... Davies, S. (2014). *Care coordination atlas version 4* (Prepared by Stanford University under subcontract to American Institutes for Research on Contract No. HHSA290-2010-00005I). AHRQ Publication No.14-0037-EF. Rockville, MD: Agency for Healthcare Research and Quality.

McManus, M., White, P., Barbour, A., Downing, B., Hawkins, K., Quion, N., ... McAllister, J.W. (2015). Pediatric to adult transition: A quality improvement model for primary care. *Journal of Adolescent Health, 56*(1), 73-78.

Naylor, M.D., & Sochalski, J.A. (2010). Scaling up: Bringing the transitional care model into the mainstream. *The Commonwealth Fund.* Retrieved from http://www.wapatientsafety.org/downloads/TCM_Forefront.pdf

Nouri, S.S., & Rudd, R.E. (2015). Health literacy in the "oral exchange": An important element of patient-provider communication. *Patient Education and Counseling, 98*(1), 565-571.

Pilcher, J., & Bradley, D.A. (2013). Best practices for learning with technology. *Journal of Nursing Professional Development, 29*(3), 133-137.

Radwin, L.E., Castonguay, D., Keenan, C.B., & Hermann, C. (2016). An expanded theoretical framework of care coordination across transitions in care settings. *Journal of Nursing Care Quality, 31*(3), 269-274.

Robert Wood Johnson Foundation (RWJF). (2013a). *Reducing avoidable readmissions through better care transitions.* Retrieved from http://www.rwjf.org/content/dam/farm/toolkits/toolkits/2013/rwjf404051

Robert Wood Johnson Foundation (RWJF). (2013b). *The revolving door: A report on U.S. hospital readmissions.* Princeton, NJ: Author.

Society of Hospital Medicine (SHM). (2013). *Project BOOST® implementation guide* (2nd ed.). Retrieved from https://shm.hospitalmedicine.org/acton/attachment/25526/f-04f0/1/-/-/-/-/BOOST%20Guide%20Second%20Edition.pdf

Swan, B., & McGinley, M. (2016). Nurse-patient communication: A catalyst for Improvement. *Nursing Management, 47*(6), 26-28.

The Joint Commission. (2010). *Advancing effective communication, cultural competence, and patient- and family-centered care: A roadmap for hospitals.* Oakbrook Terrace, IL: The Joint Commission. Retrieved from https://www.jointcommission.org/assets/1/6/ARoadmapforHospitalsfinalversion727.pdf

The Joint Commission. (2013). *Facts about the Hand-Off Communications Project.* Retrieved from http://www.centerfortransforminghealthcare.org/assets/4/6/CTH_Hand-off_commun_set_final_2010.pdf

University of Virginia Health System. (2018). *MyChart frequently asked questions.* Retrieved from https://mychart.healthsystem.virginia.edu/mychart/default.asp?mode=stdfile&option=faq#EQ_what

U.S. Department of Health & Human Services. (2017). *HITECH Act enforcement interim final rule.* Retrieved from https://www.hhs.gov/hipaa/for-professionals/special-topics/HITECH-act-enforcement-interim-final-rule/index.html

Vermeir, P., Vandijck, D., Degroote, S., Peleman, R., Verhaeghe, R., Mortier, E., ... Vogelaers, D. (2015). Communication in healthcare: A narrative review of the literature and practical recommendations. *International Journal of Clinical Practice, 69*(11), 1257-1267.

Wenger, N.S., & Young, R.T. (2007). Quality indicators for continuity and coordination of care in vulnerable elders. *Journal of the American Geriatrics Society, 5*(Suppl. 2), S285-S292.

White, P. (2015). *Transition models from pediatric to adult health care: Innovative strategies.* Retrieved from https://www.hrsa.gov/sites/default/files/hrsa/advisory-committees/heritable-disorders/meetings/20151103/white.pdf

Chapter 10

Instructions for Continuing Nursing Education Contact Hours

Continuing nursing education credit can be earned for completing the learning activity associated with this chapter. Instructions can be found at aaacn.org/CCTMCoreCNE

Population Health Management

Eileen M. Esposito, DNP, MPA, RN-BC, CPHQ
Sheila Johnson, MBA, RN
Barbara Trehearne, PhD, RN
Anne T. Jessie, DNP, RN
Jayme M. Speight, MSN, RN-BC

Learning Outcome Statement

After completing this learning activity, the learner will understand contemporary principles and key elements of population health management and will be able to describe how to apply the knowledge to inform practice.

Learning Objectives

After reading this chapter, the Care Coordination and Transition Management registered nurse (CCTM® RN) will be able to:
- Explain the purpose of population health management and how it applies to the role of the CCTM RN in care across the continuum.
- Define and describe key elements of population health management.
- Apply the principles and key elements of population health management to the CCTM RN practice.
- Describe data sources (registries, claims data, etc., for managing populations).
- Describe the value of risk stratification within a population.
- Define a gap in care within a population and articulate strategies for managing gaps.
- Understand the appropriate coaching and support methods to motivate individuals within populations to engage in preventive health behaviors.
- Define and identify wraparound services that are essential for ongoing care and support for individuals and populations.
- Discuss how informatics and decision-support tools are utilized in the provision of population health management.
- Describe elements for measuring population health management from the individual and population/group perspective.
- Interpret evolving health care policy development and appropriately implement processes for quality monitoring based on regulatory and payer expectations in the provision of care to defined populations.
- Identify the knowledge, skills, and attitudes for the CCTM RN in population health management practice (see Table 10-3 on page 218).
- Describe value-based purchasing models and how they are used in population health.

AAACN Care Coordination and Transition Management Standards:
Standard 1. Assessment
Standard 4. Planning
Standard 5. Implementation
Standard 6. Evaluation

Source: AAACN, 2016.

Competency Definition

The American Organization of Nurse Executives (AONE) population health competencies for nurse executives are organized within a framework that identifies strategies and interventions for nurses and health systems. The goal of population health management programs is "to improve the health outcomes of entire populations through the effective utilization of patient data and analyzing that data into actionable efforts that lead to improved clinical and financial outcomes" (AONE, 2015, p. 3). The competencies required to achieve this framework include:
- Identify high-risk populations and apply systems thinking to provision of care.
- Recognize and impact social determinants of health and work with other members of the health care team (e.g., social work) to address these social determinants.
- Use technology, including registries and claims data, to identify and close gaps in care.
- Interpret and utilize evidence-based practice research and guidelines to establish effective population health programs, practices, and implement population health models of care (e.g., person-centered medical and health homes).

Chapter 10

- Engage persons, families, and communities in the co-design of programs and initiatives that impact their health.
- Collaborate with stakeholders along the continuum of care to establish goals with measurable outcomes.
- Recognize and support the role of Accountable Care Organizations and value-based payment programs in management of the health of an attributed population.
- Articulate the impact of state and federal regulation and payment systems as well as commercial insurance programs on organizational finances and care to individuals and populations in a value-based environment (AONE, 2015; National Advisory Council on Nursing Education and Practice [NACNEP], 2016).

Storfjell, Winslow, and Saunders (2017) further delineate important themes for working with individuals and families in a population health or population management environment. These themes are described as:

- A holistic approach that considers mental, social, physical, and spiritual aspects within the context of an environment.
- Coordinating care across providers and sites of care.
- Collaboration with community resources, as well as other providers and professionals, to improve the health of individuals and communities.
- Advocacy for both individuals and communities (Storfjell et al., 2017).

Additional key population-focused basic and advanced nursing competencies summarized from the literature, interviews, and the Robert Wood Johnson Foundation consensus conference are listed in Table 10-1.

Definitions of the Quality and Safety Education for Nurses (QSEN) competencies are listed in Table 10-2, providing a link for the CCTM RN to connect these foundational competencies to their role in population health management.

Historically, the concept of population health has been linked to the evolution of epidemiology, aiding in the understanding of health and disease, as well as public health and its relationship between the state; and, the health and welfare of its citizens (Fawcett & Ellenbecker, 2015). While population health can certainly be linked to the science of epidemiology, distinct differences exist between the science of epidemiology and the concepts of public health, community health, and population health. Public health focuses on "the development and implementation of governmental policies, whereas community health focuses on

Table 10-1.
Key Population-Focused Nursing Competencies

Basic*	Advanced**
Wholeness (whole-person and whole-community care)	Data fluency, assessment, and analytic skills (including use of epidemiological data)
Coordination	Systems thinking
Collaboration (teamwork/partnering)	Public health science
Advocacy	Financial planning and management
Communication	Policy development/program planning
Assessment/Analysis	Ethical principles
Cultural competency/Diversity	
Attention to determinants of health	
Relationship-building	
Leadership	

*Basic population health competencies are required of all RNs.
**Advanced competencies are required for BSN and graduate-level RNs.

Sources: NACNEP, 2016; Storfjell et al., 2017.

Chapter 10

Table 10-2.
Definitions of Competencies

Patient-Centered Care	
"Recognize the patient or designee as the source of control and full partner in providing compassionate and coordinated care based on respect for the patient's preferences, values, and needs" (American Association of Colleges of Nursing [AACN] QSEN Education Consortium, 2012, p. 4).	
Teamwork and Collaboration	
"Function effectively within nursing and interdisciplinary teams, fostering open communication, mutual respect, and shared decision making to achieve quality patient care" (AACN QSEN Education Consortium, 2012, p. 4).	
Evidence-Based Practice	
"Integrate best current evidence with clinical expertise and patient/family preferences and values for delivery of optimal care" (AACN QSEN Education Consortium, 2012, p. 4).	
Quality Improvement	
"Use data to monitor the outcomes of care processes and use improvement methods to design and test changes to continuously improve the quality and safety of healthcare systems" (AACN QSEN Education Consortium, 2012, p. 4).	
Safety	
"Minimize risk of harm to patients and providers through both systems effectiveness and individual performance" (AACN QSEN Education Consortium, 2012, p. 4).	
"The overall goal for the Quality and Safety Education for Nurses (QSEN) project is to meet the challenge of preparing future nurses who will have the knowledge, skills and attitudes (KSAs) necessary to continuously improve the quality and safety of the healthcare systems within which they work" (QSEN Institute, 2014, p. 1).	
Informatics	
"Use information and technology to communicate, manage knowledge, mitigate error, and support decision making" (AACN QSEN Education Consortium, 2012, p. 4).	

specific communities at the grassroots level and population health is a broader focus on the population of a nation or worldwide population experiencing a particular health condition" (Fawcett & Ellenbecker, 2015, p. 290). Examples of differences include:
1) Determinants of health outcomes, such as education, income, and medical care, falling outside of the scope of the responsibility of public health.
2) Community health functions occurring within the boundaries of specific communities.
3) Population health existing without boundaries other than specific groups of interest (Fawcett & Ellenbecker, 2015).

Population health management (PHM) is critical to the CCTM RN role. It goes beyond traditional disease management and incorporates preventive, wellness, and chronic care needs. The CCTM RN uses PHM as a means to organize systems of care for persons and populations, identify and implement evidence-based interventions, and measure short and long-term outcomes for both the individual and the population. Person-centered care, as well as individual engagement and activation, are necessary to engage in PHM.

The terms *population health*, *population health management*, and *population management* are often used interchangeably but there are subtle differences. Population health includes not only outcomes, but includes (social) determinants of health, giving a broader definition to the collaborative activities that influence the health of persons and populations. Population health management generally refers to programs targeted to a defined population that uses a variety of individual, organizational, and societal interventions to improve health outcomes (Swarthout & Bishop, 2017). Population management focuses more narrowly on payment systems and the delivery of services for a defined population and measured by specific health care related metrics and outcomes (Robert Wood Johnson Foundation, 2017). In 2003, Kindig and Stoddart defined population health as "the health outcomes of a group of individuals, including the distribution of such outcomes within the group" (p. 380). More recently, population health has been defined as "an approach that treats the population as a whole (including the environmental and community contexts) as the patient" (Institute of Medicine, Board on Population Health Practice, & Roundtable on Population

Chapter 10

Health Improvement, 2014, p. 5). In 2019, the Centers for Disease Control and Prevention (CDC) included the following statement as written by the Healthcare Information and Management Systems Society (HIMSS) (n.d.) about population health on its website: Population health "brings significant health concerns into focus and addresses ways that resources can be allocated to overcome the problems that drive poor health conditions into the population" (para. 2).

In this chapter, a broader adaptation of the terms is used to delineate the scope of practice for the CCTM RN. PHM will be used in a holistic way to encompass the definition of population health as the work of the interprofessional team to address social determinants of health, the systems and processes that assure access to care, and the organization of care processes to address specific disease states (chronic conditions), as well as broader populations of health organized into geographic regions. Additionally, care designed and delivered by the CCTM RN in PHM will be a person-centered, integrated care delivery model based on aligned incentives and coordinated, collaborative processes built on evidence-based prevention and disease management protocols (Baehr et al., 2016).

Unlike wellness programs or disease management programs, PHM is focused on the health of a total population of individuals and encompasses the spectrum from minimal health risk through complex health conditions (Hibbard, Greene, Sacks, Overton, & Parrotta, 2017). The goal of PHM is to keep an individual population as healthy as possible, reducing the disease burden as well as minimizing the need for costly interventions such as emergency department (ED) visits, hospitalizations, imaging tests, and procedures. While PHM focuses partly on the high-risk individuals who generate most health costs, it systematically addresses the preventive and chronic care needs of every individual (Hodach, Grundy, Jain, Weiner, & Handmaker, 2016).

PHM and other value-based care models have been stimulated by state and federal policies, including the passage of the Patient Protection and Affordable Care Act (ACA) of 2009 and the Medicare Access and CHIP Reauthorization Act (MACRA) of 2015. PHM has also been driven by Accountable Care Organizations and the desire of employers to lower health care costs through the provision of primary preventive care and structured PHM strategies (National Committee for Quality Assurance [NCQA], 2018).

Key characteristics of health organizations that implement PHM are:
- An organized system of care.
- The use of interporfessional care teams.
- Coordination across care settings.
- Enhanced access to primary care.
- Centralized resource planning.
- Continuous care, both in and outside of office visits.
- Individual self-management education and coaching.
- A focus on health behavior and lifestyle changes.
- The use of health information technology for data access and reporting for communication among providers and between providers and individuals (Hodach et al., 2016).

The Population Health Conceptual Framework as published by the Population Health Alliance (2017) (see Figure 10-1) depicts the key components of PHM beginning with population monitoring/identification and refined by health assessment and risk stratification. It continues along the care continuum addressing health management interventions coordinated with risk levels and tailored to the individual inclusive of community resources that honor culture, preferences, and values to assure individual engagement. Operational and outcome measures are assessed to gauge effectiveness of care. This framework is useful in organizing the work needed to improve or maintain the physical and psychosocial well-being of individuals and populations through cost-effective and tailored health solutions.

In addition to the Population Health Process Model, Wagner's Chronic Care Model (see Figure 10-2) was developed to improve chronic illness care, a significant part of population management. The model is designed to help providers improve health outcomes by influencing the routine delivery of care through six interrelated system changes meant to make evidence-based, person-centered care easier to accomplish. Transforming the focus of care from acute and reactive to proactive, planned, and population-based is the aim of the model (Coleman, Austin, Brach, & Wagner, 2009). The key elements of the model include:
- Well-developed processes and incentives for making changes in the care delivery system.
- Self-management support that increases individuals' confidence and skills in managing their illness or condition (Higgins, Larson, & Schnall, 2017).
- Reorganized team function and practice systems (e.g., appointments and follow-up) to meet the needs of chronically ill patients.
- Evidence-based guidelines and support for those guidelines through provider education, reminders, and increased interaction between generalists and specialists.

Chapter 10

**Figure 10-1.
Population Health Conceptual Framework**

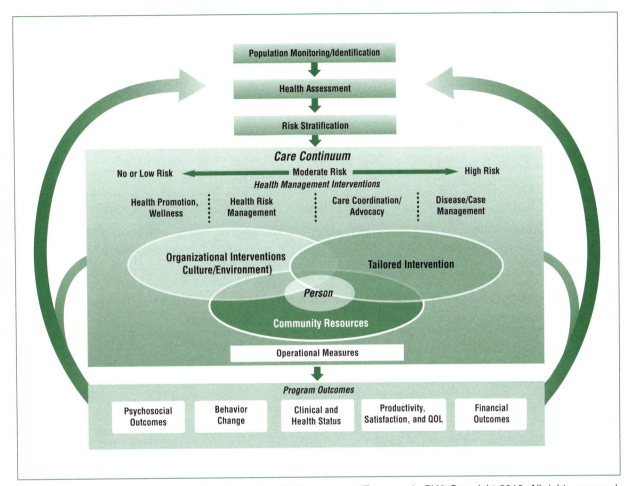

Source: Population Health Alliance – Population Health Management Framework. PHA Copyright 2010. All rights reserved. Reprinted with permission.

- Enhanced information systems to facilitate the development of disease registries, tracking systems, and reminders, and to give feedback on performance (Wagner, 1998).
- Uses a systematic approach to create partnerships between health systems and communities (Stellefson, Dipnarine, & Stopka, 2013).

The Chronic Care Model (CCM) has been in use for more than a decade in multiple organizations and countries. While its aim has been to guide practice redesign, evidence does support the CCM as an integrated framework leading to improved care and better health outcomes (Coleman et al., 2009). The six elements of the model, especially the use of registries and tracking systems to change the routine delivery of ambulatory care, speak to the need for a population approach to care. The model supports population management through identification of groups of individuals, such as those with congestive heart failure and diabetes in which practice redesign using the CCM demonstrates improved outcomes (Coleman et al., 2009).

The CCTM RN uses a comprehensive approach that utilizes principles of care coordination, case management, and population health to maximize the health outcomes and reduce resource utilization for populations and the individuals within them. The CCTM RN identifies a population for focused care and works with the interprofessional team to execute individualized care (Rushton, 2015).

I. Population Identification

To manage population health effectively, organizations, health plans, and providers must be able to track and monitor the health of individuals within a population, not just the individuals who seek care (Hibbard et al., 2017). This includes identifying subpopulations of people who might benefit from additional services including individuals who are

Figure 10-2.
The Chronic Care Model

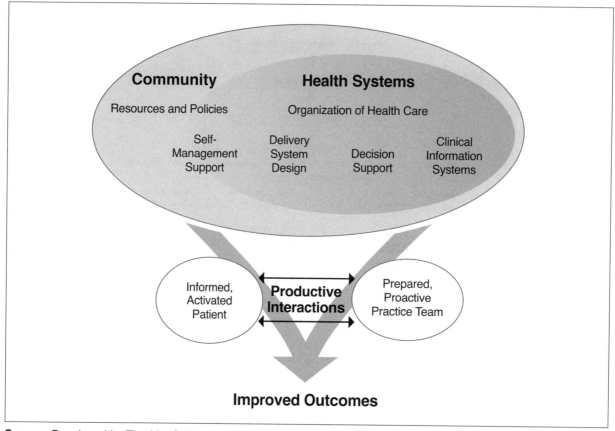

Source: Developed by The MacColl Institute.
® ACP-ASIM Journals and Books. Reprinted with permission.

due or overdue for preventive services, individuals with chronic illnesses whose measures are out of range, individuals who have experienced gaps in care, and individuals who have recently been discharged from the ED or other facility (McWilliams, Chernew, & Landon, 2017; Mullins, Mooney, & Fowler, 2013). PHM processes seek to identify individuals who would have otherwise been lost to care or follow up, working to reengage individuals with provider(s) or health care system(s). To identify individual populations for outreach and intervention tools, registries and data sets are utilized.

A. Person attribution: From a PHM perspective, clinicians are responsible for the totality of the population in their assignment, including those individuals who do not seek care in an ambulatory care practice setting (Hibbard et al., 2017).
   1. Health plan eligibility and administrative data are used to identify individual populations assigned or attributed to a given provider.
   2. Designation occurs through health plan assignment or, alternately, attribution occurs based on payer analysis of claims and utilization patterns.
   3. Health plans identify and cohort subpopulations within the member population utilizing selected chronic diseases, presence of co-morbid conditions, cost of care, as well as defining characteristics and resource needs of individuals or subpopulations including social determinants of health (NCQA, 2018).
      a. Grouping subpopulations of individuals using characteristics, utilization patterns, and commonality of chronic disease can lead to the development of effective and efficient systems to design and deliver targeted care interventions to better manage diseases and mitigate care delivery costs.
      b. Identification of subpopulations can

also drive care delivery to the most appropriate site of care based on individual or population care needs (e.g., hospice instead of hospital at end-of-life, home instead of skilled nursing facility, provider practice instead of ED).
   4. Practice management systems within the clinical setting may be used to assign individuals to clinicians (e.g., physician, advanced practice nurse, or physician assistant) (Shaljian & Nielsen, 2013).
   5. CCTM RNs, as members of the person-centered care team, play a pivotal role in understanding individual populations as they collaborate in the design and delivery of care management of a population in partnership with the interprofessional team.
B. Data systems: Include health risk assessments, registries, dashboards, and analytic reports that can assist the CCTM RN in identifying individuals and populations that may benefit from interventions (NCQA, 2018). These data warehouse applications serve as a central repository for all data allowing health care organizations to store, integrate, recall, and analyze information to provide clinicians and nurses insights that guide clinical decision-making at the point of care (Bresnick, 2016).
   1. The results of health risk assessments combined with claims data, clinical data from the electronic health record (EHR), diagnostic results, pharmacy usage, hospital activity data (e.g., admissions, emergency department usage), and evidence-based medicine parameters, provide specific information that can be used to understand the population both at the practice and individual level (Shaljian & Nielsen, 2013).
   2. Clinical data registries are databases with medical information about immunizations, cancer screenings, chronic disease prevalence, or disease-specific laboratory and diagnostic results for a panel of individuals followed by a physician, provider, or practice (Bodenheimer, Ghorob, & Margolius, 2015).
   3. Health information exchanges allow for the storage and sharing of information across payers, practice settings, health care, and tracking systems. These can include laboratory results, medications, diagnoses, care notes, discharge summaries, and procedures, but can be limited due to a lack of broad EHR interoperability (Healthcare Informatics, 2016).
   4. Registries are a critical tool used by the CCTM RN to prioritize individuals with high-risk clinical conditions, serious unmet clinical needs for outreach, and interventions to manage outcomes. Registries include EHR data, metrics for identifying multiple co-morbid chronic conditions, hospital and ED utilization, and gaps in care such as unfilled prescriptions, missed preventive screenings, and lack of post-discharge follow up after hospitalization. These registries can aid in identifying areas where necessary interventions require development. These include access to providers, the need for preventive services, chronic condition management, or individuals who are in the need of outreach (Sodihardjo-Yuen, van Dijk, Wensing, De Smet, & Teichert, 2017).
      a. Prevention.
         (1) Identifies individuals needing preventive screening/interventions/ongoing disease surveillance.
      b. At-risk individuals.
         (1) Identifies individuals at risk for chronic disease exacerbation based on lack of disease control.
            (a) Blood pressure monitoring indicates hypertension is not controlled.
            (b) Elevated hemoglobin A1C levels indicate diabetes is not controlled.
      c. High-risk individuals.
         (1) Individuals with multiple co-morbid conditions at risk for catastrophic health event, adverse disease outcome, or death.
      d. Hospital admissions/readmissions and ED visits.
C. Risk stratification: Helps target individuals or subpopulations most in need of services and resources, identifying cost drivers within the population, with the potential to reduce health care costs while improving individual outcomes. To manage population health effectively, an organization must be able to track and monitor the health of individuals and stratify a population into subgroups that require particular services at specific intervals. Individuals are stratified into risk categories using tools, including registries with embedded decision-support algorithms, to allow identification of individuals who could benefit from proactive outreach, pre-visit planning, care coordination, and identification of gaps in care

(Reddy et al., 2017).
1. Risk stratification incorporates structured data from multiple sources, applies mathematical algorithms, and utilizes predictive modeling techniques to identify groups of individuals at risk of becoming sick, those who may experience disease progression, as well as those who could receive the greatest benefit from participation in a care management program (Goldstein, Navar, Pencina, & Ionnidis, 2017; Raghupathi & Raghupathi, 2014).
2. Groups of individuals represent those who are ill enough to require ongoing support, those with less-serious chronic conditions that warrant interventions to prevent them from worsening, or those who are fairly healthy and just require preventive care and education (Health Catalyst, 2016).
3. Stratification design that applies algorithms and predictive modeling techniques in real-time can incorporate changes in diagnoses, include updated results of diagnostic tests, reflect changes in use of the ED and/or hospital admissions supporting immediate action by the CCTM RN or care team to outreach to individuals and modify the plan of care (Struijs, Drewes, Heijink, & Baan, 2015).
4. The CCTM RN uses risk-based stratification to prioritize individuals for outreach and management and to apply evidence-based protocols to implement person-specific interventions based on level of risk.
   a. Low risk: Focus on prevention and wellness.
   b. Moderate risk: Focus on education, health coaching, and self-care management.
   c. High risk: Chronic care management (The Advisory Board, 2014).
D. Clinical decision support: Also called best practice or health maintenance alerts, are prompts or reminders for preventive and chronic care interventions specific to individuals' health conditions and status that are facilitated through EHRs and integrated software applications (Reynolds, Rubens, King, & Machado, 2016).
   1. The CCTM RN utilizes decision-support tools to monitor individuals and intervene when alerted to change in status or need for a care intervention specific to individual patient needs.

E. Transitions in care: Across the continuum require closer attention of the CCTM RN. Additional person identification tools and interventions may be utilized to ensure smooth and safe transitions to the next setting of care, and to prevent readmissions.
   1. Use of the Modified LACE and assessment tool that incorporated length of stay, acuity of admission, co-morbidity, and emergency department utilization to identify individuals with a high predicted risk for readmission or death (El Morr, Ginsburg, Nam, & Woollard, 2017; Kim & Flanders, 2013).
   2. Ensure follow-up care post-hospital discharge is in place, including medication reconciliation and provider appointment scheduling (Centers for Medicare & Medicaid Services [CMS], 2016; Rennke & Ranji, 2015).
   3. Utilization of the BOOST (Better Outcomes by Optimizing Safe Transitions) tool may reduce readmissions by addressing social determinants and potential gaps in care (Society of Hospital Medicine, 2013).
   4. Pediatric consideration.
      a. PedsQL: A developmentally appropriate measurement model for the Pediatric Quality of Life Inventory (Varni, 2019).
         (1) Child Self-Reporting tool: Ages 5-7, 8-12, and 13-18.
         (2) Parent Proxy-Report tool: Ages 2-4, 5-7, 8-12, and 13-18.
         (3) Generic Core Scales and Disease-Specific Modules available.
         (4) Translated into multiple languages.

II. The Role of Big Data

With widespread adaptation of EHRs, there has been a dramatic increase in the availability of clinical data, as well as knowledge growth around broader factors that influence and contribute to the health of individuals and populations. "Advances in epidemiology have shown that policies, features of institutions, characteristics of communities, living and environmental conditions, and social relationships all contribute, together with individual behaviors and factors such as poverty and race, to the production of health" (Hu, Galea, Rosella, & Henry, 2017, p. 759). These big data sets, blended with analytic methods that go beyond traditional statistics and hypothesis testing, incorporate machine learning – artificial intelligence – to reveal information for prediction and discovery (Krumholz, 2014). In addition, both structured and non-structured data from a variety of sources allows for the study of outcomes, as well as continuous learning of large-scale population-based interventions (Andreu-Perez, Poon, Merrifield, Wong, & Yang, 2015).

Big data has been described as large in volume, high in velocity, complex, variable, and diverse requiring "advanced techniques and technologies to enable the capture, storage, distribution, management and analysis of the information" (Raghupathi & Raghupathi, 2014, p. 2). According to Hu and colleagues (2017), "the dawn of a data deluge in health…carries extraordinary promise for improving the health of populations" (p. 759).

As associations in data are discovered, data patterns are understood, trends within the data are identified, and data analytics are continuously applied, identifying opportunities to manage individuals and populations in a more focused way with the potential for cost savings (Bates, Saria, Ohno-Machado, Shah, & Escobar, 2014; Raghupathi & Raghupathi, 2014).

A. Clinical operations and research and development are two of the largest areas for savings potential with additional opportunities detailed below.
   1. Clinical operations.
      a. Comparative effectiveness research to determine more clinically relevant/cost effective strategies to diagnosis and treat.
   2. Research and development.
      a. Predictive modeling to lower attribution for a more targeted pipeline for drugs and devices.
      b. Statistical tools/algorithms to improve trial design.
      c. Clinical trial analysis to determine adverse effects before products reach the market.
   3. Public health.
      a. Analyze disease patterns and track disease outbreaks.
      b. Faster development of targeted vaccines.
      c. Use of data sets to identify needs, provide services, predict/prevent crises.
   4. Evidence-based medicine.
      a. Combine/analyze data from EHRs, financial, and operational data to match treatments with outcomes, predicting individuals at risk for disease or readmission.
   5. Genomic analytics: Incorporate as part of regular care decision-making.
   6. Pre-adjudication fraud analysis: Analyze large claims data sets to prevent fraud, waste, and abuse.
   7. Device/remote monitoring: Analyze rapidly available data from in-hospital and in-home devices to predict adverse events and monitoring safety.
   8. Person profile analytics: Identify individuals who would benefit from proactive care/lifestyle changes (Kruse, Groswamy, Raval, & Marawi, 2016; Raghupathi & Raghupathi, 2014).

B. While the possibility of new knowledge discovery exists, as massive data sets are leveraged in new ways, several challenges have been identified that may have an impact on the outcome of data use.
   1. Identifying data that matter most.
   2. Defining data standardization.
   3. Ensuring the best use of existing data, data structure, and storage and transfer.
   4. Protecting data security.
   5. Enhancing data linkage.
   6. Development of managerial skills and data governance.
   7. Extending efforts from individuals to populations by incorporating new, complex, and unstructured data sources (Hu et al., 2017; Krumholz, 2014; Kruse et al., 2016).

III. **Team-Based Interventions**

Successful population-based care requires staff and resources beyond what individual primary care providers can provide. It involves planning and implementing care for groups, working with individuals outside of the office visit, and monitoring effectiveness. Primary care providers are defined as physicians, advance practice nurses, and physician assistants.

A. Engage all team members and begin by selecting a nurse and physician leader to co-lead CCTM efforts.
   1. "Identify physician partners to co-lead care coordination and transition management strategies and to influence staff physicians" (Zangerle & Kingston, 2016, p. 172).
   2. The leaders must educate care team members on the value of CCTM RN and the achievement of health system goals of improved population health, individual experience, and increased individual engagement in self-management (Zangerle, 2015).
   3. "Team members should define their individual roles and responsibility to facilitate accountability" (Rushton, 2015, p. 232).

B. Primary care is at the heart of public health management with primary care providers

supplying the continuity required to ensure individuals receive appropriate preventive and chronic care. While there is variation in primary care provider workforce shortage projections, there is agreement on the "(a) growing gap between the population demand for primary care and the number of primary care physicians available to meet that demand and (b) nurse practitioners (NPs) and PAs that will narrow the gap" (Bauer & Bodenheimer, 2017, p. 626).
1. Other clinicians can perform much of this work, enabling physicians to focus on areas where their expertise is required.
2. Care teams led by physicians, NPs, or other professionals can manage more individuals and address more of their needs than the current primary care model.
3. Team-based care supports effective and efficient care delivery as an extension of the primary care provider, providing critical resources to ensure improved outcomes (Bodenheimer, Ghorob, Willard-Grace, & Grumbach, 2014).

C. "High-performing practices stratify the needs of their patient panels and design team roles to match those needs" (Bodenheimer et al., 2014, p. 168).
1. Panel management.
    a. Staff (medical assistant or nurse) surveys registry or health maintenance section of EHR to identify individuals with gaps in care of routine services (e.g., colorectal cancer screening, breast cancer screening, HgbA1c).
    b. 'Standard orders' are executed without having to involve the provider.
    c. Provider uses in-office visit to focus on individual concerns and interventions requiring provider expertise, plan of care, including treatment options.
2. Care teams must strive to deliver appropriate, evidence-based care during patient visits, but they must also ensure care gaps are addressed when individuals do not come into the office.
3. Teams proactively track care activities and interventions, and transparently share clinical information across the continuum with providers and individuals.
4. The primary care provider and the health care team, in full partnership with the individual and caregiver, provide "compassionate and coordinated care based on respect for patient's preferences, values, and needs" (Cronenwett et al., 2007, p. 123).

D. In team-based care, the team works together to care for a population and pursue the Triple Aim. "The team has a range of skills and expertise to care for a patient's whole continuum of needs" (Pabo, 2018, para. 1).
1. Regular communication and collaboration within the team enhances clinical and social expertise of the team, provides peer support, and allows for sharing of best practices.
2. Panels or populations are assigned to teams consisting of a provider and clinical support staff such as RNs, licensed practical nurses, medical assistants, health coach, and receptionist.
3. Smaller teams comprise a provider, clinical support staff, and a receptionist, while larger teams can have additional members such as pharmacists and therapists.
    a. Provider: Designs and directs the medical plan of care.
    b. Other members of the team: Pharmacists, social workers, behavioral health experts, dieticians, therapists, etc.

E. Characteristics of an effective team (Haas, Vlasses, & Havey, 2016).
1. RNs practice at top of licensure.
2. Full partners in care with other health professionals.
3. Wide range of clinical skills that match with needs/demands of population served.
4. Strong critical-thinking skills: Promote resolution of complex care problems.
5. Ability to engage and partner with individuals and caregivers: Activate and form meaningful relationships; person advocate.
6. Communication skills.
7. Experience in linking services.
8. Understand role and scope of other team members.

F. Activities performed by the CCTM RN.
1. Coordinates care across transitions and care settings.
    a. Facilitates access to services.
    b. Develops plan of care with primary care physician and individual/family.
    c. Oversees disease education and wellness coaching.
    d. Provides care via face-to-face and telephone.
    e. Accountable for identifying gaps in care; communicates concerns to physicians.
    f. Embedded in the primary care physician practice or can work centrally.

2. Manages referrals.
   a. To internal payer-based formalized disease management programs.
   b. To specialists.
   c. To pharmacy: Medication management support.
   d. To behavioral health, psychosocial support.
3. Tracks individual activity.
   a. Uses information technology system alerts/registries to identify inpatient, ED utilization.

G. Team role in activation.
   1. Provides education.
      a. Coaches individuals on disease management goals, monitors progress, offers encouragement, ensures understanding of necessary skills.
      b. Supports symptom management.
   2. Supports self-management.
      a. Encourages adherence to care plan, improvement through person-centric goal setting.
      b. Fosters individual and caregiver activation, offers education.
      c. Person portable health record.
   3. Encourages frequent communication.
      a. Promotes open communication through consistent monitoring, feedback, and follow-up.
      b. Forges one-on-one relationship with individual to promote two-way communication.

H. Panel size: The ratio of the CCTM RN to the volume of individuals (or panel) they are responsible for managing.
   1. Panel size or caseload can vary based on the complexity and acuity of the population served, payer contracting, and health care organization mission.
   2. Caseloads for RNs are contingent upon the model of care delivery and availability of centralized RN resources to support the team.

I. Team communication.
   1. Pre-encounter preparation: Chart review prior to the office visit, identifying preventive measures or interventions to be addressed at the time of the visit. Items are documented in the EHR for ease of communication.
   2. Decision-support alerts in the EHR notify team members of actions needed for health maintenance or chronic disease monitoring (vaccinations, lab work, preventive screenings, referrals).
   3. Daily huddles: Team gathers briefly the day of the office visit to communicate person interventions to be addressed, delegate tasks, and to ensure comprehensive care delivery.
   4. Unified care plan: Mode of documentation in the EHR that allows members of the care team across all care settings to view and edit the plan of care.

J. Electronic messaging to individuals and care team: Use of the EHR to send messages to individuals via a secure patient portal and for team members to message each other electronically with key communication regarding the plan of care.

K. Interprofessional team members (Bodenheimer et al., 2014; Tschudy et al., 2016).
   1. Primary care physician: Provides medical oversight of treatments and interventions.
   2. Mid-level or advanced clinical practitioner (NP or physician's assistant): Designs and modifies the plan of care.
   3. CCTM RN: Provides person-centered care, self-management support, education, coaching, and counseling and advocacy for individuals and families.
   4. Pharmacist: Consultant in medication management, medication reconciliation, medication assistance programs. Ensures the quality and accuracy of medication management.
   5. Social worker: Identifies and coordinates essential nonclinical services, such as housing, food, transportation.
   6. Caregiver: Family member, significant other, or person identified by the individual to participate in or provide direct care (biological family member, legal partner, case worker, care aide, church member, neighbor).
   7. Community health worker: RNs functioning in CCTM role engage community health workers as partners to address social determinants of health, such as access to care, food, housing, and community engagement/support (Biederman et al., 2016).
   8. Other team members can include medical assistants, practice nurses, hospital-based case managers, dieticians, physical and occupational therapists, community resource specialists, community care agencies, hospitalist, home care staff, palliative care and hospice nurses, skilled nursing facility nurses and discharge planners, homeless shelter staff, nonprofit community agencies, lay workers, etc.

IV. **Care Coordination**

"The Population Health Care Coordination Process utilizes principles from care coordination, case management, and population health to maximize health outcomes and resource utilization for populations and the individuals within them. The process focuses on coordinating care for the entire population, followed by an individualization of that care" (Rushton, 2015, p. 231).

The six phases of the Population Health Care Coordination Process are depicted in Figure 10-3. "While the process is generally linear, steps can be repeated as necessary particularly if additional information, assessment, or analysis is required" (Rushton, 2015, p. 231).

A. Phases 1 and 2 – Data Analysis and Selection: The use of any and all available data ranging from payer claims, clinical data from EHRs, individual self-reported data to laboratory data marts is analyzed to determine the attributes of the population including unique needs and problems.
  1. At risk for loss of life.
  2. At risk for complications.
  3. Overall needs.
  4. Most high-risk needs.
  5. Comparison to benchmarks.

B. Phase 3 – Assessment: Status and needs assessment of the high-risk group and identified subpopulation of interest (Rushton, 2015). The CCTM RN "systematically collects comprehensive and focused data relating to health needs and concerns of a patient, group, or population as they move across the care continuum" (AAACN, 2016, p. 13).
  1. Interprofessional approach.
  2. Holistic view.
  3. Defines problems and needs.

C. Phase 4 – Planning: Begin by "making decisions about how to address issues" (Rushton, 2015, p. 232). The CCTM RN "develops a patient- and/or population-centered plan of care that identifies and advocates for strategies and alternatives to attain expected outcomes" (AAACN, 2016, p. 16).
  1. Agree on goals for the subpopulation and develop care pathways.
  2. Goals are based on data, problems, and needs from analysis and assessment.
  3. Delineate individual roles for team members to foster accountability.
  4. Include the population and individual level.

D. Phase 5 – Interventions: Use evidence-based and/or best practice (Rushton, 2015). The CCTM RN "implements the identified plan of care to attain expected outcomes in selected groups or individuals" (AAACN, 2016, p. 17).
  1. Comprehensive needs of the population are targeted.
  2. Generally, three subsets: prevention, transitions of care, and chronic care.

E. Phase 6 – Evaluation: Use data to understand performance and determine next steps (Rushton, 2015). The CCTM RN "evaluates the status and progress of the patients, group, or population toward the attainment of expected outcomes and communicates the status and progress to relevant professionals across the care continuum" (AAACN, 2016, p. 21).
  1. Evaluate progress toward goals.
  2. Evaluate adherence to subpopulation care coordination process.
  3. Ensure metrics are measuring what they are intended to measure.
  4. Determine next steps.
  5. Utilize same process for individual members within the subpopulation.

V. **Preventive Care Management**

Disease prevention and health promotion rely on a proactive approach to keep persons and populations healthy. Technology is key in increasing communication regarding due or overdue care including testing and vaccinations. Use of automated outreach via telephone or push notification, such as text or email, and written reminders via mail ensure individuals are reminded to receive preventive tests and screenings, adhere with annual wellness exams, and receive immunizations appropriate to their age and medical condition (Reynolds et al., 2016).

A. Examples of preventive care management.
  1. Immunizations for flu and pneumonia prevention and pediatric immunizations (CDC, 2018): An updated schedule of vaccinations for adults and children (https://www.cdc.gov/vaccines/schedules/index.html).
  2. Cancer screenings including breast cancer screening (mammogram) and colon cancer screening (colonoscopy, sigmoidoscopy, FIT-DNA, or fecal occult blood test).

An app maintained by the U.S. Department of Health & Human Services/Agency for Healthcare Research and Quality (AHRQ) allows access to the most up-to-date recommendations published by the U.S. Preventive Services Task Force from any device (https://epss.ahrq.gov/PDA/index.jsp).
  3. Maintenance tests for HbA1c, spirometry, and metabolic lab monitoring.
  4. Medicare wellness visits and well-child checks.

B. Healthfinder.gov is a consumer-oriented website that contains health maintenance

**Figure 10-3.
The Population Care Coordination Process**

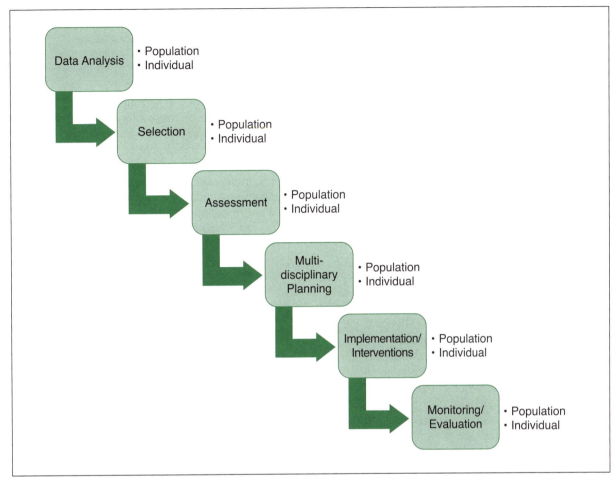

Note: A diagram of the Population Care Coordination Process outlines the six steps of the process. These steps include data analysis, selection, assessment, planning, interventions, and monitoring. These steps are completed at the population and individual levels.

Source: Rushton, 2015. Reprinted with permission from Wolters Kluwer Health, Inc.

schedules as well as supporting education and tools designed to promote preventive care (www.Healthfinder.gov).
C. Personalized preventive services recommendations are readily available and customizable by entering minimal data, such as age and gender, into the 'myhealthfinder' interactive tool (https://healthfinder.gov/myhealthfinder/).
D. Pediatric considerations: Bright Futures – a program established by the American Academy of Pediatrics established for prevention and health promotion for infants, children, adolescents, and their families – is available online (http://brightfutures.aap.org) (American Academy of Pediatrics, 2019).

VI. **Informatics and Decision-Support Systems**

Population health management processes must be supported by internal health record data and the ability to obtain, store, and analyze payer data. The ability of the CCTM RN to deploy PHM interventions focused on prevention, high-risk, and chronic disease populations is critical to the ability to have reliable and readily available data including access to decision-support tools.

As defined by the U.S. National Library of Medicine, "health informatics is the interdisciplinary study of the design, development, adoption, and application of IT-based innovations in healthcare services delivery, management, and planning" (HIMSS, 2014, para.1).

"Nursing informatics (NI) is the specialty that integrates nursing science with multiple information management and analytical sciences to identify, define, manage, and communicate data, information, knowledge, and wisdom in nursing practice. NI supports nurses, consumers, patients, the interprofessional healthcare team, and other stakeholders in their decision-making in all roles and settings to achieve desired outcomes. This support is accomplished through the use of information structures, information processes, and information technology" (American Nurses Association [ANA], 2015, pp 1-2; HIMSS, 2015).

A. Informatics systems support and facilitate person-centered care. EHRs provide a repository for individual information that is used to facilitate care and increase access to information. Information is used by care teams and individuals and families. Health information technology assists with organizing disparate data sources into one integrated record (Steichen & Gregg, 2015).
   1. Individual who are transitioning across care settings are at risk for adverse events such as insufficient follow-up and hospital readmissions (Rushton, 2015).
   2. Referrals and results from laboratory and radiologic tests, specialty consults, home health, and community-based care.
   3. Real-time monitoring of hospital admissions and ED visits that trigger the need for follow-up.
   4. Reminders/prompts regarding visits and preventive care.
   5. Decision-support tools for complex individual care (clinical pathways and guidelines).
   6. Community resource lists.
   7. Standardized evidence-based education.
   8. Support for primary care.
   9. Use of Continuity of Care Document (CCD) – a clinical information summary used for exchange of information between EHRs (Bates, 2015).
   10. Health information exchanges for data exchange including ability to access admission, discharge, and transfer information for the CCTM RN to use for transitions of care.
B. Longitudinal care plans are a best practice to support person-centered care coordination (Steichen & Gregg, 2015).
   1. Initiated by individuals and close caregivers.
   2. "Communicated, referred to and updated across organization and levels of care (Steichen & Gregg, 2015, p. 2).
   3. Enables person engagement, improves collaboration between care teams, and contributes to efficient and safe personalized care (Steichen & Gregg, 2015).
C. Registries. Refer to section "I. Population Identification," for more information.
D. Personal health records (Demiris & Kneale, 2015).
   1. The ability to access, manage, and share personal health information allows the person to be more informed of their plan of care and allows for tracking of information.
   2. Provider and clinical organization communication to the person plays a role in adoption by the person.
E. Decision-support tools.
   1. Clinical alerts.
      a. Prevention: Automated reminders and appointment systems for preventive disease care.
      b. Safety: High clinical values, potential drug interactions, allergies.
      c. Utilization: Emergency department/hospital/missed follow-up appointment/no discharge appointment, prescriptions unfilled.
F. Analytics (Demiris & Kneale, 2015; Haas et al., 2016).
   1. Predictive models: Identify individuals at increased risk early for proactive intervention.
      a. Combination of clinical data and paid medical and pharmacy claims information for a comprehensive individual snapshot.
      b. Based on predictive algorithms that rank individuals by risk profile that predicts future utilization.
   2. Risk assessment: BOOST Risk Assessment 8 P Screening tool can and should be used for CCTM RN risk assessment and stratification. It includes social determinants and can identify individuals most likely to benefit from CCTM. Scoring of modified LACE tool can be used, and includes psychosocial and clinical status, but does not include social determinants.
   3. Determines population performance against quality/service/cost goals and seeks opportunity for improvement.
   4. Uses information technology (portals and health information exchanges) to communicate data related to care of individuals and populations. See Chapter 12 for additional information.
   5. "EHR documentation screens should be developed and used by nurses and other providers doing CCTM so their care

processes and outcomes become visible and can be tracked" (Haas et al., 2016, p. 131).
G. Opportunity for continued use of health information technology for better coordination of care (Bates, 2015).
1. Interoperability is needed for communication of health information across care settings. EHRs remain in separate silos and specific to care continuum points (e.g., hospital, ambulatory care practice, home health agency, and skilled nursing facility).
2. A longitudinal plan of care is optimal for a comprehensive understanding of care for the individual; however, most EHRs do not have this specific functionality at this time.
3. Referrals for consultations, services, and transitions are 'open-loop' requests, which do not allow for knowing if the referral was acted on. Optimal use would allow for closed-loop requests and 'electronic curbsides.'
4. Electronic communication within the care team is optimal.
   a. The ability for synchronous and asynchronous communication regarding progress and barriers to progress of goals is key.
   b. Multiple providers in differing locations with different EHR platforms need to all be on same page for coordination of care.

VII. Measuring Outcomes

To describe PHM, organizations can use a variety of measures including those that detail processes (e.g., how many individuals with diabetes received an appropriate HbA1c test), intermediate outcomes (e.g., HbA1c or blood pressure levels), and long-term outcomes (e.g., quality of life). The latter requires a combination of clinical data and individual self-reported data, such as functional status and self-perceived health. It is important to consistently measure for individual experience, quality standards, quality of care, and cost effectiveness (NCQA, 2018). Examples of measures include:

A. Individual care experience.
   1. Self-perceived.
   2. Productivity (disability, absenteeism).
B. Quality of life and well-being.
   1. Functional status assessments for individuals with chronic conditions should be performed regularly by the CCTM RN to determine progression/improvement of illness.
   2. Psychosocial status assessment is necessary for individuals 12 years and older. This is particularly important for individuals with chronic conditions as depression is often a comorbidity. The PHQ-2, a two-question screening for depression, the more comprehensive PHQ-9, or other screening tool for depression, should be administered routinely to determine need for further assessment or treatment of depression (Maurer, 2012).
   3. Social determinants of health, including safe housing, socioeconomic conditions, transportation options, and social support are a few of the factors that influence individual's ability to self-manage, purchase medications and supplies (NCQA, 2018).
C. Health care utilization.
   1. Readmissions at 30 days is the key measure for conditions in which readmission is preventable.
   2. Emergency department visits that are determined to meet non-emergent status are often an indicator of the individual's ability to understand what to do when the condition is worsening.
   3. Primary care visits (face-to-face and/or telephonic/telehealth).
   4. Specialist utilization.
   5. Cost of care (claims).
   6. Other resource utilization: Lab, imaging.
D. Health behaviors.
   1. Self-management.
   2. Activation or engagement (measured with a validated tool).
   3. Treatment: Adherence to the plan including medications, follow-up visits, lifestyle changes, diet modification.
   4. Behavior change that can be measured and/or observed.
   5. Preventive care: Screening and prevention.
E. Measurement of impact on population health disparities is needed to assure equitable care across racial and ethnic groups.
F. Health status indicators can be used to measure both short and long-term progress for individuals and groups against national goals. The National Center for Health Statistics lists the following health status indicators.
   1. Race/ethnicity-specific infant mortality.
   2. Total deaths.
   3. Motor vehicle crash deaths.
   4. Work-related injury deaths.
   5. Suicides.
   6. Homicides.
   7. Lung cancer deaths.

8. Female breast cancer deaths.
9. Cardiovascular diseases deaths.
10. Reported incidence of acquired immunodeficiency syndrome.
11. Reported incidence of measles.
12. Reported incidence of tuberculosis.
13. Reported incidence of primary and secondary syphilis.
14. Prevalence of low birthweight.
15. Births to adolescents.
16. Prenatal care during the first trimester.
17. Childhood poverty.
18. Proportion of persons living in countries exceeding U.S. Environmental Protection Agency standards for air quality (CDC, 2015).

G. Clinical indicators or measures can be structure, process, and outcome oriented (AHRQ, 2011).
1. Structure: The ratio of providers to individuals.
2. Process: The number of individuals with diabetes who had their hemoglobin A1C tested.
3. Outcome: The number of individuals with Hemoglobin A1C levels less than 9.

H. Displaying data using person dashboards or reports can be done in a variety of ways depending on the need, including:
1. Payer requirements.
2. Person care activities.
3. By provider.
4. By health condition.
5. Identified care gap.

VIII. Population Health and Policy Development

Health care policy development is a dynamic process influenced by legislation, governmental agencies, health care organizations, payer entities, academia, lobbyists, and public opinion. The CCTM RN must stay current with emerging trends, new legislation, and payment and reimbursement models in the provision of care design and delivery in the populations managed.

A. "Prioritizes early detection, treatment, and mitigation of, and rehabilitation following, disease among at-risk and symptomatic individuals and takes into account social determinants of health" (Bhattacharya & Bhatt, 2017, p. 384, 386).
1. Public health agencies taking on a larger role to assure outcomes at a population level (Bhattacharya & Bhatt, 2017, p. 384).
2. Emphasis on early detection.
3. Identification of vulnerable populations.
4. Treatment of persons with symptoms.
5. Supports sustainable population health policy.

B. Health care quality measures.
1. NCQA (n.d.a) Healthcare Effectiveness Data and Information Set (HEDIS) measures (http://www.ncqa.org/hedis-quality-measurement).
2. CMS 5-star quality ratings (CMS, 2018a).
3. CMS (2018b) and Centers for Medicare & Medicaid Innovation (CMMI) Accountable Care Organization models.
4. America's Health Insurance Plans (2016) and CMS Core Sets of Quality Measures.

C. Required compliance activities.
1. Occupational Safety and Health Administration (OSHA) (n.d.).
2. The Joint Commission (n.d.).
3. CMS.
4. State health department.

D. Emerging reimbursement models and federal regulations.
1. CMS, CMMI, Medicaid, and commercial payers.
2. Medicare Access and CHIP Reauthorization Act of 2015 (MACRA).
3. As we continue to transition from volume to value, more reimbursement models will be based on indicators felt to convey quality and care experience.

E. Regulations regarding electronic health record utilization and security.
1. Health Insurance Portability and Accountability Act (HIPAA) (https://www.hhs.gov/hipaa/index.html).
2. Health Information Technology for Economic and Clinical Health Act (HITECH) (https://www.healthit.gov/).
3. Agency for Healthcare Policy and Research and the National Library of Medicine (Bates, 2015).
4. Office of National Coordinator for Health Information Technology (https://www.healthit.gov/).

F. Disease certification programs and quality designations.
1. NCQA (n.d.b) Patient-Centered Medical Home recognition.
2. NCQA (n.d.c) Disease Management.
3. The Joint Commission (n.d.) Disease Management Recognition Programs.
4. American Nurses' Credentialing Center (ANCC) (n.d.) Magnet® designation for nursing excellence.

G. Persons, providers, payers, and purchasers.
1. Health Care Transformation Task Force (https://hcttf.org/).

H. State physician and nursing licensing agencies.

Chapter 10

1. Nursing scope of practice revision for expanded role.
2. Other care team members including, but not limited to, unlicensed assistive personnel scope.

I. Professional organizations.
   1. Political action committees.
   2. Advocacy and legislative efforts.

IX. **Value-Based Care and Purchasing**

Value-based health care is a model in which hospitals and physicians are paid for outcomes of care versus the quantity of care. More than 10 years ago, CMS created value-based programs that support incentive payments for the quality of care to Medicare beneficiaries (CMS, 2016). Value-based purchasing refers to the linking of financial reimbursement for performance based on agreed-upon measures of quality and cost/resource use (Damberg et al., 2014)

The original CMS value-based programs included:
- End stage renal disease.
- Hospital Value-Based Purchasing Program.
- Hospital Readmission Reduction Program.
- Value Modifier Program (also called the Physician Value-Based Modifier).
- Hospital-Acquired Conditions Reduction Program.

The CMS programs provide financial incentives to hospitals and physicians for improving care based on an approved set of *measures* and *dimensions* grouped into specific quality domains. The CMS domains include safety, clinical care, efficiency and cost reduction, individual and caregiver centeredness with experience of care/care coordination (CMS, 2016).

Pay for performance is the more common of the models for value-based purchasing and is a primary tool to support overall health care reform by focusing on incentives for improving quality (Van Herck et al., 2010). The focus of pay for performance is to improve outcomes for both the individual and the population. This may, for example, include improving the management of diabetes for an individual as well as a group or population of individuals under the care of a system/physician. Financial incentives are used by both private and public payers to drive improvement (Damberg et al., 2014).

Damberg and colleagues (2014) provide the following definitions of value-based purchasing models:

- **Pay-for-performance (P4P)** refers to a payment arrangement in which providers are rewarded (bonuses) or penalized (reductions in payments) based on meeting pre-established targets or benchmarks for measures of quality and/or efficiency.
- **Accountable Care Organization (ACO)** refers to a health care organization comprising doctors, hospitals, and other health care providers who voluntarily come together to provide coordinated care and agree to be held accountable for the overall costs and quality of care for an assigned population of individuals. The payment model ties provider reimbursements to performance on quality measures and reductions in the total cost of care. Under an ACO arrangement, providers in the ACO agree to take financial risk and are eligible for a share of the savings achieved through improved care delivery provided they achieve quality and spending targets negotiated between the ACO and the payer.
- **Bundled payments** are a method in which payments to health care providers are based on the expected costs for a clinically defined episode or bundle of related health care services. The payment arrangement includes financial and quality performance accountability for the episode of care.

A. Most P4P programs focus on clinical effectiveness through other metrics, such as safety, efficiency, access, and experience.
   1. The P4P interventions use a proportion of hospital or physician renumeration to support quality improvement to achieve results on specified quality indicators.
   2. P4P may also be used for improving clinical effectiveness, access, equity, coordination and continuity, patient centeredness, and cost effectiveness.
   3. Variables that influence P4P include program design, care setting, patient population size, payer, the nature of the health care setting, and measurement (Van Herck et al., 2010).
   4. Various models of value-based purchasing exist. These include, but are not limited to:
      a. P4P, which includes pay for quality and pay for efficiency and/or costs.
      b. Shared savings models often deployed in ACOs.
      c. Bundled payments for episodes of care (Damberg et al., 2014).

B. Current data and studies demonstrate mixed results on P4P (Asch & Werner, 2010).
   1. There is insufficient evidence that financial incentives improve performance; however, more recent studies are demonstrating improvement when program design and identification of the population are clear (Damberg et al., 2014).

2. Performance improvement is also contingent on internal alignment, clear communication to providers, the ability to measure, and available data.
3. There is a general agreement that paying for outcomes versus quantity while assuring cost effectiveness is the right direction, assuming organizations/providers can deliver value through the appropriate population health interventions (Jacobson, Isham, & Rutten, 2015).
4. Literature contains additional consensus that population outcomes associated with P4P are impacted by more than medical care. Social-economic variables and individual behavior may be just as important (Kindig, 2006).
5. Value-based purchasing relies on changes in practice patterns in order to achieve improved performance (VanLare & Conway, 2012).
6. CMS programs are primarily focused on clinical care processes, safety, and individual experience. The scope of measurement is expanding to include better health for communities, care coordination, and lower costs (VanLare & Conway, 2012).
7. Current programs in ambulatory care settings focus more on preventive care, and management of heart disease and diabetes. The focus for hospital programs is more on congestive heart failure, heart attack, pneumonia, and surgical infection prevention (Damberg et al., 2014).
8. P4P programs should include:
    a. Targets based on improvement from baseline performance.
    b. Use of both process and outcome indicators as measures.
    c. Involvement of stakeholders and clear communication to teams/providers.
    d. Uniform program design across payers.
    e. Focus on quality improvement.
    f. Distribution of incentives to the individual or team (Van Herck et al., 2010).
C. P4P programs offer tremendous opportunity for the CCTM RN.
   1. Most P4P process measures involve interventions usually deployed by RNs (e.g., hypertension control, diabetes HbA1c levels, cholesterol levels, etc.).
   2. The CCTM RN provides patient education and counseling on medical conditions in which improvement is often a function of lifestyle changes.
   3. P4P reinforces the need to assure team members function at top of licensure and that CCTM RNs and medical assistants as well as physicians have a critical role.
   4. Appropriate measurement of CCTM program interventions in chronic conditions is needed to improve performance. Both the clinical process measure must be tracked as well as the processes used by the CCTM team to achieve improvements.
   5. In one study, HbA1c levels less than 8% improved 2.3% in less than 1 year due to RN interventions in a defined population (Trehearne & McGrann, 2017-2018).
   6. CCTM RNs can be included in the financial incentives of P4P programs when the incentives are distributed at the team level and not only the individual physician level.
   7. Characteristics of high-performing physician groups.
      a. Greater engagement in care management processes.
      b. Use of order sets.
      c. Use of clinical pathways.
      d. Nursing support for quality improvement (Damberg et al., 2014).

Chapter 10

Case Study 10-1.
Exemplar – Big Data for Population Health – Fostering Accountable Care

In the U.S., the estimated cost for readmissions is $25 billion annually and readmission rates continue to rise (Datafloq, 2018). With increased emphasis on creating and strengthening ACOs, a large health system is faced with increased pressure to reduce unplanned readmissions. Historical practices of using individual risk prediction tools failed to provide sustained improvement owing in part to the two-dimensional nature of such tools. Additionally, gaps in care related to suboptimal care coordination and limited patient engagement exacerbated this growing problem. To that end, traditional methods of data collection and statistical analysis were no longer sufficient to achieve desired outcomes.

To address the larger problem of all cause readmissions, the health system leveraged the power of the existing electronic health records coupled with big data analytics. The health system was able to use hundreds of disparate clinical measures, updated multiple times per day, to develop new predictive models. Additionally, using data from multiple payer sources, trends with readmissions were identified including utilization of clinics and emergency rooms both within the system and external to the system. Merging these two data sources provided a multi-dimensional view of patient risk that allowed data analysts to identify patterns among different groups of patients and to highlight populations at risk for unplanned readmission.

Following identification of at-risk groups, the CCTM team was able to design and implement inter-professional intervention bundles to address common causes for readmission that were previously undetected using traditional methods for risk prediction. Increased precision and accuracy in identification of patients at risk ultimately led to a significant reduction in readmission rates for several high-risk populations representing the largest percentage of the health system's overall readmissions.

Case Study 10-2.
A Population Care Example

An example demonstrates how the Population Care Coordination Process might be applied. Suppose that you are working as a care coordinator in a family practice, which is a patient-centered medical home. In the analysis phase, you would review the practice's electronic health record and registry data and conclude that your asthmatic patients are your highest risk subpopulation based on the number of patients involved, the severity of disease, and frequency of utilization.

A comprehensive assessment of the asthmatic subpopulation members should include demographics, social determinants of health, ability to self-manage, severity of disease, asthma knowledge, medication adherence, asthma triggers, etc. What do the aggregated data of the subpopulation reveal in terms of patterns or commonalities? Is there evidence of adherence to established evidence-based guidelines on asthma and documentation of deviations, existing referral processes, models of care, and office practices? In the larger community, what are the existing local, state, and federal laws and other relevant factors related to the environment, health policy, community resources, school resources, educational programs, materials, or access to care of patients with asthma? The two most pressing problems identified by the team might be lack of knowledge related to asthma and lack of recommended primary care follow-up on the part of the patient.

In the planning phase, the care team might set a numerical goal for education of a 20% increase in the number of subpopulation members who were able to correctly identify their asthma triggers. A directional goal for the lack of follow-up might be that there will be an increase in the percentage of the subpopulation, who received follow-up care at the recommended time. The team might choose to implement the care plan within the electronic health record. The communication route would also be secure e-mail with phone calls for urgent concerns. The roles and responsibilities of each team member should be included.

When developing interventions for an asthmatic subpopulation, the care team should develop a list of options available to providers interacting with patients with asthma over time. In practice, all interventions related to asthma management should be included, but for this example only a sample of interventions related to the two problems will be included (see Case Study Table). The plan could include specific modifications or adjustments to each intervention that may arise as the plan is implemented for subpopulation members. If you have a large number of patients who speak Russian in your population, you might include educational materials in Russian. Another example might relate to community specifics, such as the development and dissemination of a list of local restaurants that allow smoking, so that asthmatic patients are able to avoid a known trigger.

The next step requires evaluation of the process. Change in knowledge level of patients with asthma might be evaluated with the Asthma Knowledge Questionnaire for Consumers (Kritikos, Krass, Chan, & Bosnic-Anticevich, 2005). The questionnaire could be administered prior to a specific educational intervention, then again after the intervention to assess for improvement. The results of each subpopulation members' scores should be aggregated to see how the entire subpopulation has changed. To assess improvement in the percentage of the asthma-affected subpopulation who attended scheduled follow-up appointments, the team could focus on measuring the number of patients who attended a follow-up appointment (based on documentation) divided by the total number in subpopulation who had a recommended follow-up appointment.

As mentioned previously, the process should be repeated for each patient. This is a process with which most care coordinators are familiar. In brief, care coordinators gather data on the patient, select what aspects make him or her high-risk, assess for problems and needs, plan care, implement interventions, and evaluate. Some key steps for individualization will be the assessment, care planning, and implementation. As with the population, assessment of an individual patient is a critical step. Most patients will come with more than one comorbid condition that will need to be factored into the care plan. In addition, unique circumstances need to be considered. For example, if a patient has low literacy, then educational interventions will need to be modified with materials written at appropriate literacy level or provided in their preferred learning style. In terms of care planning, the patient and family should be fully involved to ensure a patient-centered approach (Rushton, 2015).

Source: Rushton, 2015. Reprinted with permission from Wolters Kluwers Health, Inc.

Chapter 10

Case Study 10-2 Table.
Sample Asthmatic Subpopulation Interventions

Problem Addressed with Goal	Subpopulation Interventions
P: Problem	
G: Goal	

P: Knowledge deficit
G: The subpopulation will have an increase in their knowledge related to asthma.
	Literacy Assessment
	    Review of literacy assessment tools
	    Select health literacy tool for use in practice
	Assessment of asthma knowledge
	    Review options for asthma knowledge assessment
	    Select option to use
	Assessment of available educational programs
	Review of available evidence
	Evidence-based programs available through
	    Professional organizations
	    Government
	    Local
	Implementation of selected formal asthma education program including disease process, symptoms, triggers, management, medications, nebulizers, peak flow meters, action plans
	Delivery formats
	    One on one
	    Group education courses
	    Written materials
	    Videos
	    Referral to existing community educational program

P: Lack of follow-up
G: The percentage of the subpopulation who attends scheduled follow-up appointments will increase.
	Community resource referral
	    Health Insurance Portability and Accountability Act (HIPAA) approved process
	    School programs if member is a student
	Assessment of barriers
	    Unable to get off work to get to appointment
	    Transportation
	    Cost
	    Forgetting appointments
	Redesign office practices
	    Create a formal procedure for addressing follow-up
	    Extend hours
	    Reminder phone calls
	Social work consult
	    Transportation arrangements (make a list of options)
	    Insurance (Department of Social Services Referral when appropriate; review of benefits)
	    Childcare
	    Social determinants

Source: Rushton, 2015. Reprinted with permission from Wolters Kluwers Health, Inc.

Table 10-3.
Population Health Management: Knowledge, Skills, and Attitudes for Competency

Knowledge	Skills	Attitudes	Sources
Person/Population-Centered Care			
Analyze and integrate multiple dimensions of person-centered care and the care needs of identified populations: • Individual/family/community preferences, values • Coordination and integration of care • Information, communication, and education • Physical comfort and emotional support • Involvement of family and friends • Transition and continuity	Elicit individual values, preferences, and expressed needs as part of clinical interview, diagnosis, implementation of care plan, and evaluation of care. Communicate individual and group values, preferences, and expressed needs to other members of health care team. Provide person-centered care with sensitivity, empathy, and respect for the diversity of human experience.	Value seeing health care situations "through patients' eyes." Respect and encourage individual expression of patient values, preferences, and expressed needs. Honor learning opportunities with individuals and populations who represent all aspects of human diversity. Seek to understand one's personally held attitudes about working with individuals from different ethnic, cultural, and social backgrounds.	Cronenwett et al., 2007
Analyze how diverse cultural, ethnic, spiritual, and social backgrounds of both individuals and populations function as sources of individual, family, and community values. Analyze social, political, economic, and historical dimensions of individual care processes and the implications for person-centered care and the care of populations.	Ensure the systems within which one practices support person-centered care for individuals and populations whose values differ from the majority or one's own.	Willingly support person-centered care for individuals and groups whose values differ from own.	Cronenwett et al., 2009
Analyze ethical and legal implications of caring for populations of individuals. Describe the limits and boundaries of therapeutic person-centered care.	Respect the boundaries of therapeutic relationships. Acknowledge the tension that may exist between individuals and population preferences and organizational and professional responsibilities for ethical care. Facilitate informed patient consent for care.	Value shared decision making with empowered individuals, families, and communities even when conflicts occur.	Cronenwett et al., 2007 Cronenwett et al., 2009

continued on next page

**Table 10-3. (continued)
Population Health Management: Knowledge, Skills, and Attitudes for Competency**

Knowledge	Skills	Attitudes	Sources
Person/Population-Centered Care (continued)			
Analyze strategies that empower individuals, families, or communities in all aspects of the health care process. Analyze reasons for common barriers to active involvement of individuals, families, and groups in their own health care processes.	Engage individuals, designated surrogates, or groups in active partnerships along the health-illness continuum.	Respect individual preferences for degree of active engagement in care process. Honor active partnerships with individuals, designated surrogates or groups in planning, implementation, and evaluation of care.	Cronenwett et al., 2007
Analyze features of physical facilities that support or pose barriers to person-centered care.	Create or change organizational cultures so that individual, family, and community preferences are assessed and supported.	Respect individual's right to access personal health records.	Cronenwett et al., 2009
	Assess level of individual's decisional conflict and provide access to resources.		Cronenwett et al., 2007
	Eliminate barriers to presence of families and other designated surrogates based on individual preferences.	Value system changes that support person-centered and population-based care.	Cronenwett et al., 2009
Analyze principles of consensus building and conflict resolution.	Communicate care provided and needed at each transition in care.	Value continuous improvement of own communication and conflict-resolution skills.	Cronenwett et al., 2007
Describe nursing's role in assuring coordination, integration, and continuity of care. Integrate principles of effective communication with knowledge of quality and safety competencies.	Continuously analyze and improve own level of communication skill in encounters with individuals, families, and teams. Provide leadership in building consensus or resolving conflict in the context of a person's care.	Value consensus.	Cronenwett et al., 2009
"Describe the characteristics of a population-based health problem (e.g., health care equity, social determinants, and environmental barriers)."	Identify population characteristics that influence the effectiveness of care delivery, such as age, demographics, ethnicity, financial status, psychosocial challenges.	Appreciate the impact of social determinants on individual engagement in self-care and outcomes of care interventions.	Council on Linkages Between Academia and Public Health Practice, 2014, p. 7 Jessie, Johnson, & Trehearne, 2014

continued on next page

Table 10-3. (continued)
Population Health Management: Knowledge, Skills, and Attitudes for Competency

Knowledge	Skills	Attitudes	Sources
Person/Population-Centered Care (continued)			
"Identify the health literacy of populations served."	Demonstrate the ability to determine levels of individual and population health literacy. Ensure sensitivity to unique characteristics of populations in the evaluation of health literacy.	Value the diversity in population education levels, experiences, and backgrounds that influence health literacy.	Council on Linkages Between Academia and Public Health Practice, 2014, p. 11 Jessie et al., 2014
"Incorporate strategies for interacting with persons from diverse backgrounds (e.g., cultural, socioeconomic, educational, racial, gender, age, ethnic, sexual orientation, professional, religious affiliation, mental and physical capabilities)."	"Describe the role of cultural, social, and behavioral factors in the accessibility, availability, acceptability, and delivery of health care." "Respond to diverse needs that are the result of cultural differences."	Value the diversity of individuals and populations. Seek to understand one's personally held attitudes about working with individuals from different ethnic, cultural, and social backgrounds.	Council on Linkages Between Academia and Public Health Practice, 2014, p. 12 Jessie et al., 2014
Teamwork and Collaboration			
Analyze own strengths, limitations, and values as a member of a team. Analyze impact of own nursing practice role and its contributions to team functioning.	Demonstrate awareness of own strengths and limitations as a team member. Continuously plan for improvement in use of self in effective team development and functioning.	Acknowledge own contributions to effective or ineffective team functioning.	Cronenwett et al., 2007 Cronenwett et al., 2009
Analyze strategies for identifying and managing overlaps in team member roles and accountabilities.	Function competently within own scope of practice as a member of the health care team. Solicit input from other team members to improve individual, as well as team, performance. Assume role of team member or leader based on the situation. Guide the team in managing areas of overlap in team member functioning.	Respect the unique attributes that members bring to a team, including variation in professional orientations, competencies, and accountabilities. Respect the centrality of the patient/family as core members of any health care team.	Cronenwett et al., 2007 Cronenwett et al., 2009

continued on next page

Table 10-3. (continued)
Population Health Management: Knowledge, Skills, and Attitudes for Competency

Knowledge	Skills	Attitudes	Sources
Teamwork and Collaboration (continued)			
"Describe the process of team development and practices of effective teams." "Share accountability with other professions, patients, and communities for outcomes relevant to prevention and health care." "Apply leadership practices that support collaborative practice and team effectiveness."	Empower "contributions of others who play a role in helping patients/ families achieve health goals."		Interprofessional Education Collaborative (IPEC), 2016, p. 16
		Value the contributions of all members of the care team in population care planning and health care management.	Jessie et al., 2014
Analyze strategies that influence the ability to initiate and sustain effective partnerships with members of nursing and interprofessional teams. Analyze impact of cultural diversity on team functioning. Engage diverse health care professionals who complement one's own professional expertise, as well as associated resources, to develop strategies to meet specific patient care needs.	Communicate with team members, adapting own style of communicating to needs of the team and situation.		Cronenwett et al., 2007
	Initiate and sustain effective health care teams.	Appreciate importance of interprofessional collaboration. Value collaboration with nurses and other members of the nursing team.	Cronenwett et al., 2009
	Communicate respect for team member competence in communication.	Value different styles of communication.	Cronenwett et al., 2007 Cronenwett et al., 2009

continued on next page

Table 10-3. (continued)
Population Health Management: Knowledge, Skills, and Attitudes for Competency

Knowledge	Skills	Attitudes	Sources
Teamwork and Collaboration (continued)			
"Recognizes relationships that are affecting health in a community (e.g., relationships among health departments, hospitals, community health centers, primary care providers, schools, community-based organizations, and other types of organizations)."			Council on Linkages Between Academia and Public Health Practice, 2014, p. 15
"Facilitates communication among individuals, groups, and organizations."			Council on Linkages Between Academia and Public Health Practice, 2014, p. 12
"Communicate information with patients, families, and health care team members in a form that is understandable, avoiding discipline-specific terminology when possible."	"Engage self and others to constructively manage disagreements about values, roles, goals, and actions that arise among health care professionals and with patients, families, and community members."		IPEC, 2016, p. 13
Describe examples of the impact of team functioning on safety and quality of care.	Follow communication practices that minimize risks associated with hand-offs among providers and across transitions in care.	Appreciate the risks associated with hand-offs among providers and across transitions in care.	Cronenwett et al., 2007
	Choose communication styles that diminish the risks associated with authority gradients among team members.		
	Initiate actions to resolve conflict.		
	Assert own position/perspective and supporting evidence in discussions about an individual's care.		
	Act with integrity, consistency, and respect for differing views.		
		Value the solutions obtained through systematic, interprofessional collaborative efforts.	Cronenwett et al., 2009
		Appreciate and value the effectiveness of diverse communication techniques.	Jessie et al., 2014

continued on next page

Table 10-3. (continued)
Population Health Management: Knowledge, Skills, and Attitudes for Competency

Knowledge	Skills	Attitudes	Sources
Teamwork and Collaboration (continued)			
Identify system barriers and facilitators of effective team functioning. Examine strategies for improving systems to support team functioning.			Cronenwett et al., 2007
	Lead or participate in the design and implementation of systems that support effective teamwork. Engage in state and national policy initiatives aimed at improving teamwork and collaboration.	Value the influence of system solutions in achieving team functioning.	Cronenwett et al., 2009
	"Use the full scope of knowledge, skills, and abilities of professionals from health and other fields to provide care that is safe, timely, efficient, effective, and equitable."		IPEC, 2016, p. 12
Evidence-Based Practice			
Demonstrate knowledge of basic scientific methods and processes. Describe evidence-based practice to include the components of research evidence, clinical expertise, and individual/family values.		Appreciate strengths and weaknesses of scientific bases for practice. Value the need for ethical conduct of research and quality improvement.	Cronenwett et al., 2007
	Use health research methods and processes, alone or in partnership with scientists, to generate new knowledge for practice.	Value all components of evidence-based practice.	Cronenwett et al., 2009
	Base evidence-based interventions on individualized care plan based on individual/population values and nursing expertise.		Jessie et al., 2014
Identify efficient and effective search strategies to locate reliable sources of evidence.	Employ efficient and effective search strategies to answer focused clinical questions.	Value development of search skills for locating evidence for best practice.	Cronenwett et al., 2009

continued on next page

Table 10-3. (continued)
Population Health Management: Knowledge, Skills, and Attitudes for Competency

Knowledge	Skills	Attitudes	Sources
Evidence-Based Practice (continued)			
Differentiate clinical opinion for research and evidence and identify sources for locating evidence-based reports and clinical practice guidelines.	Locate evidence-based reports and clinical practice guidelines.	Appreciate the importance of regularly reading professional journals and attending educational conferences.	Cronenwett et al., 2007
Summarize current evidence regarding major diagnostic and treatment actions within the practice specialty.	Exhibit contemporary knowledge of best evidence related to practice specialty.	Value knowing the evidence-base for practice specialty.	Cronenwett et al., 2009
Determine evidence gaps within the practice specialty.	Promote research agenda for evidence that is needed in practice specialty.	Value public policies that support evidence-based practice.	
	Initiate changes in approaches to care when new evidence warrants evaluation of other options for improving outcomes or decreasing adverse events.		
		Acknowledge own limitations in knowledge and clinical expertise before determining when to deviate from evidence-based best practices.	Cronenwett et al., 2007
		Value the need for continuous improvement in clinical practice based on new knowledge.	
Analyze how the strength of available evidence influences the provision of care (assessment, diagnosis, treatment, and evaluation).	Develop guidelines for clinical decision-making regarding departure from established protocols/ standards of care.		Cronenwett et al., 2009
Evaluate organizational cultures and structures that promote evidence-based practice.	Participate in designing systems that support evidence-based practice.		

continued on next page

Table 10-3. (continued)
Population Health Management: Knowledge, Skills, and Attitudes for Competency

Knowledge	Skills	Attitudes	Sources
Quality Improvement			
Describe strategies for improving outcomes of care for identified populations.	Use a variety of sources of information to review outcomes of care and identify potential areas for improvement. Propose appropriate goals for quality improvement activities.		Cronenwett et al., 2009
Analyze the impact of context and social determinants (e.g., access, cost, team functioning, age, demographics) on improvement efforts.		Appreciate that continuous quality improvement is an essential role of the CCTM RN.	Jessie et al., 2014
Analyze ethical issues associated with quality improvement.	Assure ethical oversight of quality improvement projects.	Value the need for ethical conduct of quality improvement.	Cronenwett et al., 2009
	Use databases as sources of information for improving an individual's care.	Appreciate the importance of data as a tool to measure and/or estimate the quality of care.	Cronenwett et al., 2009
Understand the benefits and limitations of quality improvement data sources and measurement.	Select and use population-relevant benchmarks.		Jessie et al., 2014
Explain common causes of variation in outcomes.	Select and use tools (such as control charts and run charts) that are helpful for understanding variation. Identify gaps between local and best practice.	Appreciate how unexpected variation affects outcomes of care processes.	Cronenwett et al., 2009

continued on next page

Table 10-3. (continued)
Population Health Management: Knowledge, Skills, and Attitudes for Competency

Knowledge	Skills	Attitudes	Sources
Quality Improvement (continued)			
	Use measures to evaluate the effect of change. Design, implement, and evaluate tests of change in daily work (using an experiential learning method such as Plan-Do-Study-Act).	Appreciate the value of what individuals and teams can to do to improve care.	Cronenwett et al., 2007
Analyze the differences between micro-system and macro-system change. Understand principles of change management. Analyze the strengths and limitations of common quality improvement methods.	Use principles of change management to implement and evaluate care processes at the micro-system level. Align the aims, measures, and changes involved in improving care.	Value local systems improvement (in individual practice, team practice on a unit, or in the macro-system) and its role in professional job satisfaction. Appreciate that all improvement is change but not all change is improvement.	Cronenwett et al., 2009
Safety			
Describe the benefits and limitations of selected safety-enhancing technologies (health maintenance alerts, individual reminder systems, computer provider order entry, and electronic prescribing).		Value the contributions of standardization and reliability to safety.	Cronenwett et al., 2007
Describe human factors and other basic safety design principles as well as commonly used unsafe practices (such as work-arounds, lack of consistent communication across care delivery settings, and in complete follow-up).	Participate in the design, promotion, and effective use of technology and standardized practices that support safety and quality. Participate as a team member to design, promote, and model effective use of strategies to reduce risk of harm to self and others. Promote a practice culture conducive to highly reliable processes. Utilize automated reminder systems to prompt future actions required.	Appreciate the importance of safety consciousness both in the provision of care and in the work environment.	Cronenwett et al., 2009

continued on next page

Table 10-3. (continued)
Population Health Management: Knowledge, Skills, and Attitudes for Competency

Knowledge	Skills	Attitudes	Sources
Safety (continued)			
Describe factors that create a just culture and culture of safety.	Communicate observations or concerns related to hazards and errors to individuals, families, and the health care team.	Value own role in reporting and preventing errors.	Cronenwett et al., 2007
Describe best practices that promote individual and provider safety in the practice specialty.		Value systems approaches to improving individual safety in lieu of blaming individuals.	Cronenwett et al., 2009
Identify categories of potential errors and hazards in care delivery.	Participate in identifying and correcting system failures and hazards in care.	Value the use of organizational error-reporting systems.	
Identify best practices for organizational responses to error.	Engage in system-focused problem solving.	Value an organizational just culture.	Jessie et al., 2014
Informatics			
Evaluate the strengths and weaknesses of information systems used in individual care and population management.	Communicate the integral role of information technology in nurses' work. Assist team members to adopt information technology by piloting and evaluating proposed workflows and technologies. Demonstrate the appropriate use of electronic health records and technology in the care of individuals and populations.	Value the use of information and communication technologies in individual, population care, and transition management.	Cronenwett et al., 2009 Jessie et al., 2014
	Promote access to patient care information through use of standardized documentation tools for all professionals who provide care to individuals and populations. Serve as a resource for how to document nursing care at basic and advanced levels. Develop safeguards for protected health information.	Appreciate the need for consensus and collaboration in developing systems to manage information for individual and population-based care. Value the confidentiality and security of all individual records.	Cronenwett et al., 2007

continued on next page

Table 10-3. (continued)
Population Health Management: Knowledge, Skills, and Attitudes for Competency

Knowledge	Skills	Attitudes	Sources
Informatics (continued)			
"Identify essential information that must be available in a common database to support patient and population care delivery." Evaluate benefits and limitations of different communication technologies and their impact on safety, quality, and effective care management.	Champion communication technologies that support clinical decision making, error prevention, care coordination, and protection of a person's privacy.		Cronenwett et al., 2009
Demonstrate understanding of large data sets including how to manage and manipulate data. Identify a variety of data management tools (including Excel).	Data professionals need to demonstrate the ability to interpret data through both visualization and use of electronic analytics tools.	Appreciate the importance of thinking beyond traditional data analysis.	Verma, 2018
Identify the health status of populations and their related determinants of health and illness using electronic decision-support tools (e.g., factors contributing to health promotion and disease prevention; the quality, availability, and use of health services).			Council on Linkages Between Academia and Public Health Practice, 2014
	Use basic statistical analysis and quality improvement techniques to review population characteristics, variation, health risks.	Value the use of decision-support tools in identifying individuals and populations for interventions, preventive services, chronic disease management, and health care delivery design.	Jessie et al., 2014 NCQA, 2018

continued on next page

Table 10-3. (continued)
Population Health Management: Knowledge, Skills, and Attitudes for Competency

Knowledge	Skills	Attitudes	Sources
Informatics (continued)			
	Using decision-support tools, demonstrate the ability to identify factors that facilitate or impede care coordination at both a systems and individual level depending on the complexity of specific circumstances (resources available, payment structure, person complexity, capacity).		
"Uses information technology in accessing, collecting, analyzing, using, maintaining, and disseminating data and information." Use electronic reporting to identify variables that measure public health conditions, gaps in care.	Navigate the electronic health record. Seek education about how information is managed in care settings before providing care. Apply technology and information management tools to support safe processes of care. Respond appropriately to clinical decision-making supports and alerts. Use information management tools to monitor outcomes of care processes. Use high-quality electronic sources of health care information	Value technologies that support clinical decision making, error prevention, and care coordination. Appreciate the necessity for all health professionals to seek lifelong, continuous learning of information technology skills. Value nurses' involvement in design, selection, implementation, and evaluation of information technologies to support an individual's care.	Cronenwett et al., 2007 Council on Linkages Between Academia and Public Health Practice, 2014, p. 5 Jessie et al., 2014 NCQA, 2018

continued on next page

Table 10-3. (continued)
Population Health Management: Knowledge, Skills, and Attitudes for Competency

Knowledge	Skills	Attitudes	Sources
Informatics (continued)			
Choose effective communication tools and techniques, including information systems and communication technologies, to facilitate discussions and interactions that enhance team function.			

Source Notes: Cronenwett et al. (2007). *Nursing Outlook, 55*(3), 122-131. Reprinted with permission from Elsevier. Cronenwett et al. (2009). *Nursing Outlook, 57*(6), 338-348. Reprinted with permission from the author.

Editors' Note: Population Health Management is so new there are not always full KSA statements; therefore, the chapter authors, as experts, developed needed skills and attitudes.

Chapter 10

References

Agency for Healthcare Research and Quality (AHRQ). (2011). *Types of health care quality measures.* Retrieved from http://www.ahrq.gov/professionals/quality-patient-safety/talkingquality/create/types.html

American Academy of Ambulatory Care Nursing (AAACN). (2016). *Scope and standards of practice for registered nurses in care coordination and transition management.* Pitman, NJ: Author.

American Academy of Pediatrics. (2019). *Bright Futures.* Retrieved from https://brightfutures.aap.org/Pages/default.aspx

American Association of Colleges of Nursing (AACN) QSEN Education Consortium. (2012). *Graduate-level QSEN competencies: Knowledge, skills and attitudes.* Retrieved from https://www.aacnnursing.org/Portals/42/AcademicNursing/CurriculumGuidelines/Graduate-QSEN-Competencies.pdf

American Nurses Association (ANA). (2015). *Nursing informatics: Scope and standards of practice* (2nd ed.). Silver Spring, MD: Author.

American Nurses' Credentialing Center (ANCC). (n.d.). *ANCC Magnet Recognition Program®.* Retrieved from https://www.nursingworld.org/organizational-programs/magnet/

American Organization of Nurse Executives (AONE). (2015). *Nurse executive competencies: Population health.* Retrieved from http://www.aone.org/resources/population-health-competencies.pdf

America's Health Insurance Plans. (2016). *AHIP, CMS collaborative announces core sets of quality measures.* (2017). Retrieved from https://www.ahip.org/ahip-cms-collaborative-announces-core-sets-of-quality-measures/

Andreu-Perez, J., Poon, C.C.Y., Merrifield, R.D., Wong, S.T.C., & Yang, G.Z. (2015). Big data for health. *IEEE Journal of Biomedical and Health Informatics, 19*(4), 1193-1208. doi:10.1109/JBHI.2015.2450362

Asch, D.A., & Werner, R.M. (2010). Paying for performance in population health: Lessons from health care settings. *Preventing Chronic Disease, 7*(5), A98. Retrieved from https://www.ncbi.nlm.nih.gov/pmc/articles/PMC2938414/

Baehr, A., Holland, T., Biala, K., Margolis, G.S., Wiebe, D.J. & Carr, B.G. (2016). Describing total population health: A review and critique of existing units. *Population Health Management, 19*(5), 306-314.

Bates, D.W. (2015). Health information technology and care coordination: The next big opportunity for informatics? *Yearbook of Medical Informatics, 10*(1), 11-14. doi:10.15265/iy-2015-020

Bates, D.W., Saria, S., Ohno-Machado, L., Shah, A., & Escobar, G. (2014). Big data in health care: Using analytics to identify and manage high-risk and high-cost patients. *Health Affairs, 33*(7), 1123-1131. doi:10.1377/hlthaff.2014.0041

Bauer, L., & Bodenheimer, T. (2017). Expanded roles of registered nurses in primary care delivery of the future. *Nursing Outlook, 65*(5), 624-632. doi:10.1016/j.outlook.2017.03.011

Bhattacharya, D., & Bhatt, J. (2017). Seven foundational principles of population health policy. *Population Health Management, 20*(5), 383-388. doi:10.1089/pop.2016.0148

Biederman, D.J., Gamble, J.C., Wilson, S., Duff, L.K., Bristow, E., & Wiederhoeft, L.M. (2016). Transitional care for homeless persons: An opportunity for nursing leadership, innovation, and creativity. *Creative Nursing, 22*(2), 76-81. doi:10.1891/1078-4535.22.2.76

Bodenheimer, T., Ghorob, A.M., & Margolius, D. (2015*).* Panel management: Focus on providing proactive, preventive care to improve the health of your patients. Retrieved from https://www.stepsforward.org/modules/panel-management#downloadable

Bodenheimer, T., Ghorob, A., Willard-Grace, R., & Grumbach, K. (2014). The 10 building blocks of high-performing primary care. *The Annals of Family Medicine, 12*(2), 166-171. doi:10.1370/afm.1616

Bresnick, J. (2016). Defining the basics of healthcare big data warehouse. *HIT Infrastructure.* Retrieved from https://hitinfrastructure.com/news/defining-the-basics-of-the-healthcare-big-data-warehouse

Centers for Disease Control and Prevention (CDC). (2015). *Healthy People 2000: Health status indicators.* https://www.cdc.gov/nchs/healthy_people/hp2000/hp2000_indicators.htm

Centers for Disease Control & Prevention (CDC). (2018). *Immunization schedules.* Retrieved from https://www.cdc.gov/vaccines/schedules/index.html

Centers for Medicare & Medicaid Services (CMS). (2016). *Transitional care management services.* Retrieved from https://www.cms.gov/Outreach-and-Education/Medicare-Learning-Network-MLN/MLNProducts/Downloads/Transitional-Care-Management-Services-Fact-Sheet-ICN908628.pdf

Centers for Medicare & Medicaid Services (CMS). (2018a). *Five-star quality rating system.* Retrieved from https://www.cms.gov/medicare/provider-enrollment-and-certification/certificationandcomplianc/fsqrs.html

Centers for Medicare & Medicaid Services (CMS). (2018b*).* *Accountable care organizations.* Retrieved from https://www.cms.gov/Medicare/Medicare-Fee-for-Service-Payment/ACO/index.html

Coleman, K., Austin, B.T., Brach, C., & Wagner, E.H. (2009). Evidence on the chronic care model in the new millennium: Thus far, the evidence on the chronic care model is encouraging, but we need better tools to help practices improve their systems. *Health Affairs (Project Hope), 28*(1), 75-85. doi:10.1377/hlthaff.28.1.75

Council on Linkages Between Academia and Public Health Practice. (2014). *Core competencies for public health professionals.* Retrieved from www.phf.org/programs/corecompetencies/Pages/About_the_Core_Competencies_for_Public_Health_Professionals.aspx

Cronenwett, L., Sherwood, G., Barnsterner, J., Disch, J., Johnson, J., Mitchell, P., ... Warren, J. (2007). Quality and safety education for nurses. *Nursing Outlook, 55*(3), 122-131.

Cronenwett, L., Sherwood, G., Pohl, J., Barnsteiner, J., Moore, S., Sullivan, D.T., ... Warren, J. (2009). Quality and safety education for advanced nursing practice. *Nursing Outlook, 57*(6), 338-348.

Damberg, C.L., Sorbero, M.E., Lovejoy, S.L., Marstaff, G.R., Raaen, L., & Mandel, D. (2014). Measuring success in health care value-based purchasing programs. Findings from an environmental scan, literature review, and expert panel discussion. *Rand Health Quarterly, 4*(3), 9.

Datafloq. (2018). *Could big data reduce hospital readmission rates?* Retrieved from https://datafloq.com/read/could-big-data-reduce-hospital-readmission-rates/2540

Demiris, G., & Kneale, L. (2015). Informatics systems and tools to facilitate patient-centered care coordination. *Yearbook of Medical Informatics, 10*(1), 15-21. doi:10.15265/iy-2015-003

El Morr, C., Ginsburg, L., Nam, S., & Woollard, S. (2017). Assessing the performance of a modified LACE index (LACE-rt) to predict unplanned readmission after discharge in a community teaching hospital. *Interactive Journal of Medical Research, 6*(1), e2. doi:10.2196/ijmr.7183

Fawcett, J., & Ellenbecker, C.H. (2015). A proposed conceptual model of nursing and population health. *Nursing Outlook, 63*(3), 288-298. doi:10.1016/j.outlook.2015.01.009

Goldstein, B.A., Navar, A.M., Pencina, M.J., & Ionnidis, J.P. (2017). Opportunities and challenges in developing risk prediction models with electronic health records data: A systematic review. *Journal of the American Medical Informatics Association, 24*(1), 198-208.

Haas, S.A., Vlasses, F., & Havey, J. (2016). Developing staffing models to support population health management and quality outcomes in ambulatory care settings. *Nursing Economic$, 34*(3), 126-133.

Healthcare Information and Management Systems Society (HIMSS). (2014). *Health informatics defined.* Retrieved from https://www.himss.org/health-informatics-defined

Healthcare Information and Management Systems Society (HIMSS). (2015). *What is nursing informatics?* Retrieved from https://www.himss.org/what-nursing-informatics

Healthcare Information and Management Systems Society (HIMSS). (n.d.). *Population health.* Retrieved from https://www.himss.org/population-health

Healthcare Informatics. (2016). *A roadmap for population health management*. Retrieved from http://ihealthtran.hs-sites.com/a-roadmap-for-population-health-management

Health Catalyst. (2016). *Care management: A critical component of effective population health management*. Retrieved from https://www.healthcatalyst.com/success_stories/care-management-program

Hibbard, J., Greene, J., Sacks, R., Overton, V., & Parrotta, C. (2017). Improving population health management strategies: Identifying patients who are more likely to be users of avoidable costly care and those more likely to develop a new chronic disease. *Health Services Research, 52*(4). 1297-1309. doi:10.1111/1475-6773.12545

Higgins, T., Larson, E., & Schnall, R. (2017). Unraveling the meaning of patient engagement: A concept analysis. *Patient Education and Counseling, 100*(1), 30-36. doi:10.1016/j.pec.2016.09.002

Hodach, R., Grundy, P., Jain, A., Weiner, M., & Handmaker, K.E. (2016). *Provider-led population health management: Key strategies for health care in the cognitive era* (2nd ed.). Indianapolis, IN: John Wiley & Sons, Inc.

Hu, H., Galea, S., Rosella, L., & Henry, D. (2017). Big data and population health: Focusing on the health impacts of the social, physical, and economic environment. *Epidemiology, 28*(7), 759-762. doi:10.1097/EDE.0000000000000711

Institute of Medicine, Board on Population Health Practice, & Roundtable on Population Health Improvement. (2014). *Population health implications of the Affordable Care Act*. Washington, DC: The National Academies Press.

Interprofessional Education Collaborative (IPEC). (2016). *Core competencies for interprofessional collaborative practice*. Retrieved from https://www.aacom.org/docs/default-source/insideome/ccrpt05-10-11.pdf?sfvrsn=77937f97_2

Jacobson, R.M., Isham, G.J. & Rutten, L.J.F. (2015). Population health as a means for health care organizations to deliver value. *Mayo Clinic Proceedings, 90*(11), 1465-1470.

Jessie, A.T., Johnson, S.A., & Trehearne, B.E. (2014). Population health management. In S.A. Haas, B.A. Swan, & T.S. Haynes (Eds.), *Care coordination and transition management core curriculum* (pp. 113-140). Pitman, NJ: American Academy of Ambulatory Care Nursing.

Kim, C.S., & Flanders, S A. (2013). In the clinic: Transitions of care. *Annals of Internal Medicine, 158*(5, Pt. 1); ITC3-1. doi:10.7323/0003-4819-158-5-20130305-01003

Kindig, D., & Stoddart, G. (2003). What is population health? *American Journal of Public Health, 93*(3), 380-383. doi:10.2105/AJPH.93.3.380

Kindig, D.A. (2006). A pay-for-population health performance system. *JAMA. 296*(21), 2611-2613. doi:10.1001/jama.296.21.2611

Kritikos, V., Krass, I., Chan, H.S., & Bosnic-Anticevich, S.Z. (2005). The validity and reliability of two asthma knowledge questionnaires. *The Journal of Asthma, 42*(9), 795-801.

Krumholz, H.M. (2014). Big data and new knowledge in medicine: The thinking, training, and tools needed for a learning health system. *Health Affairs, 33*(7), 1163-1170. doi:10.1377/hlthaff.2014.0053

Kruse, C.S., Goswamy, R., Raval, Y., & Marawi, S. (2016). Challenges and opportunities of big data in health care: A systematic review. *JMIR Medical Informatics, 4*(4), e38. doi:10.2196/medinform.5359

Maurer, D. (2012). Screening for depression. *American Family Physician, 85*(2), 139-144. Retrieved from https://www.aafp.org/afp/2012/0115/p139.html

McWilliams, J.M., Chernew, M.E., & Landon, B.E. (2017). Medicare ACO Program savings not tied to preventable hospitalizations or concentrated among high-risk patients. *Health Affairs, 36*(12), 2085-2093. doi:10.1377/hlthaff.2017.0814

Mullins, A., Mooney, J., & Fowler, R. (2013). The benefits of using care coordinators in primary care: A case study. *Family Practice Management, 20*(6), 18-21.

National Advisory Council on Nursing Education and Practice (NACNEP). (2016). *Preparing nurses for new roles in population health management*. Retrieved from https://www.hrsa.gov/advisorycommittees/bhpradvisory/nacnep/Reports/fourteenthreport.pdf

National Committee for Quality Assurance (NCQA). (2018). *Population Health Management Resource Guide*. Retrieved from: http://www.ncqa.org/programs/accreditation/health-plan-hp/population-health-management-resource-guide

National Committee for Quality Assurance (NCQA). (n.d.a). *HEDIS and performance measurement*. Retrieved from http://www.ncqa.org/hedis-quality-measurement

National Committee for Quality Assurance (NCQA). (n.d.b). *Patient-centered medical home (PCMH)*. Retrieved from http://www.ncqa.org/programs/recognition/practices/patient-centered-medical-home-pcmh

National Committee for Quality Assurance (NCQA). (n.d.c). *Disease management*. Retrieved from https://www.ncqa.org/programs/health-plans/disease-management-dm/

Occupational Safety and Health Administration (OSHA). (n.d.). *Online OSHA training*. Retrieved from https://www.osha.com/

Pabo, E. (2018). *Is team-based care the key to successful population management?* Retrieved from http://www.ihi.org/communities/blogs/is-team-based-care-the-key-to-successful-population-management

Population Health Alliance. (2017). *PHA framework*. Retrieved from https://populationhealthalliance.org/research/understanding-population-health/

QSEN Institute. (2014). *QSEN competencies*. Retrieved from http://qsen.org/competencies/pre-licensure-ksas.

Raghupathi, W., & Raghupathi, V. (2014). Big data analytics in healthcare: Promise and potential. *Health Information Science and Systems, 2*(3). doi:10.1186/2047-2501-2-3

Reddy, A., Sessums, L., Gupta, R., Jin, J., Day, T., Finke, B., & Bitton, A. (2017). Risk stratification methods and provision of care management services in comprehensive primary care initiative practices. *Annals of Family Medicine, 15*(5), 451-454. doi:10.1370/afm.2124

Rennke, S., & Ranji, S.R. (2015). Transitional care strategies from hospital to home: A review for the neurohospitalist. *The Neurohospitalist, 5*(1), 35-42. doi:10.1177/1941874414540683

Reynolds, A., Rubens, J., King, R., & Machado, P. (2016). *Technology and engagement: How digital tools are reshaping population health*. Retrieved from https://populationhealthalliance.org/technology-and-engagement-how-digital-tools-are-reshaping-population-health/

Robert Wood Johnson Foundation. (2017). *Catalysts for change: Harnessing the power of nurses to build population health in the 21st century*. Retrieved from https://www.rwjf.org/en/library/research/2017/09/catalysts-for-change--harnessing-the-power-of-nurses-to-build-population-health.html

Rushton, S. (2015). The population care coordination process. *Professional Case Management, 20*(5), 230-238.

Shaljian, M., & Nielsen, M. (2013). *Managing populations, maximizing technology: Population health management in the medical neighborhood*. Retrieved from https://www.pcpcc.org/resource/managing-populations-maximizing-technology

Society of Hospital Medicine. (2013). *Project BOOST implementation guide* (2nd ed.). Retrieved from www.hospitalmedicine.org/BOOST

Sodihardjo-Yuen, F., van Dijk, L., Wensing, M., De Smet, P.A., & Teichert, M. (2017). Use of pharmacy dispensing data to measure adherence and identify nonadherence with oral hypoglycemic agents. *European Journal of Clinical Pharmacology, 73*(2), 205-213. doi:10.1007/s00228-016-2149-3

Steichen, O., & Gregg, W. (2015). Health information technology coordination to support patient-centered care coordination. *Yearbook of Medical Informatics, 10*(1), 34-37. doi:10.15265/iy-2015-027

Stellefson, M., Dipnarine, K., & Stopka, C. (2013). The chronic care model and diabetes management in US primary care settings: A systematic review. *Preventing Chronic Disease, 10*, E26. doi:10.5888/pcd10.120180

Storfjell, J.J., Winslow, B.W., & Saunders, J.S.D. (2017). *Catalysts for change: Harnessing the power of nurses to build population health in the 21st century*. Retrieved from https://www.rwjf.org/content/dam/farm/reports/reports/2017/rwjf440276

Struijs, J.N., Drewes, H.W., Heijink, R., & Baan, C.A. (2015). How to evaluate population management? Transforming the Care Continuum Alliance population health guide toward a broadly applicable analytical framework. *Health Policy, 119*(4), 522-529. doi:10.1016/j.healthpol.2014.12.003

Swarthout, M., & Bishop, M.A. (2017). Population health management: Review of concepts and definitions. *American Journal of Health-System Pharmacy, 74*(18), 1405-1411.

The Advisory Board. (2014). *Three steps to prioritize population health interventions.* Retrieved from https://www.advisory.com/research/health-care-advisory-board/resources/2014/posters/three-steps-to-prioritize-population-health-interventions

The Joint Commission. (n.d.). *Types of disease-specific care programs certified.* Retrieved from https://www.jointcommission.org/certification/diseasespecific_care_programs.aspx

Trehearne, B. & McGrann, G. (2017-2018). *Measuring the impact of RN interventions as outcomes for the diabetic in ambulatory care* [Unpublished study]. Seattle, WA: Kaiser Permanente Washington.

Tschudy, M.M., Raphael, J.L., Nehal, U.S., O'Connor, K.G., Kowalkowski, M.A., & Stille, C.J. (2016). Barriers to care coordination and medical home implementation. *Pediatrics, 138*(3), e20153458-e20153458. doi:10.1542/peds.2015-3458

Van Herck, P., De Smedt, D., Annemans, L., Remmen, R., Rosenthal, M.B., & Sermeus, W. (2010). Systematic review: Effects, design choices, and context of pay-for-performance in health care. *BMC Health Services Research.* doi:10.1186/1472-6963-10-247

VanLare, J.M., & Conway, P.H. (2012). Value-based purchasing – National programs to move from volume to value. *New England Journal of Medicine, 367*(4), 292-295. doi:10.10556/NEJMp1204939

Varni, J.W. (2019). *The PedsQL™ Measurement Model for the Pediatric Quality of Life Inventory™.* Retrieved from http://pedsql.org/about_pedsql.html

Verma, A. (2018). *Top 10 big data skills to get big data jobs.* Retrieved from https://www.whizlabs.com/blog/big-data-skills/

Wagner, K. (2016). *Risk stratification for better population health management.* Retrieved from http://www.hfma.org/Leadership/Archives/2016/Summer/Risk_Stratification_for_Better_Population_Health_Management/

Zangerle, C., & Kingston, M.B. (2016). Managing care coordination and transitions: The nurse leader's role. *Nurse Leader, 14*(3), 171-173. doi:10.1016/j.mnl.2016.04.002

Zangerle, C.M. (2015). Nurses as navigators. *Nursing Management, 46*(10), 27-28. doi:10.1097/01.numa.0000471587.08691.ba

Additional Readings

The Advisory Board. (2018). *Partner to create comprehensive wraparound support services.* Retrieved from https://www.advisory.com/research/health-care-advisory-board/studies/2013/playbook-for-population-health/creating-the-high-risk-patient-care-team/6

Agency for Healthcare Research and Quality (AHRQ). (2012). *Guide to patient and family engagement in hospital safety and quality.* Retrieved from http://www.ahrq.gov/professionals/systems/hospital/engagingfamilies/guide.html

Ahmed, O.I. (2016). Disease management, case management, care management, and care coordination: A framework and a brief manual for care programs and staff. *Professional Case Management, 21*(3), 137-146. doi:10.1097/ncm.0000000000000147

Babiker, A., El Husseini, M., Al Nemri, A., Al Frayh, A., Al Juryyan, N., Faki, M.O., ... Al Zamil, F. (2014). Health care professional development: Working as a team to improve patient care. *Sudanese Journal of Paediatrics, 14*(2), 9-16.

Boyle, J., Speroff, T., Worley, K., Cao, A., Goggins, K., Dittus, R.S., & Kripalani, S. (2017). Low health literacy is associated with increased transitional care needs in hospitalized patients. *Journal of Hospital Medicine, 12*(11), 918-924. doi:10.12788/jhm.2841

Carman, K.L., Dardess, P., Maurer, M., Sofaer, S., Adams, K., Bechtel, C., & Sweeney, J. (2013). Patient and family engagement: A framework for understanding the elements and developing interventions and policies. *Health Affairs, 32*(2), 223-231.

Carman, K.L., & Workman, T.A. (2017). Engaging patients and consumers in research evidence: Applying the conceptual model of patient and family engagement. *Patient Education and Counseling, 100*(1), 25-29.

Center for Advancing Health. (2010). *A new definition of patient engagement: What is engagement and why is it important?* Retrieved from http://www.cfah.org/file/CFAH_Engagement_Behavior_Framework_current.pdf

Center for Connected Health Policy. (2018). *What is telehealth?* Retrieved from http://www.cchpca.org/about/about-telehealth

Centers for Disease Control and Prevention (CDC). (2019). *What is population health?* Retrieved from https://www.cdc.gov/pophealthtraining/whatis.html

Chambers, P., & Laughlin, C. (2013). Transcultural nursing care. In C.B. Laughlin (Ed.), *Core curriculum for ambulatory care nursing* (3rd ed.). Pitman, NJ: American Academy of Ambulatory Care Nursing.

Esposito, E.M., Rhodes, C.A., Besthoff, C.M., & Bonuel, N. (2016). Patient engagement as a nurse-sensitive indicator in ambulatory care. *Nursing Economic$, 34*(6), 303-306.

Heath, S. (2016). Better health IT interoperability needed to close gaps in care. *Patient Engagement HIT.* Retrieved from https://hitinfrastructure.com/news/better-health-it-interoperability-needed-to-close-gaps-in-care

Heath, S. (2018). What is the patient activation measure in patient-centered care? *Patient Engagement HIT.* Retrieved from https://patientengagementhit.com/news/what-is-the-patient-activation-measure-in-patient-centered-care

Hibbard, J.H. (2009). Using systematic measurement to target consumer activation strategies. *Medical Care Research and Review, 66*(1, Suppl.), 9S-27S. doi:10.1177/1077558708326969

Hibbard, J.H. (2017). Commentary on "Refining Consumer Engagement Definitions and Strategies." *Journal of Ambulatory Care Management, 40*(4), 265-269.

Hibbard, J.H., & Gilburt, H. (2014). *Supporting people to manage their health: An introduction to patient activation.* Retrieved from http://www.kingsfund.org.uk/sites/files/kf/field/field_publication_file/supporting-people-manage-health-patient-activation-may14.pdf

Hibbard, J.H., & Greene, J. (2013). What the evidence shows about patient activation: Better health outcomes and care experiences; fewer data on costs. *Health Affairs, 32*(2), 207-214.

Hibbard, J.H., & Lorig, K. (2012). The do's and don'ts of patient engagement in busy office practices. *Journal of Ambulatory Care Management, 35*(2), 129-132.

Hibbard, J.H., & Mahoney, E. (2010). Toward a theory of patient and consumer activation. *Patient Education and Counseling, 78*(3), 377-388. doi:10.1016/j.pec.2009.12.015

Hibbard, J.H., Mahoney, E.R., Stockard, J., & Tusler, M. (2005). Development and testing of a short form of the Patient Activation Measure. *Health Services Research, 40*(6, Pt. 1), 1918-1930. doi:10.1111/j.1475-6773.2005.00438.x

Lamb, G., & Newhouse, R. (2018) *Care coordination: A blueprint for action for RNs.* Silver Springs, MD: American Nurses Association.

Lee, C.H., & Yoon, H.J. (2017). Medical big data: Promise and challenges. *Kidney Research and Clinical Practice, 36*(1), 3-11. doi:10:23876/j.krcp.2017.36.1.3

Mehlsen, M., Hegaard, L., Ørnbøl, E., Jensen, J.S., Fink, P., & Frostholm, L. (2017). The effect of a lay-led, group-based self-management program for patients with chronic pain. *Pain, 158*(8), 1437-1445. doi:10.1097/j.pain.0000000000000931

mHealth Intelligence (2018). *How mHealth Technology improved population health messaging.* Retrieved from https://

mhealthintelligence.com/features/how-mhealth-technology-improves-population-health-messaging

National Quality Registry Network. (2014). *What is a clinical data registry?* Retrieved from: https://www.abms.org/media/1358/what-is-a-clinical-data-registry.pdf

National Wraparound Initiative. (2018). *Wraparound basics or what is wraparound: An introduction.* Retrieved from https://nwi.pdx.edu/wraparound-basics/

Rich, E., Lipson, D., Libersky, J., & Parchman, M. (2012). *Coordinating care for adults with complex care needs in the patient-centered medical home: Challenges and solutions.* Retrieved from https://pcmh.ahrq.gov/sites/default/files/attachments/Coordinating%20Care%20for%20Adults%20with%20Complex%20Care%20Needs.pdf

Sofaer, S., & Schumann, M.J. (2013). *Fostering successful patient and family engagement: Nursing's critical role.* Retrieved from http://www.naqc.org/WhitePaper-Patient Engagement

Sortedahl, C. (2017). The "human side" of care coordination: A whole-person approach. *Professional Case Management, 22*(3), 142-143. doi:10.1097/ncm.0000000000000221

U.S. Department of Health and Human Services. (n.d.). *Health information privacy.* Retrieved from https://www.hhs.gov/hipaa/index.html

Wagner, E.H. (1998). Chronic disease management: What will it take to improve care for chronic conditions? *Effective Clinical Practice, 1*(1), 2-4.

Wasson, J., & Coleman, E.A. (2014). Health confidence: A simple, essential measure for patient engagement and better practice. *Family Practice Management, 21*(5), 8-12.

Chapter 11

Care Coordination and Transition Management Between Acute Care and Ambulatory Care

Jacqueline Adams, MSN, RN, CORLN, CCCTM®
Anne M. Delengowski, MSN, RN, AOCN, CCCTM®
Bonnie Robertson, MSN, RN-BC, CRNP, CCCTM®

Learning Outcome Statement

After completing this learning activity, the learner will be able to understand the outcomes of a mutually developed, implemented, and continuously evaluated transition of care plan and the impact it has on quality of care, individual and family satisfaction, and person-centered outcomes. In addition, recognizing the financial impact and understanding the importance of integrating evidence-based practice guidelines into a transition of care plan are essential components of care coordination and transition management (CCTM®) and the role of the registered nurse (RN).

Learning Objectives

After reading this chapter, the CCTM RN will be able to:
- Identify opportunities for transition management within the continuum of care.
- Identify key elements of successful transition planning including identification of vulnerable populations and effective communication techniques.
- Review the most common factors influencing poor transitions of care.
- Describe components of an evidence-based transition plan that includes engagement of the individual, family, and health care team.
- Discuss examples of transition of care models.
- Apply an evidence-based format to coordinate information transfer between sites of care, focusing on the role of the RN within these transitions.
- Demonstrate the knowledge, skills, and attitudes required for transitions in care (see Table 11-1 on page 244).

AAACN Care Coordination and Transition Management Standards
Standard 5a.   Coordination of Care
Standard 11.   Communication
Standard 12.   Leadership
Standard 13.   Collaboration
Standard 15.   Resource Utilization

Source: AAACN, 2016.

Competency Definition

Transition of care is the movement of an individual from one setting of care (hospital, ambulatory primary care practice, ambulatory specialty care practice, long-term care, home health, rehabilitation facility) to another (Centers for Medicare & Medicaid Services [CMS], 2013).

"It comprises a range of time-limited services that complement primary care and are designed to ensure health care continuity and avoid preventable poor outcomes among at-risk populations as they move from one level of care to another, among multiple providers and across settings" (Naylor, Aiken, Kurtzman, Olds, & Hirschman, 2011, p. 747).

Transitional care is "a set of actions designed to ensure the coordination and continuity of health care as patients transfer between different locations or different levels of care within the same location" (Coleman & Boult, 2003, p. 555).

Until recently, much of the research conducted on transition of care events emphasized hospitals and the discharge planning process. It has become apparent there are numerous instances along the continuum of care during which the progress toward positive clinical outcomes has the potential to derail. It is also becoming apparent that responsibility for a person's care does not end when that person enters or exits another care setting. Through active involvement of the

Chapter 11

individual and caregiver, and participation of providers of care from environments outside the hospital, in concert with transition and discharge planning occurring during hospitalization, opportunities for preventing errors will be uncovered, preventable readmissions will be decreased, and more conscientious use of the shrinking health care dollar will occur.

The coordination of care is an established standard of nursing practice, regardless of the practice environment. Engaging the individual and family to participate in determining the needs and preferences surrounding their care and providing education and securing essential equipment, supplies, and community resources to manage their care has long been part of the scope of the practicing RN. The American Nurses Association (ANA) released a position statement regarding the essential role of RNs in this endeavor.

"Patient-centered care coordination is a core professional standard and competency for all registered nursing practice. Based on a partnership guided by the health care consumer's and family's needs and preferences, the registered nurse is integral to patient care quality, satisfaction, and the effective and efficient use of health care resources. Registered nurses are qualified and educated for the role of care coordination, especially with high risk and vulnerable populations" (ANA, 2012, para. 2).

In October 2012, Medicare began linking hospital reimbursement to the quality of care. This increased focus on quality places more emphasis on better preparation of individuals for managing their illness at home. The goal is to promote quality and cost savings through the reduction of after-hospital adverse events and prevent readmissions. In particular, the RN plays a critical role in care coordination and transition management by focusing on prevention of illness, management of specific high-risk conditions, reduction or elimination of preventable complications, as well as promotion of healthy lifestyle changes and careful use of valuable health care resources. Management of a care transition generally begins when a person is identified as having a status change (deterioration or improvement) that makes it appropriate to move to another setting or level of care (American Medical Directors Association, 2010).

I. **Standards Guiding Care Coordination and Transition Management Between Acute and Ambulatory Care**

There are many standards from AAACN's *Scope and Standards of Practice for Registered Nurses in Care Coordination and Transition Management* (2016) that are encompassed within the transition of an individual from acute to ambulatory care. The following are a list of standards that apply to this topic, and some of the competencies that directly pertain to it.

A. Standard 5a: Coordination of Care (AAACN, 2016). "The RN practicing CCTM coordinates the delivery of care within the practice setting and across health care settings" (p.18).
   1. Demonstrate accountability across care settings in maintaining continuity of care.
   2. Facilitate individual and/or population progress toward positive person-centered clinical outcomes.
   3. Facilitate the transition of individual/population to the appropriate level of care.
   4. Recognize and maximize opportunities to increase the quality of care.
   5. Manage high-risk individuals with the aim of preventing/delaying adverse outcomes.
   6. Communicate relevant information to the individual, caregiver, and interprofessional health care team across the care continuum.

B. Standard 11: Communication (AAACN, 2016). "The RN practicing CCTM communicates effectively using a variety of formats, tools, and technologies to build professional relationships and deliver care across the continuum" (p. 26).
   1. Promote active communication using a method or manner that enhances learning and the sharing of information.
   2. Maintain professional communication with members of the health care team, families, and stakeholders to promote effective interactions.
   3. Share with the health care team hazards or barriers that could have a negative effect on individuals and/or caregivers.

C. Standard 12: Leadership (AAACN, 2016). "The RN practicing CCTM acquires and utilizes leadership behaviors in practice settings, within the profession, and across the care continuum" (p. 27).
   1. Demonstrate respect for human dignity and worth by valuing people as the central asset of the work setting, the profession, and the community.
   2. Serve as a mentor for new staff, colleagues, and students by identifying and engaging in learning opportunities.

3. Initiate and/or participate in continuous quality health and improvement activities as a means to advance individual, community, and population wellness.
4. Lead and actively participate in projects, community education, committees, and councils by serving in key roles in the practice and community settings.
D. Standard 13: Collaboration (AAACN, 2016). "The RN practicing CCTM interacts with the individual, family members, caregivers, and health care professionals to foster professional relationships that improve population health" (p. 28).
   1. Partner with interprofessional team members in diverse settings regarding the promotion, prevention, and restoration of health in populations.
   2. Provide outreach to individuals and their caregivers to identify health or psychosocial issues used in the development of an appropriate plan of care.
   3. Coordinate with local and community resources to improve the health of populations or individuals.
   4. Communicate recommended intervention(s) and plan(s) of care with expected outcomes with individuals or caregivers and applicable members of the interprofessional team.
E. Standard 15: Resource Utilization (AAACN, 2016). "The RN practicing CCTM utilizes appropriate resources to plan and facilitate services that are safe, effective, and fiscally responsible" (p. 30).
   1. Partner with individuals and caregivers to assess individual health care needs and target the resources available to achieve desired outcomes, and assist with access to necessary resources.
   2. Evaluate resources for potential harm, complexity of the task, cost effectiveness, and desired outcome when considering resource allocation.
   3. Identify evidence-based practices when evaluating resource allocation.
   4. Modify CCTM practice when necessary to promote optimal interaction between health care consumers, care providers, and the usage of technology.
   5. Educate and support individuals and caregivers to become informed consumers about the options, costs, risks, and benefits of health care services.

II. Defining Transition of Care
A. Care transitions refer to the movement of individuals from health care practitioners and settings as their care needs change during the course of an illness (Coleman & Boult, 2003).
B. Transition of care should always incorporate potential issues with language barriers, health literacy, and culture.
C. Plans of care should be collaborative among the individual, family, and health care providers. They should include clearly defined goals, individual's preferences, and be culturally appropriate.
D. There are multiple opportunities for transition of care to occur (Kansagara et al., 2016; Naylor et al., 2017):
   1. Acute care to ambulatory care.
   2. Acute care to long-term care.
   3. Ambulatory care, or extended care, to acute care.
   4. Primary care to specialty care.
   5. Pediatric care to young adult care.

III. Transition of Care Opportunities
A. Acute care to ambulatory care (Hirschman et al., 2017; Scott et al., 2017).
   1. Transition.
      a. One of the most common transitions.
      b. Research has established best practices.
   2. Communication.
      a. Necessitates the need for effective hand-off communication to avoid communication gaps.
         (1) I-PASS Handoff Bundle (Starmer et al., 2014).
            (a) **I**: Illness severity.
            (b) **P**: Patient summary.
            (c) **A**: Action list.
            (d) **S**: Situation awareness and contingency planning.
            (e) **S**: Synthesis by receiver.
   3. Factors influencing poor outcomes.
      a. When not done correctly, length of stay and 30-day readmissions increase.
      b. Health care providers seeing discharge as the end of the process.
      c. System-related issues.
         (1) Communication gaps between settings.
         (2) Lack of consistent and intraoperative documentation systems.
         (3) Inadequacy of insurance coverage.

Chapter 11

                (4) Preauthorization for medications or supplies not complete.
                (5) Discharge instructions different from prescription instructions.
                (6) Follow-up appointments not made prior to transition or timely appointments not made.
                (7) Lack of follow-up with pending results.
                (8) Lack of transportation to appointments (Scott et al., 2017).
         4. Factors influencing positive outcomes.
            a. When transition is done correctly, length of stay and 30-day readmissions decrease.
            b. Assuring the individual is prepared for discharge.
                (1) PREPARED (Cibulskis, Giardino, & Moyer, 2011).
                    (a) **P:** Presenting history.
                    (b) **R:** Received therapies.
                    (c) **E:** Existing baseline.
                    (d) **P:** Pending test for discharge.
                    (e) **A:** Anticipated needs.
                    (f) **R:** Records to be sent.
                    (g) **E:** End of life preferences.
                    (h) **D:** Discussion with family and provider.
            c. Early identification of persons at risk for readmission.
                (1) LACE (Robinson & Hudali, 2017).
                    (a) **L:** Length of stay.
                    (b) **A:** Acuity of admission.
                    (c) **C:** Condition.
                    (d) **E:** Emergency department visit.
                (2) Better Outcomes by Optimizing Safe Transitions (BOOST) (Society of Hospital Medicine, 2014).
                (3) HOSPITAL: Score uses seven readily available clinical predictors to accurately identify individuals at high risk of potentially avoidable hospital readmission within 30 days (Robinson & Hudali, 2017).
         5. Role of the CCTM RN in transition.
            a. RN-RN handoff from acute care to ambulatory care.
            b. Early education utilizing "teach back."
            c. Early assessment of post-acute care needs.
                (1) Identification of new medications.
                    (a) Is there a need for preauthorization?
                    (b) Assuring the person has ability to access the medication.
                (2) Assessing transportation needs.
      B. Acute to long-term care (Jusela, Struble, Gallagher, Redman, & Ziemba, 2017; Toles, Colon-Emeric, Asafu-Adjei, Moreton, & Hanson, 2016).
         1. Transition.
            a. This transition often exposes older adults to:
                (1) Medication errors.
                (2) Decreased quality of care.
                (3) Overuse of acute health care services.
            b. Care in long-term and post-acute care (LTPAC) provides care to persons with more complex conditions than historically seen.
            c. Persons in this setting are often the elderly, frail, and disabled.
         2. Communication.
            a. Can be challenging due to lack of consistent electronic health record (EHR).
            b. Transmission options for care summary.
                (1) Provision of hard copy of medical record.
                (2) Fax.
                (3) Health information exchange (HIE).
                (4) Direct secure messaging (National Learning Consortium, n.d.).
         3. Factors influencing poor outcomes.
            a. Individuals being admitted with more acute health issues.
            b. Inadequate communication of critical information.
            c. Lack of medication reconciliation.
            d. Lack of communication regarding goals of care.
         4. Factors influencing positive outcomes (National Learning Consortium, n.d.).
            a. Care coordination.
            b. Assure communication of:
                (1) Durable power of attorney for health care (DPOAH).
                (2) Goals of care.
                (3) Advance directives.
            c. Transition of appropriate health care information to receiving area, including but not limited to:
                (1) Demographics.
                (2) Person-specific health/medical information.
                (3) Physical findings.
                (4) Cognition.
                (5) Functional status.
                (6) Immunizations.
                (7) Medications including allergies.

(8) Pain assessment and treatments.
(9) Pressure injuries/skin conditions.
(10) Summary of expectations for care.
5. Role of the CCTM RN in transition.
    a. Assure medication reconciliation.
    b. RN-RN handoff from acute care to LTPAC.
C. Ambulatory care, or extended care, to acute care.
    1. Transition.
        a. This is an important transition as it often represents a significant change in the person's condition.
        b. Should represent an opportunity to address goals of care.
    2. Communication.
        a. Assess if clinical information available through HIE and if not, how the information is to be sent and received.
    3. Factors influencing poor outcomes.
        a. Information from person's ambulatory care or extended stay plan of care is seldom shared with the acute care team.
        b. Often the care team retrieves information from individual or family leading to incomplete information.
    4. Factors influencing positive outcomes.
        a. Identification of accountable provider on receiving and sending areas.
        b. Communication of active care plan from sending area to receiving area with clearly defined goals.
    5. Role of the CCTM RN in transition.
        a. Transition to RN-RN handoff from ambulatory care/long-term care to acute care.
        b. Assure medication reconciliation.
D. Transition to specialty care: This transition might represent the person is now receiving care from a new provider such as a primary care provider to an oncologist.
    1. Transition.
        a. Oncology.
        b. Palliative care.
        c. Hospice.
    2. Communication.
        a. Need to assure all pertinent health history is received by specialist.
        b. Need to assess goals of care.
    3. Factors influencing poor outcomes.
        a. Incomplete hand-off communication.
        b. Person not understanding the transition to a specialist.
        c. Specialist often focusing on a specific issue, not the whole person.
        d. Stress related to new diagnosis impacting the person's ability to receive information.
        e. Lack of access to pending results.
    4. Factors influencing positive outcomes.
        a. Complete communication handoff.
        b. Person utilizing "PREPARED" for the visit (Cibulskis et al., 2011).
    5. Role of RN in transition.
        a. Assure proper handoff.
        b. Assure medication reconciliation.
E. Pediatric care to young adult care (Mallory et al., 2017).
    1. Transition.
        a. This is often an overlooked transition.
        b. It often represents a culture change for the individual and family as prior to 18 years of age, or emancipation, the parent/guardian makes the health/medical decisions.
    2. Communication.
        a. Ascertain, without parent/guardian present, if the individual continues to want parent/guardian part of the communication with the health care providers.
        b. Assess who the individual would want to be the DPOAH/medical power of attorney.
    3. Factors influencing poor outcomes.
        a. Inability for the individual to navigate the health care system.
        b. Poor or lack of handoff between pediatric providers and new primary/specialty team.
        c. Management of follow-up left to individual/family to navigate (Swan, 2012).
        d. Lack of clear direction as to who to call with problems or concerns.
    4. Factors influencing positive outcomes.
        a. Support and empowerment of the individual as he or she transitions to adult care.
    5. Role of the CCTM RN in transition.
        a. Proper and complete handoff.
        b. Assisting the young adult to navigate the new health system.
        c. Continual assessment of needs.
        d. Assisting the family in transition.

IV. **Evidence-Based Transition Models**

A. Nearly one in five Medicare recipients discharged from a hospital – approximately 2.6 million seniors – are readmitted within 30 days, at a cost of over $26 billion every year (CMS, 2018).

B. Community-based Care Transitions Program (CCTP) was developed by the CMS to test care transition interventions for currently enrolled Medicare persons who are at high-risk for admission following hospitalization (CMS, 2018).
  1. Provides framework for community-based organizations to partner with hospitals to address needs of this high-risk population.
C. CCTP sites, which included community-based organizations and hospitals, as well as other organizations, used evidence-based care transition models to:
  1. Improve transitions from inpatient to other settings.
  2. Reduce costs.
  3. Improve quality.
  4. Improve individual experience (CMS, 2018).
D. CCTP ended in 2017; however, key findings support the continued need for partnerships and continuity of care from one care transition to another.
E. Various care models currently being used include:
  1. BOOST (Society of Hospital Medicine, 2014).
    a. Provides hospitals with core metrics for improvement as well as a set of tools to help enhance discharge for facilities.
    b. Nationally recognized quality improvement program from the Center for Medicare and Medicaid Innovation for reducing readmissions (Coffey, Greenwald, Budnitz, & Williams, 2013).
    c. Focus of Project BOOST is to:
      (1) Identify high-risk individuals on admission and target risk-specific interventions through use of 8P screening tool (see Appendix 11-1).
      (2) Reduce 30-day readmission rates for general medicine.
      (3) Reduce length of stay.
      (4) Improve facility individual satisfaction and Hospital Consumer Assessment of Healthcare Providers and Systems (HCAHPS) scores.
      (5) Improve information flow between inpatient and outpatient providers.
      (6) Since its launch in 2008, BOOST has helped more than 180 hospitals and health care institutions improve their care transition processes (Coffey et al., 2013).
    d. Project BOOST 8Ps screening tool.
      (1) Includes assessment of social determinants such as social support and health literacy.
      (2) Incorporated into discharge planning to predict an individual's risk of adverse event post discharge.
      (3) Comprised of risk-specific interventions that are evidence-based and allow for accountability and signoff by providers when intervention is done.
  2. Transitional Care Model (TCM) (Naylor, 2012; Naylor et al., 1999, 2004, 2011, 2017).
    a. Led by a master's-prepared nurse to treat chronically ill, high-risk older adults before, during, and after hospitalization.
    b. Comprised of 10 key elements:
      (1) Advanced practice RN serves as primary coordinator of care.
      (2) In-hospital assessment and development of plan of care takes place.
      (3) Home visits by the advanced practice RN (APRN) coupled with ongoing telephone follow-ups.
      (4) Transitions between acute and primary care facilitated by APRN (may be present at follow-up primary care appointments).
      (5) Individualized needs as focal point of care.
      (6) Engagement of both individuals and support systems with primary focus on education and supportive services.
      (7) Early identification of health care risks and symptom management.
      (8) Interprofessional collaborative approaches to care.
      (9) Provider-nurse collaboration.
      (10) Open, effective communication between all involved persons.
    c. A study performed by Naylor and colleagues (2011) found that implementation of TCM provided for improvements in all health status and quality of life measures post intervention and allowed for a significant decrease in readmissions (45 vs. 60, $p<0.041$) and length of stay (252 vs. 351, $p<0.032$) at 3 months post implementation (Naylor, 2011, 2012).

3. Care Transitions Intervention® (Coleman, Parry, Chalmers, & Min, 2006).
   a. Also known as CTI® Skill Transfer Model, The Coleman Transitions Intervention Model®, and Coleman Model®.
   b. Utilizes Transitions Coach® to coordinate the care of an assigned group of individuals with complex care needs over a 4-week period.
   c. A "self-management model" that utilizes principles of adult learning and simulation to enhance skill transfer and self-management.
   d. Comprised of the following components:
      (1) Personal health record.
      (2) Discharge preparation checklist.
      (3) Individual self-activation and management session with a Transitions Coach.
      (4) Transitions Coach follow-up visits and phone calls.
   e. Intervention focuses on four conceptual areas (The Four Pillars®) (Coleman, 2007).
      (1) Medication self-management.
      (2) Individual understands and uses the personal health record to communicate.
      (3) Primary care and specialist follow-up.
      (4) Knowledge of red flags.
         (a) Understanding of indications that condition is worsening.
         (b) Awareness of how to respond.
   f. Individuals who underwent the intervention were significantly less likely to be readmitted at 30-, 60-, and 90-day intervals post discharge (Coleman et al., 2006).
   g. Another study done by Coleman, Roman, Hall, and Min (2015) found, "The enhanced family caregiver CTI significantly improved activation, quality, goal achievement, satisfaction, and medication safety. The enhanced family caregiver CTI may have application in improving the hospital discharge experience" (p. 2).
4. Project Re-Engineered Discharge (RED) (Jack, Paasche-Orlow, Mitchell, Forsythe, & Martin, J. 2013).
   a. Developed by a research group at Boston University Medical Center.
   b. Focus is on standardized discharge process to ensure individuals are prepared when leaving the hospital, with a specific focus on safety and reduced readmission rates.
   c. Endorsed by the National Quality Forum; provides comprehensive safe practice for the discharge process.
   d. In 2008, researchers found individuals discharged using Project RED had a 30% lower rate of hospital utilization 30 days post-discharge, and readmission or emergency department visit was prevented for every 7.3 subjects receiving the intervention (National Transitions of Care Coalition [NTOCC], n.d.).
   e. Additionally, individuals who received intervention had a 33.9% lower cost than those who did not receive intervention, which equated to a savings of $412 per person (NTOCC, n.d.).
   f. Composed of 12 components:
      (1) Language assistance.
      (2) Prescheduled discharge appointments for individuals, including labs and radiology testing.
      (3) Planned follow-up and discussion of labs and radiology testing following discharge.
      (4) Organization of post discharge equipment and services.
      (5) Medication reconciliation with administration plans for individuals.
      (6) Reconciliation of the discharge plan with established national guidelines.
      (7) Utilization of a home care plan that the individual can understand and follow.
      (8) Education about individual's diagnosis.
      (9) "Teach back" of the discharge plan to be completed by individual.
      (10) Symptom/emergency management review with the individual prior to discharge.
      (11) Transmission of discharge summary to all providers caring for the individual.
      (12) Telephone follow-up of the discharge plan with the individual/caregiver within 3 days (Jack et al., 2013).
5. State Action on Avoidable Rehospitalizations (STAAR) (Boutwell, Jencks, Nielsen, & Rutherford, 2009).

a. Institute for Healthcare Improvement (IHI)-partnered initiative to improve transitions in care, reduce hospitalizations, and share best practices, from May 2009 to June 2013.
b. Three states participated in STAAR initiative, including Massachusetts, Michigan, and Washington (IHI, 2018a).
c. A study performed by Carter and colleagues (2015) using the STAAR model showed a decrease in hospital readmissions on a general medical surgical unit by 30% (from 21% to 14.5%).

6. Geriatric Resources for Assessment and Care of Elders (GRACE) (Counsell, Callahan, Buttar, Clark, & Frank, 2006).
    a. A model that provides interprofessional team care and home-based management.
    b. Team is usually comprised of a social worker and APRN.
    c. Study found that this model improved quality of care, reduced admissions and readmissions, and positively impacted cost of care.
    d. Foundational principles include:
        (1) Specific targeting of older people at risk.
        (2) Availability of collaborative expertise in geriatrics.
        (3) Integration of program into primary care.
        (4) Coordination of care across all sites of care.
        (5) Use of EHR to support physician practices and facilitate monitoring of clinical parameters.
        (6) Institutionally endorsed clinical practice guide.

V. **Engagement of the Individual, Family, and Interprofessional Team**

A. Engagement of the individual, family, and health care team (physician, RN, pharmacy, social work, allied health providers, care coordinator, etc.) to discuss, coordinate, and communicate the individual's goals and plan of care is essential. Elements identified as significant in transitioning between the acute care setting and the ambulatory care setting include:
    1. Completion of checklists that will ensure effective communication has occurred between individual and provider in terms of discharge preparedness. This includes the General Assessment of Preparedness (GAP) checklist and a patient discharge checklist such as the BOOST discharge checklist (Society of Hospital Medicine, 2014).
    2. Identification of barriers to care with potential resolutions implemented. Barriers include psychosocial needs, social support, economic, cognitive, and physical.
    3. Evaluation of medication management including reconciliation of medication at discharge and postdischarge to identify adherence and resolve problems.
    4. Individual and caregiver education regarding self-management, assessing and acknowledging functional and cognitive status, and assessment of learning through "teach back" and "Ask Me 3" (IHI, 2018b).
        a. Teach back.
        b. Ask Me 3.
            (1) What is my main problem?
            (2) What do I need to do?
            (3) Why is it important for me to do this?
    5. Education of individuals and caregivers regarding signs and symptoms that indicate a worsening condition and steps to take (red flags).
    6. Education of individuals and caregivers on communication skills that include how to speak with physicians to relay care needs.
    7. Coordination of follow-up appointments with primary physician and specialists that include questions to ask and information to provide physicians. Remember the PREPARED tool (Cibulskis et al., 2011).
    8. Discussion regarding incomplete test and imaging results; when and how information will be communicated.
    9. Communication and handoff to all providers regarding plans of care, which reflects individual and caregiver goals.
    10. Arrangements for post-discharge home visit or follow-up via telephone within 72 hours for reinforcement of teaching, problem identification, and validation of receipt of medical/social services and equipment identified at discharge.
    11. Incorporation of disease-specific care guideline into plan of care (coronary heart failure, myocardial infarction, hypertension, asthma, diabetes management) (Agency for Healthcare Research and Quality, n.d.). Due to overlap of guidelines for care of individuals with multiple chronic conditions,

the CCTM RN needs to help guide the individual and caregiver through the health care maze to determine which guideline(s) are best suited based on the individual's goals.

VI. Application of Evidence-Based Tools

A. Case Study 1: Lymphoma (Appendix 11-1).
B. Case Study 1: BOOST Tool CCTM RN to Acute Care Oncology, Universal Discharge Checklist with GAP (Appendix 11-2).
C. Case Study 1 Patient PASS: A Transition Record (Appendix 11-3).
D. Case study 2: Type 2 Diabetes (see Appendix 11-4).
E. Case Study 2: BOOST Tool CCTM RN in PCMH Diabetes, Universal Discharge Checklist with GAP (Appendix 11-5).
F. Case study 2: Patient PASS: A Transition Record (Appendix 11-6).

Table 11-1.
CCTM® Between Acute Care and Ambulatory Care: Knowledge, Skills, and Attitudes for Competency

Person-Centered Care			
Recognize the individual or designee as the source of control and full partner in providing compassionate and coordinated care based on respect for individual's preferences, values, and needs (Cronenwett et al., 2007).			
Knowledge	**Skills**	**Attitudes**	**Sources**
Analyze multiple dimensions of person-centered care including individual/family/community preferences and values, as well as social, cultural, psychological, and spiritual contexts. *Types of transitions:* • Acute to home • Acute to subacute • Home to acute • Acute care to long-term acute care	Identify individual and caregiver main concerns regarding care after discharge, management of symptoms, attainable goals related to disease and prognosis. Identify and create plans to address barriers in care settings that prevent fully integrating person-centered care. Engage individuals or designated surrogates in active partnerships along the health-illness continuum.	Commit to the individual as the source of control and full partner in his/her care. Commit to person-centered, collaborative care planning. Appreciate physical and other barriers to person-centered care. Value the involvement of individuals and families in care decisions. Respect preferences of individuals related to their level of engagement in health care decision-making.	Cronenwett et al., 2007
Analyze person-centered care in the context of care coordination, individual education, physical comfort, emotional support, and care transitions.	Work to address ethical and legal issues related to individuals' rights to determine their care. Work with individuals to create plans of care that are defined by the individual.	Commit to respecting the rights of individuals in determining their plan of care. Recognize the need to work with family members to accept the individual's right for self-determination. Value the decisions of individual and family in choosing best next level of care based on individual's goals.	National POLST Paradigm, 2018
Analyze strategies that empower individuals and/or families involved in the health care process.	Engage individuals and/or caregivers in developing active partnerships at all levels of care. Eliminate barriers to family or other caregiver's presence during care discussions per individual's request.	Value the involvement of individuals and families in care decisions. Respect individual preferences for degree of active engagement in care process. Honor active partnership with individuals or their designated participants in planning, implementing, and evaluating care provided.	Cronenwett et al., 2007

continued on next page

**Table 11-1. (continued)
CCTM® Between Acute Care and Ambulatory Care: Knowledge, Skills, and
Attitudes for Competency**

Safety			
Minimize risk of harm to individuals and providers through both system effectiveness and individual performance (Cronenwett et al., 2007).			
Knowledge	**Skills**	**Attitudes**	**Sources**
Identify best practices that promote individual, community, and provider safety in the practice setting.	Integrate strategies and safety practices to reduce risk of harm to individuals, self, and others. Essential elements of communication between providers during care handoff to include: • Readmission risk. • Overview of individual. • Current problems. • Outstanding tests. • Individual preferences. • Medication and allergies.	Commit to being a safety mentor and role model. Value a systems approach to improving individual care instead of blaming individuals.	Cronenwett et al., 2007
Describe evidence-based practices when responding to errors and good catches.	Use evidence-based best practices to create policies and processes to manage medical care.	Commit to identifying errors and potential risks to improve quality and systems. Value open and honest communication with individuals and families about errors and hazards.	Cronennett et al., 2007
Teamwork and Collaboration			
Function effectively within nursing and interprofessional teams, fostering open communication, mutual respect, and shared decision-making to achieve quality care (Cronenwett et al., 2007).			
Knowledge	**Skills**	**Attitudes**	**Sources**
Understand the roles and scope of practice of each interprofessional team member including individuals, in order to work effectively to provide the highest level of care possible.	Work with team members to identify goals for individuals based on personal decisions for care. Ensure inclusion of individuals and family members as part of the team based on the individual and families' preference to be included. "Explain the roles and responsibilities of other providers and how the team works together to provide care, promote health, and prevent disease" (p.12). "Use the full scope of knowledge, skills, and abilities of professionals from health and other fields to provide care that is safe, timely, efficient, effective, and equitable" (p. 12).	Respect the role of the individual within the family group. Appreciate cultural differences and integration into care of the individual. Value individuals and families as the source of control for their health care. "Engage health and other professionals in shared patient-centered and population-focused problem-solving" (p.14). "Integrate the knowledge and experience of health and other professions to inform health and care decisions, while respecting patient and community values and priorities/preferences for care" (p.14).	Cronenwett et al., 2007 Interprofessional Education Collaborative (IPEC), 2016

continued on next page

Table 11-1. (continued)
CCTM® Between Acute Care and Ambulatory Care: Knowledge, Skills, and Attitudes for Competency

Teamwork and Collaboration (continued)			
Knowledge	**Skills**	**Attitudes**	**Sources**
Describe appropriate hand-off communication practices.	Use communication practices that minimize risks associated with hand-offs among providers and across transitions of care. At a minimum, communication at handoff should include: • Medication management. • Timely primary care/specialist follow-up. • Knowledge of red flags or warnings. • Copy or access to person-centered health record.	Appreciate the risks associated with missing information during hand-offs among providers and across transitions in care.	Cronenwett et al., 2007
	"Listen actively, and encourage ideas and opinions of other team members" (p.13).	"Communicate information with patients, families, community members, and health team members in a form that is understandable, avoiding discipline-specific terminology when possible" (p. 13).	IPEC, 2016
	"Recognize how one's uniqueness (experience level, expertise, culture, power, and hierarchy within the health team) contributes to effective communication, conflict resolution, and positive interprofessional working relationships" (p. 13).	"Use respectful language appropriate for a given difficult situation, crucial conversation, or conflict" (p. 13).	
"Choose effective communication tools and techniques, including information systems and communication technologies, to facilitate discussions and interactions that enhance team function" (p. 13).	"Use process improvement to increase effectiveness of interprofessional teamwork and team-based services, programs, and policies" (p. 14).	"Share accountability with other professions, patients, and communities for outcomes relevant to prevention and health care" (p. 14). "Reflect on individual and team performance for individual, as well as team, performance improvement" (p. 14).	IPEC, 2016
Analyze the impact of team-based practice.	Act with integrity, consistency, and respect for differing views. Continuously plan for improvement in self and others for effective transition management development and functioning. Elicit input from other team members to improve individual and team performance.	Commit to being an effective team member. Be open to continual assessment and improvement of skills as a team member. Support the development of a safe team environment where issues can be addressed between team members and conflict can be resolved.	Cronenwett et al., 2007 Mitchell et al., 2012

continued on next page

Chapter 11

Table 11-1. (continued)
CCTM® Between Acute Care and Ambulatory Care: Knowledge, Skills, and Attitudes for Competency

Evidence-Based Practice			
Integrate best current evidence with clinical expertise and individual/family preferences and values for delivery of optimal health care (Cronenwett et al., 2007).			
Knowledge	**Skills**	**Attitudes**	**Sources**
Identify efficient and effective search strategies to locate reliable sources of evidence.	Employ efficient and effective search strategies to answer focused clinical or health system practices.	Value development of search skills for locating evidence for best practice.	Cronenwett et al., 2007
Summarize current evidence regarding major diagnostic and treatment actions within the practice specialty and health care delivery system.	Exhibit contemporary knowledge of best evidence related to practice and health care systems. "Use available evidence to inform effective teamwork and team-based practices" (p.14).	Value cutting-edge knowledge of current practice. "Place interests of patients and populations at center of interprofessional health care delivery and population health programs and policies, with the goal of promoting health and health equity across the life span" (p. 11). "Work in cooperation with those who receive care, those who provide care, and others who contribute to or support the delivery of prevention and health services and programs" (p. 11).	Cronenwett et al., 2007 IPEC, 2016

Source: Cronenwett et al., 2007. Reprinted with permission from Elsevier.

Chapter 11

Case Study 11-1.
Clinical Interactions and Implementation for Older Adult (Male) with Lymphoma and a History of Hypertension and Type 2 Diabetes

Introduction

Mr. F, age 74, originally from Puerto Rico, presented to a community hospital emergency department after a fall. He was found to have a fractured clavicle. Upon work up, it was found to be a pathologic fracture and Mr. F was ultimately diagnosed with lymphoma. He had a history of hypertension and type 2 diabetes. He was transferred to an academic medical center for aggressive treatment of his lymphoma. Upon further workup, he was found to have other areas of bone disease, which made him non-weight bearing on right upper extremity and left lower extremity. It was recommended that he go to a skilled nursing facility.

Mr. F is the primary caregiver for his wife, who is bedbound with many chronic illnesses. He became tearful when talking about his inability to care for his wife. He lives in a row home with multiple steps to get into the house. He is on multiple medications and has difficulty remembering when to take his medications. He identified minimal social supports. He has difficulty getting to appointments due to lack of transportation.

Clinical Interactions

- Nursing Process includes plan for:
- Continued education for lymphoma
- Identification of barriers for successful care transition including social support, transportation, and physical limitations
- Follow-up for hypertension and diabetes care – primary care
- Follow-up for continued therapy for lymphoma – oncology
- Medication management

Clinical Implementation

- Multiple clinical assessments required on an ongoing basis
- Assess need to reach out for social support
- Extended family
- Wraparound services
- Meals on Wheels
- Leukemia & Lymphoma Society
- American Cancer Society for assistance with transportation
- Transition from skilled nursing facility to home
- Home assessment
- Evaluation of outcomes and individual satisfaction

Note: Refer to Appendices 11-1 through 11-3.

Chapter 11

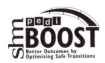

Appendix 11-1.
Tool for Addressing Risk: A Geriatric Evaluation for Transitions CCTM RN to Acute Care Oncology
Note: Bold/italic areas apply to Case Study 11-1.

Risk Assessment: 8P Screening Tool (Check all that apply.)		Risk-Specific Intervention	Signature of individual responsible for insuring intervention administered
Problem medications (anticoagulants, insulin, aspirin & clopidogrel dual therapy, digoxin, narcotics) ☒	☒	Medication-specific education using teach back provided to patient and caregiver ***Identified by niece and nephew that individual had a difficult time remembering when and how to take medications. Niece verbalized willingness to assist with this issue post discharge*** ***Niece and/or nephew verbalized understanding of the medication education using teach back.***	L. Davis, RN
	☒	Monitoring plan developed and communicated to patient and aftercare providers, where relevant (e.g., warfarin, digoxin, and insulin) ***Individual, using teach back, verbalized that he will be able to follow the oncology treatment plan post discharge***	
	☐	Specific strategies for managing adverse drug events reviewed with patient/caregiver	
	☒	Follow-up phone call at 72 hours to assess adherence and complications ***Will be discharged to skilled nursing facility (SNF) and will be followed by nursing staff at SNF and a follow-up call will be made to the SNF in 72 hours.***	
Psychological (depression screen positive or h/o depression diagnosis) ☒	☐	Assessment of need for psychiatric aftercare if not in place	L. Davis, RN
	☐	Communication with aftercare providers, highlighting this issue if new	
	☒	Involvement/awareness of support network insured ***Individual is the primary caretaker for wife. Identified niece and nephew as part of his support network.***	
Principal diagnosis (cancer, stroke, DM, COPD, heart failure)	☐	Review of national discharge guidelines, where available	L. Davis, RN
	☒	Disease specific education using teach back with patient/caregiver ***Individual educated about lymphoma and its treatment using teach back.***	
	☒	Action plan reviewed with patient/caregivers regarding what to do and who to contact in the event of worsening or new symptoms ***Individual transitioning from ambulatory care to specialty care. Educated as to how to communicate with this specialty.***	
	☒	Discuss goals of care and chronic illness model discussed with patient/caregiver ***Individual goal is to return home after rehab to his wife with assistance of niece and nephew and wrap-around services.***	

continued on next page

Chapter 11

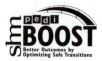

Appendix 11-1. (continued)
Tool for Addressing Risk: A Geriatric Evaluation for Transitions CCTM RN to Acute Care Oncology
Note: Bold/italic areas apply to Case Study 11-1.

Risk Assessment: 8P Screening Tool (Check all that apply.)	Risk-Specific Intervention	Signature of individual responsible for insuring intervention administered
Polypharmacy (≥5 more routine meds) ☒	☐ Elimination of unnecessary medications ☒ Simplification of medication scheduling to improve adherence ***Arranged with niece a method via phone call to assure individual takes correct medications at the correct time, including the new oncology medications.*** ☒ Follow-up phone call at 72 hours to assess adherence and complications ***Follow-up call scheduled to address and review medication questions after stay at SNF.***	L. Davis, RN
Poor health literacy (inability to do Teach Back) ☒	☒ Committed caregiver involved in planning/administration of all general and risk-specific interventions ***Identified niece and nephew as committed caregivers to this process.*** ☐ Aftercare plan education using teach back provided to patient and caregiver ☒ Link to community resources for additional patient/caregiver support ***Meals on Wheels*** ***Leukemia & Lymphoma Society*** ***American Cancer Society (ACS) for assistance with transportation***	L. Davis, RN
Patient support (absence of caregiver to assist with discharge and home care) ☒	☐ Follow-up phone call at 72 hours to assess condition, adherence, and complications ☒ Follow-up appointment with aftercare medical provider within 7 days ***Arrangement made for American Cancer Society (ACS) to provide ongoing transportation and to ensure that 7-day post discharge appointment is scheduled.*** ☒ Involvement of home care providers of services with clear communications of discharge plan to those providers ***Disposition to SNF.***	L. Davis, RN
Prior hospitalization (non-elective; in last 6 months) ☒	☒ Review reasons for re-hospitalization in context of prior hospitalization ***Signs and symptoms related to complications of diagnosis reviewed using teach back with support network.*** ☐ Follow-up phone call at 72 hours to assess condition, adherence, and complications ☒ Follow-up appointment with aftercare medical provider within 7 days ***Appointments made, transportation arranged, and follow-up with ACS navigator scheduled.***	L. Davis, RN

continued on next page

Chapter 11

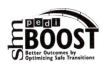

**Appendix 11-1. (continued)
Tool for Addressing Risk: A Geriatric Evaluation for
Transitions CCTM RN to Acute Care Oncology**

Note: Bold/italic areas apply to Case Study 11-1.

Risk Assessment: 8P Screening Tool (Check all that apply.)	Risk-Specific Intervention	Signature of individual responsible for insuring intervention administered
Palliative care (Would you be surprised if this patient died in the next year? Does this patient have an advanced or progressive serious illness?) Yes to either: ☒	☐ Assess need for palliative care services ☐ Identify goals of care and therapeutic options ☐ Communicate prognosis with patient/family/caregiver ☐ Assess and address bothersome symptoms ☐ Identify services or benefits available to patients based on advanced disease status ☒ Discuss with patient/family/caregiver role of palliative care services and benefits and services available *Advanced directives were discussed, currently, a full code, no need for palliative care at this time, and niece and nephew present during discussion.*	L. Davis, RN

Source: Adapted with permission from the Society of Hospital Medicine (SHM). © 2014. All rights reserved.

Chapter 11

Appendix 11-2.
Universal Patient Discharge Checklist and General Assessment of Preparedness (GAP)

Note: Bold/italic areas apply to Case Study 11-1.

	Universal Patient Discharge Checklist – **COMPLETED BY ACUTE CARE RN**			Initials
1.	GAP assessment (see below) completed with issues addressed.	☒ YES	☐ NO	LD
2.	Medications reconciled with pre-admission list.	☒ YES	☐ NO	LD
3.	Medication use/side effects reviewed using "teach back" with patient/caregiver(s).	☒ YES	☐ NO	LD
4.	"Teach back" used to confirm patient/caregiver understanding of disease, prognosis, and self-care requirements. *Completed with niece.*	☒ YES	☐ NO	LD
5.	Action plan for management of symptoms/side effects/complications requiring medical attention established and shared with patient/caregiver using "teach back."	☒ YES	☐ NO	LD
6.	Discharge plan (including educational materials; medication list with reason for use and highlighted new/changed/discontinued drugs; follow-up plans) taught with written copy provided to patient/caregiver at discharge.	☒ YES	☐ NO	LD
7.	Discharge communication provided to principal care provider(s).	☒ YES	☐ NO	LD
8.	Documented receipt of discharge information from principal care provider(s).	☒ YES	☐ NO	LD
9.	Arrangements made for outpatient follow-up with principal care provider(s).	☒ YES	☐ NO	LD
	For increased-risk patients, consider:			
1.	Interdisciplinary rounds with patient/caregiver prior to discharge to review after-care plan.	☒ YES	☐ NO	LD
2.	Direct communication with principal care provider before discharge.	☒ YES	☐ NO	LD
3.	Phone contact with patient/caregiver arranged within 72 hours post-discharge to assess condition, discharge plan comprehension and adherence, and to reinforce follow-up.	☒ YES	☐ NO	LD
4.	Follow-up appointment with principal care provider within 7 days of discharge.	☒ YES	☐ NO	LD
5.	Direct contact information for hospital personnel familiar with patient's course provided to patient/caregiver to address questions/concerns *if unable to reach principal care provider* prior to first follow-up.	☒ YES	☐ NO	LD

Confirmed by: _____Lynn Davis, RN_____   _____Lynn Davis, RN_____   4/15/2019
                        Signature   Print Name   Date

General Assessment of Preparedness (GAP)
Prior to discharge, evaluate the following areas with the patient/caregiver(s). Communicate concerns identified as appropriate to principal care providers.
A = beginning upon Admission; **P** = Prior to discharge; **D** = at Discharge

	Logistical Issues			
1.	Functional status assessment completed (P). *Non-weight bearing right upper extremity and left lower extremity.*	☒ YES	☐ NO	☐ N/A
2.	Access (e.g., keys) to home ensured (P) for after SNF stay.	☒ YES	☐ NO	☐ N/A
3.	Home prepared for patient's arrival (P) *Meals on Wheels arranged.*	☒ YES	☐ NO	☐ N/A
4.	Financial resources for care needs assessed (P). *Home care covered by insurance previously.*	☒ YES	☐ NO	☐ N/A
5.	Ability to obtain medications confirmed (P).	☒ YES	☐ NO	☐ N/A
6.	Responsible party for ensuring medication adherence. Identified/prepared; if not patient (P) *(niece/nephew).*	☒ YES	☐ NO	☐ N/A
7.	Transportation to initial follow-up arranged (D).	☒ YES	☐ NO	☐ N/A
8.	Transportation home arranged (D). *ACS navigator*	☒ YES	☐ NO	☐ N/A

continued on next page

Chapter 11

Appendix 11-2.
Universal Patient Discharge Checklist and
General Assessment of Preparedness (GAP)

Note: Bold/italic areas apply to Case Study 11-1.

General Assessment of Preparedness (GAP)				
Prior to discharge, evaluate the following areas with the patient/caregiver(s). Communicate concerns identified as appropriate to principal care providers. **A** = beginning upon Admission; **P** = Prior to discharge; **D** = at Discharge				
Psychosocial Issues				
1. Substance abuse/dependence evaluated (A).		☒ *YES*	☐ NO	☐ N/A
2. Abuse/neglect presence assessed (A).		☒ *YES*	☐ NO	☐ N/A
3. Cognitive status assessed (A); makes own decisions.		☒ *YES*	☐ NO	☐ N/A
4. Advanced care planning documented (A).		☒ *YES*	☐ NO	☐ N/A
5. Support circle for patient identified (P).		☐ YES	☒ *NO*	☐ N/A
6. Contact information for home care services. Obtained and provided to patient (D) *(niece/nephew).* *Son, limited availability; can't get out much to see church friends*		☐ YES	☐ NO	☐ N/A
Confirmed by: _____*Lynn Davis, RN*_____ Signature	_____*Lynn Davis, RN*_____ Print Name		_____*5/13/2018*_____ Date	

Source: Adapted with permission from the Society of Hospital Medicine (SHM). © 2008. All rights reserved.

Chapter 11

**Appendix 11-3.
Patient PASS: A Transition Record**

**Patient Preparation to Address Situations
(after discharge) Successfully**

Note: Patient PASS applies to Case Study 11-1.

I was in the hospital because I fell and hurt my shoulder, but they told me I have cancer.		
If I have the following problems	**I should…**	**Important contact information:**
1. Fractured clavicle	1. Take pain medication as needed	1. My primary doctor: Dr. Smith (555) 111-2222
2. Lymphoma (Cancer of the lymph system)	2. Follow doctor and physical therapy orders	2. My hospital doctor: Dr. Jones (555) 333-9999
3. Diabetes	3. Go to follow-up with oncologist	3. My visiting nurse: Mary House, RN (555) 444-7777
4. High blood pressure	4. Monitor blood sugars and eat better	4. My pharmacy: (555) 666-8888
5. Difficulty taking care of myself and my wife		5. Other: Dr. Palermo
6. Poor medication compliance		
My appointments: 1. Dr. Smith On: 12/05/18 at 2:00pm For: blood sugar check 2. Dr. Jones On: 12/08/18 at 2:00pm For: oncology plan 3. Dr. Palmero On: 11/29/18 at 1:00pm For: routine follow-up of fracture	**Tests and issues I need to talk with my doctor(s) about at my clinic visit:** 1. A1C 2. My blood pressure 3. Oncology regimen and lab tests needed 4. Any scans needed for clavicle fracture 5. PT/OT after skilled nursing stay	
Other instructions: 1. Ice clavicle and take pain mediation as needed 2. Monitor for any signs and symptoms of infection 3. Call office if needed		I understand my treatment plan. I feel able and willing to participate actively in my care: _____ Patient/Caregiver

Source: Adapted with permission from the Society of Hospital Medicine (SHM). © 2014. All rights reserved.

Chapter 11

Case Study 11-2.
Clinical Interactions and Implementation for an Older Adult (Male) Presenting to ER with "Stomach Bug"

Introduction

Mr. R, a 75-year-old African American, presented to the emergency department with nausea, vomiting, increased urination, and generalized weakness. He reported having a "stomach bug" for 3 days prior to presenting to the emergency department and, as a result, had limited intake and inability to take his medications. Upon workup, he was found to have a glucose of 550, beta hydroxybutyrate of 4, and a hemoglobin A1c of 11.5. He presented physically deconditioned.

Review of his records revealed that Mr. R had three admissions within the last 6 months for elevated blood sugars and did not follow up with his primary care provider after discharge from acute care. In addition, Mr. R has a past medical history of hypertension and depression.

Mr. R lives with his wife, who is presently hospitalized with an acute myocardial infarction. His wife is his support for both medical and emotional help. Additionally, he identified a neighbor who could assist him after discharge. He and his wife are very involved in their faith community. He became tearful when he talked about his wife as he did not know how to help or support her. He is on multiple medications, including antihypertensive medications and insulin. He has difficulty remembering when to take his medications and lacks insight into diabetic care despite having all the necessary supplies. The CCTM® RN is notified of the potential discharge barriers and gaps in care Mr. R will face upon discharge. The CCTM RN is working to ensure Mr. R is set up with the local community health center for follow-up care planning.

Clinical Interactions

Nursing Process includes plan for:
- Continued education for diabetes
- Identification of barriers for successful care transition including social support, transportation, and physical limitations
- Follow-up for hypertension and diabetes care – primary care
- Medication management

Clinical Implementation

- Multiple clinical assessments required on an ongoing basis
- Assess need to reach out for social support
- Neighbors
- Parish nurses
- Wrap-around services
- Meals on Wheels
- Corporation for the Aging
- Transportation services
- Local senior centers
- Transition from acute care to home
- Home assessment
- Establish PT/OT in the home
- Visiting nurses
- Evaluation of outcomes and individual satisfaction

Note: Refer to Appendices 11-4 through 11-6.

Chapter 11

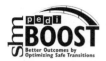

Appendix 11-4.
Tool for Addressing Risk: A Geriatric Evaluation for Transitions
Handoff Tool – Acute Care to CCTM® RN in PCMH Diabetes

Note: Bold/italic areas apply to Case Study 11-2.

Risk Assessment: 8P Screening Tool (Check all that apply.)		Risk-Specific Intervention	Signature of individual responsible for insuring intervention administered
Problem medications (anticoagulants, insulin, aspirin and clopidogrel dual therapy, digoxin, narcotics) ☒	☒	Medication specific education using teach back provided to patient and caregiver ***During hospitalization, "teach back" provided to ensure correct administration of insulin, including programming insulin pen and correct injection technique. Individual has no caregiver currently as wife is admitted in the hospital, relying on neighbor for assistance.***	T. Smith, RN
	☒	Monitoring plan developed and communicated to patient and aftercare providers, where relevant (e.g., warfarin, digoxin, and insulin) ***Individual taught to monitor and record blood sugar with each meal, and bring to follow-up appointment with primary care provider (PCP) and CCTM-RN. Individual and PCP aware that individual's insulin regimen has changed and that they are taking glargine 20 units daily and aspart 5 units with meals.***	
	☒	Specific strategies for managing adverse drug events reviewed with patient/caregiver ***Individual aware if experiencing hypo/hyperglycemia greater than x3 episodes he is to call PCP or CCTM RN.***	
	☒	Follow-up phone call at 72 hours to assess adherence and complications ***CCTM RN to follow-up with patient 72 hours post discharge. Individual was able to fill prescription for new medications at hospital pharmacy prior to discharge.***	
Psychological (depression screen positive or h/o depression diagnosis) ☒	☒	Assessment of need for psychiatric aftercare if not in place ***Individual has a history of depression, controlled well on sertraline and PCP has been following individual for years for this diagnosis.***	T. Smith, RN
	☒	Communication with aftercare providers, highlighting this issue if new ***Phone call placed by medical team to CCTM RN regarding change in insulin regimen, follow-up appointment scheduled with PCP.*** Involvement/awareness of support network insured	
	☒	***Individual's wife is in the hospital, a neighbor will be assisting the individual with grocery shopping, cleaning, and transportation to appointments.***	

continued on next page

Chapter 11

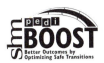

Appendix 11-4. (continued)
Tool for Addressing Risk: A Geriatric Evaluation for Transitions
Handoff Tool – Acute Care to CCTM® RN in PCMH Diabetes

Note: Bold/italic areas apply to Case Study 11-2.

Risk Assessment: 8P Screening Tool (Check all that apply.)		Risk-Specific Intervention	Signature of individual responsible for insuring intervention administered
Principal diagnosis (cancer, stroke, DM, COPD, heart failure) ☒	☒	Review of national discharge guidelines, where available	T. Smith, RN
	☒	Disease specific education using teach back with patient/caregiver	
		Registered dietician provided education to individual regarding meal planning, maintaining a food diary. Nursing reinforced meal planning, as well as use of glucometer and finger sticks, and how to manage sick days, using teach back.	
	☒	Action plan reviewed with patient/caregivers regarding what to do and who to contact in the event of worsening or new symptoms	
		Individual aware to contact CCTM RN or PCP regarding symptoms. Taught also to utilize urgent care if needed.	
Polypharmacy (≥5 more routine meds) ☒	☐	Elimination of unnecessary medications	T. Smith, RN
	☒	Simplification of medication scheduling to improve adherence	
		Individual's long-acting insulin was changed from BID administration to daily administration. Aspart insulin was simplified to same unit dosing with meals – 5 units with each meal (rather than 10 units with breakfast and 14 units with lunch and dinner).	
	☒	Follow-up phone call at 72 hours to assess adherence and complications	
		Individual was informed that a follow-up call will be made in 72 hours and confirmed contact number for the individual and neighbor.	
Poor health literacy (inability to do teach back) ☒	☒	Committed caregiver involved in planning/administration of all general and risk-specific interventions	T. Smith, RN
		As wife is unavailable, individual's neighbor will be acting as the caregiver. The neighbor is aware of follow-up appointments and to monitor the individual for mental status changes.	
	☒	Aftercare plan education using teach back provided to patient and caregiver	
	☒	Link to community resources for additional patient/caregiver support	
		Individual will have home physical therapy (PT) and has connected with a senior-group for individuals with diabetes that meets locally in the community.	
	☒	Follow-up phone call at 72 hours to assess adherence and complications	

continued on next page

Chapter 11

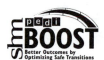

Appendix 11-4. (continued)
Tool for Addressing Risk: A Geriatric Evaluation for Transitions
Handoff Tool – Acute Care to CCTM® RN in PCMH Diabetes

Note: Bold/italic areas apply to Case Study 11-2.

Risk Assessment: 8P Screening Tool (Check all that apply.)	Risk-Specific Intervention	Signature of individual responsible for insuring intervention administered
Patient support (absence of caregiver to assist with discharge and home care) ☒	☒ Follow-up phone call at 72 hours to assess condition, adherence, and complications ☒ Follow-up appointment with aftercare medical provider within 7 days ***Individual has PCP appointment already scheduled for 5 days post discharge.*** ☒ Involvement of home care providers of services with clear communications of discharge plan to those providers ***Home PT has been set up. The neighbor is aware of follow-up appointments and the individual will also follow-up with a registered dietician. Both the PCP and CCTM RN are aware of follow-ups.***	T. Smith, RN
Prior hospitalization (non-elective; in last 6 months) ☒	☒ Review reasons for re-hospitalization in context of prior hospitalization ***Individual is aware to monitor for signs and symptoms of hypo/hyperglycemia, and is aware of sick day management.*** ☒ Follow-up phone call at 72 hours to assess condition, adherence and complications ☒ Follow-up appointment with aftercare medical provider within 7 days	T. Smith, RN
Palliative care (Would you be surprised if this patient died in the next year? Does this patient have an advanced or progressive serious illness?) Yes to either: ☒	☐ Assess need for palliative care services ☐ Identify goals of care and therapeutic options ☐ Communicate prognosis with patient/family/caregiver ☐ Assess and address bothersome symptoms ☐ Identify services or benefits available to patients based on advanced disease status ☐ Discuss with patient/family/caregiver role of palliative care services and benefits and services available ***Advanced directives were discussed, currently, a full code, no need for palliative care at this time, and family not available.***	T. Smith, RN

Source: Adapted with permission from the Society of Hospital Medicine (SHM). © 2014. All rights reserved.

Appendix 11-5.
Universal Patient Discharge Checklist and General Assessment of Preparedness (GAP)

Note: Bold/italic areas apply to Case Study 11-2.

	Universal Patient Discharge Checklist – *COMPLETED BY ACUTE CARE RN*			Initials
1.	GAP assessment (see below) completed with issues addressed.	☒ YES	☐ NO	TS
2.	Medications reconciled with pre-admission list.	☒ YES	☐ NO	TS
3.	Medication use/side effects reviewed using "teach back" with patient/caregiver(s).	☒ YES	☐ NO	TS
4.	"Teach back" used to confirm patient/caregiver understanding of disease, prognosis, and self-care requirements. *Completed with niece.*	☒ YES	☐ NO	TS
5.	Action plan for management of symptoms/side effects/complications requiring medical attention established and shared with patient/caregiver using "teach back."	☒ YES	☐ NO	TS
6.	Discharge plan (including educational materials; medication list with reason for use and highlighted new/changed/discontinued drugs; follow-up plans) taught with written copy provided to patient/caregiver at discharge.	☒ YES	☐ NO	TS
7.	Discharge communication provided to principal care provider(s).	☒ YES	☐ NO	TS
8.	Documented receipt of discharge information from principal care provider(s).	☒ YES	☐ NO	TS
9.	Arrangements made for outpatient follow-up with principal care provider(s).	☒ YES	☐ NO	TS
For increased-risk patients, consider:				
1.	Interdisciplinary rounds with patient/caregiver prior to discharge to review after-care plan.	☒ YES	☐ NO	TS
2.	Direct communication with principal care provider *before* discharge.	☒ YES	☐ NO	TS
3.	Phone contact with patient/caregiver arranged within 72 hours post-discharge to assess condition, discharge plan comprehension and adherence, and to reinforce follow-up.	☒ YES	☐ NO	TS
4.	Follow-up appointment with principal care provider within 7 days of discharge.	☒ YES	☐ NO	TS
5.	Direct contact information for hospital personnel familiar with patient's course provided to patient/caregiver to address questions/concerns *if unable to reach principal care provider* prior to first follow-up.	☒ YES	☐ NO	TS

Confirmed by: _____T. Smith, RN_____   _____T. Smith, RN_____   _____4/15/2019_____
                              Signature   Print Name   Date

General Assessment of Preparedness (GAP)
Prior to discharge, evaluate the following areas with the patient/caregiver(s). Communicate concerns identified as appropriate to principal care providers.
A = beginning upon Admission; **P** = Prior to discharge; **D** = at Discharge

	Logistical Issues			
1.	Functional status assessment completed (P). *Yes PT/OT to see patient*	☒ YES	☐ NO	☐ N/A
2.	Access (e.g., keys) to home ensured (P).	☒ YES	☐ NO	☐ N/A
3.	Home prepared for patient's arrival (P)	☒ YES	☐ NO	☐ N/A
4.	Financial resources for care needs assessed (P). *Patient insurance to cover health care visits Home care covered by insurance previously.*	☒ YES	☐ NO	☐ N/A
5.	Ability to obtain medications confirmed (P). *Will have filled prior to discharge*	☒ YES	☐ NO	☐ N/A
6.	Responsible party for ensuring medication adherence. Identified/prepared; if not patient (P). *Patient is aware about meds*	☒ YES	☐ NO	☐ N/A
7.	Transportation to initial follow-up arranged (D). *Neighbor to transport patient*	☒ YES	☐ NO	☐ N/A
8.	Transportation home arranged (D). *Neighbor to transport patient*	☒ YES	☐ NO	☐ N/A

continued on next page

**Appendix 11-5. (continued)
Universal Patient Discharge Checklist and
General Assessment of Preparedness (GAP)**

Note: Bold/italic areas apply to Case Study 11-2.

General Assessment of Preparedness (GAP)
Prior to discharge, evaluate the following areas with the patient/caregiver(s). Communicate concerns identified as appropriate to principal care providers.
A = beginning upon Admission; **P** = Prior to discharge; **D** = at Discharge

Psychosocial Issues			
1. Substance abuse/dependence evaluated (A).	☒ **YES**	☐ NO	☐ N/A
2. Abuse/neglect presence assessed (A).	☒ **YES**	☐ NO	☐ N/A
3. Cognitive status assessed (A); makes own decisions.	☒ **YES**	☐ NO	☐ N/A
4. Advanced care planning documented (A).	☒ **YES**	☐ NO	☐ N/A
5. Support circle for patient identified (P). (neighbor)	☐ YES	☒ **NO**	☐ N/A
6. Contact information for home care services. Obtained and provided to patient (D). *Son, limited availability; can't get out much to see church friends*	☐ YES	☐ NO	☐ N/A

Confirmed by: _____T. Smith, RN_____   _____T. Smith, RN_____   _____4/15/2019_____
              Signature   Print Name   Date

Source: Adapted with permission from the Society of Hospital Medicine (SHM). © 2008. All rights reserved.

Chapter 11

Appendix 11-6.
Patient PASS: A Transition Record
Patient Preparation to Address Situations (after discharge) Successfully

Note: Patient PASS applies to Case Study 11-2.

I was in the hospital because I had a stomach virus and elevated blood sugars.		
If I have the following problems...	**I should...**	**Important contact information:**
1. Diabetes	1. Check my blood sugars with my machine 3 times a day.	1. **My primary doctor:** Dr. Smith (555) 111-2222
2. High blood pressure	2. Take my medications. Decrease salt in my diet.	2. **My hospital doctor:** Dr. Jones (555) 333-9999
3. Problems taking my medication	3. Contact my physician's office to speak with nurse or doctor about my medications.	3. **My visiting nurse:** Mary House, RN (555) 444-7777
4. Use my glucometer	4. Work with visiting nurse to learn functionality of glucometer.	4. **My pharmacy:** (555) 666-8888
My appointments: 1. Dr. Smith On: 10/20/18 at 2:00pm For: blood sugar check 2. On: __/__/__ at __:__ am/pm For: _____ 3. On: __/__/__ at __:__ am/pm For: _____ 4. On: __/__/__ at __:__ am/pm For: _____	**Tests and issues I need to talk with my doctor(s) about at my clinic visit:** 1. A1C 2. My blood pressure 3. _____ 4. _____ 5. _____	5. Other: _____
Other instructions: 1. _____ 2. _____ 3. _____		I understand my treatment plan. I feel able and willing to participate actively in my care: _____ Patient/Caregiver

Source: Adapted with permission from the Society of Hospital Medicine (SHM). © 2014. All rights reserved.

Chapter 11

References

Agency for Healthcare Research and Quality. (n.d.). *Guidelines and measures.* Retrieved from http://www.guideline.gov/

American Academy of Ambulatory Care Nursing (AAACN). (2016). *Scope and standards of practice for registered nurses in care coordination and transition management.* Pitman, NJ: Author.

American Medical Directors Association. (2010). *Transitions of care in the long-term care continuum: Practice guideline.* Columbia, MD: AMDA. Retrieved from https://www.nhqualitycampaign.org/files/Transitions_of_Care_in_LTC.pdf

American Nurses Association (ANA). (2012). *Care coordination and registered nurses' essential role.* [Position statement]. Silver Spring, MD: Author.

Boutwell, A., Jencks, S., Nielsen, G.A., & Rutherford, P. (2009). *STate Action on Avoidable Rehospitalizations (STAAR) initiative: Applying early evidence and experience in front-line process improvements to develop a state-based strategy.* Cambridge, MA: Institute for Healthcare Improvement.

Carter, J.A., Carr, L.S., Collins, J., Petrongolo, J.D., Hall, K., Murray, J., ... Tata, L.A. (2015). STAAR: Improving the reliability of care coordination and reducing hospital readmissions in an academic medical centre. *BMJ Innovations, 1*(3), 75-80. doi:10.1136/bmjinnov-2015-000048

Centers for Medicare & Medicaid Services (CMS). (2013). *Partnership for patients: Readmissions and care transitions.* Retrieved from http://partnershipforpatients.cms.gov/p4p_resources/tsp-preventablereadmissions/toolpreventablereadmissions.html

Centers for Medicare & Medicaid Services (CMS). (2018). *Community-based care transitions program.* Retrieved from http://innovation.cms.gov/initiatives/CCTP/?itemID=CMS1239313

Cibulskis, C.C., Giardino, A.P., & Moyer, V.A. (2011). Care transitions from inpatient to outpatient settings: Ongoing challenges and emerging best practices. *Hospital Practice, 39*(3), 128-139. doi:10.3810/hp.2011.08.588

Coffey, C., Greenwald, J., Budnitz, T., & Williams, M.V. (2013). *Project BOOST® implementation guide (2nd ed.).* Philadelphia, PA: Society of Hospital Medicine.

Coleman, E.A. (2007). *The Care Transitions Program®.* Retrieved from https://caretransitions.org

Coleman, E.A., & Boult, C. (2003). Improving the quality of transitional care for persons with complex care needs. *Journal of the American Geriatrics Society, 51*(4), 556-557. doi:10.1046/j.1532-5415.2003. 51186.x

Coleman, E.A., Parry, C., Chalmers, S., & Min, S.J. (2006). The care transitions intervention: Results of a randomized controlled trial. *Archives of Internal Medicine, 166*(17), 1,822-1,828.

Coleman, E.A., Roman, S.P., Hall, K.A., & Min, S.J. (2015). Enhancing the care transitions intervention protocol to better address the needs of family caregivers. *Journal for Healthcare Quality, 37*(1), 2-11. doi:10.1097/01.JHQ.0000460118.60567.fe

Counsell, S.R., Callahan, C.M., Buttar, A.B., Clark, D.O., & Frank, K.I. (2006). Geriatric Resources for Assessment and Care of Elders (GRACE): A new model of primary care for low-income seniors. *Journal of the American Geriatric Society, 54*(7), 1,136-1,141.

Cronenwett, L., Sherwood, G., Barnsteiner, J., Disch, J., Johnson, J., Mitchell, P., ... Warren, J. (2007). Quality and safety education for nurses. *Nursing Outlook, 55*(3), 122-131. doi:10.1016/j. outlook.2007.02.006

Hirschman, K.B., Shaid, E., Bixby, M.B., Badolato, D.J., Barg, R., Byrnes, M.B., ... Naylor, M.D. (2017). Transitional care in the patient-centered medical home: Lessons in adaptation. *Journal for Healthcare Quality, 39*(2), 67-77. doi:10.1097/01.JHQ.0000462685.78253.e8

Institute for Healthcare Improvement (IHI). (2018a). *STate Action on Avoidable Rehospitalizations (STAAR).* Retrieved from http://www.ihi.org/Engage/Initiatives/Completed/STAAR/Pages/default.aspx

Institute for Healthcare Improvement (IHI). (2018b). *Ask me 3: Good questions for your good health.* Retrieved from http://www.npsf.org/?page=askme3

Interprofessional Education Collaborative (IPEC). (2016). *Core competencies for interprofessional collaborative practice: 2016 update.* Retrieved from https://hsc.unm.edu/ipe/resources/ipec-2016-core-competencies.pdf

Jack, B., Paasche-Orlow, M., Mitchell, S., Forsythe, S., & Martin, J. (2013). *Re-Engineered Discharge (RED) toolkit.* AHRQ Publication No. 12(13)-0084. Rockville, MD: Agency for Healthcare Research and Quality. Retrieved from https://www.ahrq.gov/professionals/systems/hospital/red/toolkit/index.html

Jusela, C., Struble, L., Gallagher, N.A., Redman, R.W., & Ziemba, R.A. (2017). Communication between acute care hospitals and skilled nursing facilities during care transitions: A retrospective chart review. *Journal of Gerontological Nursing, 43*(3), 19-28. doi:10.3928/00989134-20161109-03

Kansagara, D., Chiovaro, J.C., Kagen, D., Jencks, S., Rhyne, K., O'Neil, M., ... Englander, H. (2016). So many options, where do we start? An overview of the care transitions literature. *Journal of Hospital Medicine, 11*(3), 221-230. doi:10.1002/jhm.2502

Mallory, L.A., Osorio, S.N., Prato, B.S., DiPace, J., Schmutter, L., Soung, P., ... Cooperberg, D. (2017). Project IMPACT pilot report: Feasibility of implementing a hospital-to-home transition bundle. *Pediatrics, 139*(3). doi:10.1542/peds.2015-4626

Mitchell, P., Wynia, M., Golden, R., McNellis, B., Okun, S., Webb, C.E., ... Kohorn, I.V. (2012). *Core principles & values of effective team-based health care.* [Discussion paper]. Washington, DC: Institute of Medicine. doi:10.31478/201210c

National Learning Consortium. (n.d.). *Care coordination tool for transition to long-term and post-acute care.* Retrieved from https://www.healthit.gov/sites/default/files/nlc_ltpac_carecoordinationtool.pdf

National POLST Paradigm. (2018). *For patients and families.* Retrieved from http://www.polst.org/advance-care-planning/

National Transitions of Care Coalition (NTOCC). (n.d.). *Improved transitions of patient care yield tangible savings.* Retrieved from http://www.ntocc.org/portals/0/pdf/resources/TangibleSavings.pdf

Naylor, M.D. (2012). *Making transitional care more effective & efficient: APRNs ensure smooth transition from hospital to home, cutting re-hospitalization rates for geriatric patients.* Retrieved from https://higherlogicdownload.s3.amazonaws.com/AANNET/c8a8da9e-918c-4dae-b0c6-6d630c46007f/UploadedImages/docs/Edge%20Runners/rtv_making-transitional-care-more%20effective-efficient%20aprn_web.pdf

Naylor, M.D., Aiken, L.H., Kurtzman, E.T., Olds, D.M., & Hirschman, K.B. (2011). The care span: The importance of transitional care in achieving health reform. *Health Affairs, 30*(4), 746-754. doi:10.1377/hlthaff.2011.0041

Naylor, M.D., Brooten, D., Campbell, R., Jacobsen, B.S., Mezey, M.D., Pauly, M.V., & Schwartz, J.S. (1999). Comprehensive discharge planning and home follow-up of hospitalized elders: A randomized clinical trial. *Journal of the American Medical Association, 281*(7), 613-620.

Naylor, M.D., Brooten, D.A., Campbell, R.L., Maislin, G., McCauley, K.M., & Schwartz, J.S. (2004). Transitional care of older adults hospitalized with heart failure: A randomized, controlled trial. *Journal of the American Geriatrics Society, 52*(5), 675-684.

Naylor, M.D., Shaid, E.C., Carpenter, D., Gass, B., Levine, C., Li, J., ... Williams, M.V. (2017). Components of comprehensive and effective transitional care. *Journal of the American Geriatrics Society, 65*(6), 1119-1125. doi:10.1111/jgs.14782

Robinson, R., & Hudali, T. (2017). The HOSPITAL score and LACE index as predictors of 30 day readmission in a retrospective study at a university-affiliated community hospital. *PeerJ, 5*. doi:10.7717/peerj.3137

Scott, A.M., Li, J., Oyewole-Eletu, S., Nguyen, H.Q., Gass, B., Hirschman, K.B, ... Williams, M.V. (2017). Understanding facilitators and barriers to care transitions: Insights from

Project ACHIEVE site visits. *Joint Commission Journal on Quality and Patient Safety, 43*(9), 433-447. doi:10.1016/j.jcjq.2017.02.012

Society of Hospital Medicine. (2014). *The 8 Ps: Assessing your patient's risk for adverse events after discharge.* Philadelphia, PA: Author.

Starmer, A.J., Spector, N.D., Srivastava, R., West, D.C., Rosenbluth, G., Allen, A.D., ... Landrigan, C.P. (2014). Changes in medical errors after implementation of a handoff program. *The New England Journal of Medicine, 371*(5), 1803-1812.

Swan, B.A. (2012). A nurse learns firsthand that you may fend for yourself after a hospital stay. *Health Affairs, 31*(11), 2,579-2,582. doi:10.1377/hlthaff.2012.0516

Toles, M., Colon-Emeric, C., Asafu-Adjei, J., Moreton, E., & Hanson, L.C. (2016). Transitional care of older adults in skilled nursing facilities: A systematic review. *Geriatric Nursing, 37*(4), 296-301. doi:10.1016/j.gerinurse.2016.04.012

Additional Readings

Coleman, E.A., & Boult, C. (2007). Improving the quality of transitional care for persons with complex care needs. *Assisted Living Consult, 3*(2), 30-32.

Grimmer, K., Moss, J., Falco, J., & Kindness, H. (2006). Incorporating patient and carer concerns in discharge plans: The development of a practical patient-centered checklist. *The Internet Journal of Allied Health Sciences and Practice, 4*(1), 1-8. Retrieved from https://nsuworks.nova.edu/cgi/viewcontent.cgi?article=1095&context=ijahsp/

Hughes, R.G. (Ed.). (2008). *Patient safety and quality: An evidence-based handbook for nurses.* Rockville, MD: Agency for Healthcare Research and Quality.

Kim, C.S., & Flanders, S.A. (2013). Transitions of care. *Annals of Internal Medicine, 158*(5). doi:10.7326/0003-4819-158-5-201303050-01003

Leff, B., Reider, L., Frick, K.D., Scharfstein, D.O., Boyd, C.M., Frey, K., ... Boult, C. (2009). Guided care and the cost of complex healthcare: A preliminary report. *The American Journal of Managed Care, 15*(8), 555-559.

Manheim, J., & Rifkin, J. (2010). *Transitions of care: Physician to physician communication.* Denver, CO: The Colorado Health Foundation. Retrieved from http://www.ucdenver.edu/academics/colleges/medicalschool/departments/medicine/gim/education/continuingeducation/documents/3_9_10_manheimandrifkinpdf.pdf

National Transitions of Care Coalition (NTOCC). (2011). *Care transition bundle: Seven essential intervention categories.* Retrieved from http://www.ntocc.org/Portals/0/PDF/Compendium/SevenEssentialElements.pdf

Chapter 12

Instructions for Continuing Nursing Education Contact Hours
Continuing nursing education credit can be earned for completing the learning activity associated with this chapter. Instructions can be found at aaacn.org/CCTMCoreCNE

Informatics Competencies to Support Nursing Practice

Robin Austin, PhD, DNP, RN-BC
Naomi Mercier, DNP, MSN, RN-BC
Rosemary Kennedy, PhD, RN, MBA, FAAN
Sharon Bouyer-Ferullo, DNP, RN, MHA, CNOR
Rachel Start, MSN, RN, NE-BC
Diane Storer-Brown, PhD, RN, CPHQ, FNAHQ, FAAN

Learning Outcome Statement

After completing this learning activity, the learner will be able to demonstrate the elements of competency in informatics to support nursing practice that are required for the Care Coordination and Transition Management registered nurse (CCTM® RN) role.

The competencies that will be addressed in this chapter include:
- Competency 1: Integrates health information technology that is aligned with the CCTM RN Model.
- Competency 2: Explains why information and technology skills are essential for safe patient care (Cronenwett et al., 2007).
- Competency 3: Integrates the Centers for Medicare and Medicaid Services (CMS) Meaningful Measures Framework within use of health information technology to identify the highest priorities for quality measurement and improvement in CCTM (CMS, 2018).

Competency Definitions

Although nursing informatics is a highly specialized area of practice, there are fundamental competencies that all practicing nurses need to achieve for safe, quality, and competent CCTM in the current technological environment. A nursing informatics competency is defined as "adequate knowledge, skills, and the ability to perform specific informatics tasks" (McGonigle, Hunter, & Hebda, 2013, p. 239). Information systems that support nursing practice require the incorporation of clinical knowledge/clinical content within health information technology (HIT) that will assist in determining errors that are technology induced. This includes an understanding of nursing workflow, clinical decision support mechanisms, and support for nursing documentation in an effort to streamline nursing care for efficiency and effectiveness.

Nursing informatics (NI) is defined by the American Nurses Association (ANA) (2015) as a "specialty that integrates nursing science, with multiple information and analytical sciences to identify, define, manage, and communicate data, information, knowledge, and wisdom in nursing practice. NI supports nurses, consumers, individuals, the interprofessional healthcare team and other stakeholders in their decision-making in all roles and settings to achieve desired outcomes. This support is accomplished through the use of information structures, information processes, and information technologies" (p. 65). HIT is a tool used to facilitate care coordination by analyzing, collecting, and sharing data that communicates person-centered information among individuals, families, and care providers across communities (Cipriano et al., 2013). Because HIT plays a critical role in communication, frequently the terms information and communications technology are used along with HIT and may be used interchangeably with HIT. The increasing integration of HIT and communications technology provides an opportunity to gather meaningful data to generate patient-reported outcomes (PROs). PROs are defined as any report of the status of a patient's condition that is derived directly from the patient, without interpretation by a clinician or anyone else (National Quality Forum [NQF], 2012.

There are numerous technologies that are included under the umbrella term of HIT. One of national importance is the electronic health record (EHR), which includes comprehensive and longitudinal information about the individual, and supporting care across all settings (acute, post-acute, home, ambulatory, clinic, etc.). The Healthcare Information and Management Systems

Society (HIMSS) defines an EHR as a longitudinal electronic record of an individual's health information and can include one or more encounters across multiple health settings. Information collected in the EHR includes individual demographics, progress notes, health problems, current and past medications, vital signs, previous medical history, immunizations, laboratory data, and radiology reports (HIMSS, 2018). The EHR automates and streamlines the clinician's workflow. The EHR has the ability to generate a complete record of a clinical encounter and can facilitate interprofessional collaboration and coordination of care activities to support evidence-based decisions, quality care management, and health outcomes reporting (HIMSS, 2018). Personal health records (PHRs) originated from EHRs and are defined as an integrated health record that can be used by health care providers and individuals (Roehrs, da Costa, da Rosa Righi, & de Oliveira, 2017). PHRs typically contain patient-reported care outcomes and clinical information that is needed for effective care coordination. A difference between PHR and EHR is in the PHR, the individual has more control of the type of information included in the records and who may have access to the data versus an EHR is driven by the health system. Connecting both EHR and PHR records may improve the care coordination process to support person-centered goals and individual self-management and potentially avoid unwanted care or unnecessary cost (Cipriano et al., 2013). An individual can access the information if their health system EHR is enabled with the use of patient portals. Patient portals are stored on a secure server, which communicates with the server, and is encrypted. It provides secure online 24-hour access to personal health information, such as medications, laboratory results, allergies, appointments, immunizations, and care plans, from any location via the Internet.

Mobile technology and cloud computing play a major role in CCTM. The major advantage of cloud computing for care coordination is 'on demand' access to information without requiring human interaction with individual service providers. Mobile applications have been targeting individual engagement, and are useful tools for supporting person-centered care coordination by improving the interaction between providers and individuals (Baysari & Westbrook, 2015). With the appropriate security and individual privacy software, cloud computing can be a tool to facilitate information exchange across geographic settings, providers, and individuals. As nurses advise and educate individuals, it is important to assess the internet sources of education using criteria ensuring the entity posting the information is a valid and reliable source of evidence-based content, that original sources of publication are provided, and that the information is reviewed by someone with the appropriate credentials before it is posted.

The proliferation of smartphone use combined with FDA approval of wearable devices that monitor and transmit individual data, whether the individual is in the hospital, home, or clinic, enables nurses to detect deterioration or a change in an individual's condition from any location. Through advances in alarm algorithms, nurses in clinics can receive alarms on smartphones indicating that an individual at home is at risk of deterioration. The wearable devices include built-in sensors that capture body movement, immobility, vital signs, ECG, SpO2, and heart rate variability. The wearable devices can communicate information through wireless interfaces to smartphones and EHRs (Lu, Zhang, Zhang, Xiao, & Yu, 2017).

The flow of health information across numerous and disparate electronic systems and health care facilities can enable collaboration and coordination of care to improve outcomes, reduce redundant tests, and lower costs. Individual information follows the patient regardless of institution, vendor software, or geographical setting. In essence, the electronic systems interoperate with each other to send data that is received in a manner useful for both the individual and the clinician. This interoperability refers to messaging standards that make it possible for diverse electronic systems and applications to communicate with each other. This exchange occurs both within and between provider settings across broad geographical settings forming information networks that combine different vendor systems. This enables the formation of health information exchanges (HIEs) which are organizations that electronically transfer individual health and insurance data (such as diagnoses, test results, plans of care, insurance information) between providers to enable valid and reliable CCTM (Langabeer & Champagne, 2016). Information for an individual discharged from Hospital A is sent to the clinic/office, post-acute care facility, home care agency, nurse-led urgent care clinic, and subsequently this outpatient information is sent to Hospital B's emergency room when the individual arrives for care.

Nursing informatics practice is directly aligned with the CCTM Scope and Standards. Specifically, Standard 5A states, "The RN practicing CCTM coordinates the delivery of care within the practice setting and across health care settings" (American Academy of Ambulatory Care Nursing [AAACN], 2015, p. 18). This is evident as the RN uses technology to facilitate care coordination across multiple health settings. Informatics nursing practice is reflected in Standard 11 as the RN uses

Chapter 12

technology to communicate effectively and enhance relationships to deliver effective care (AAACN, 2018). Through use of informatics tools, the CCTM RN incorporates Standard 15 to identify appropriate resources to plan and facilitate services that are safe, effective, and fiscally responsible (AAACN, 2018).

I. Competency 1: The Use of Health Information Technology that Is Aligned with the CCTM RN Model

Learning Outcome Statement

- Integrate the application of information science within the CCTM RN Model to manage data, information, and knowledge during CCTM.
- Describe the use of HIEs to support nursing practice related to CCTM while also facilitating coordinated individual care, avoiding duplication in treatment, and increasing individual/consumer satisfaction.
- Describe the functionalities that patient portals need to have as a foundation for individual engagement and empowerment in their care.
- Describe the application of standardized terminologies to support all aspects of the nursing process including documentation of assessments, diagnoses, interventions, goals, and outcomes as described in the CCTM RN Model.
- Understand the importance of using messaging standards to communicate information during CCTM across providers and geographical settings.
- Describe the application of data analytics to measure CCTM outcomes correlated with nursing practice and the associated impact on individual outcomes.
- Describe the integration of the knowledge, skills, and attitudes between the CCTM RN Model and nursing informatics (see Table 12-1 on page 276).
- Integrate various HIT solutions, such as EHRs, PHRs, the Internet, smartphones, body-worn sensors, and HIEs into CCTM using the CCTM RN Model as the foundation.

Learning Objectives

- Show knowledge, skills, and the ability to perform specific informatics tasks as described here in this chapter to support nursing practice within CCTM.
- Describe the data, information, and knowledge required within HIT databases to support data analytics, outcomes measurement, and coordination of care associated with CCTM.
- Describe the role of standardized terminologies in supporting communication of information between disparate electronic systems across providers and geographical settings.
- Show how the CCTM RN Model can be used to identify the requirements for HIT to support CCTM.
- Evaluate requirements for the electronic care plan that support the CCTM RN Model to support self-care management, cross-setting communication, and identification of high-risk individuals and population management.
- Recognize the importance of the entire clinical team, including the individual/family/caregiver, in defining requirements for HIT to support CCTM.
- Show knowledge in the use of HIE's to advance both nursing practice and individual outcomes within the context of CCTM.
- Describe how to optimize individual portals to increase patient engagement around CCTM.

The Technology Informatics Guiding Education Reform (TIGER), formed in 2006, developed informatics recommendations for all practicing nurses and graduating nursing students. The TIGER Informatics Competency Collaborative performed an extensive review of literature for informatics, which resulted in over 1,000 individual competency statements. This body of work was then synthesized to create the TIGER Informatics Competency Model. In September 2014, TIGER looked to broaden its mission towards acceptance of HIT, and transitioned to HIMSS with an interprofessional focus (Blake & Shaw, 2017).

The 2012 Quality and Safety Education for Nurses (QSEN) competencies for informatics focus on the use of information and technology to communicate, manage knowledge, mitigate error, and support decision-making. These competencies are closely aligned with the competencies in the CCTM RN Model, which evolved from an effort to standardize work that nurses do using evidence from the interprofessional literature on CCTM.

HIT can support activities and decision-making related to CCTM in real-time. Communication technologies, combined with HIT, have the potential to reduce cost, support data capture to measure performance, and improve outcomes for all populations in all health care settings. RNs in CCTM, require basic knowledge of the importance of data standards, EHRs, HIEs, data analytics, and communication technologies as they apply to CCTM.

HIT solutions capture large data sets as a byproduct of care delivery. These data sets can be analyzed to improve individual care such as identification of nursing interventions which have the greatest impact on outcomes. This helps individuals and informs nursing practice by generating evidence-based interventions personalized to the individual. For example, reducing pressure ulcers has been informed by big data analysis using nursing data sets that include documented nursing interventions and this has generated evidence to inform nursing practice (Raju, Su, Patrician, Loan, & McCarthy, 2015). The inquiry into these large data sets starts with a question/hypothesis and nurses involved in CCTM are best positioned to develop these questions for data science inquiry. Nursing needs big data to advance practice (Brennan & Bakken, 2015).

When data from an electronic clinical documentation source such as an EHR is extracted or "mined" it can be analyzed to help create new knowledge and improve individual care. For example, surgical site infections (SSIs) are costly and far too common for individuals, and account for 20% of all hospital acquired infections (HAIs) – an estimated national cost of $3- to $5-billion (Merkow et al., 2015). As surgeries become increasingly complex, the approach to reducing SSI must continue to implement practices to reflect updated technique and supporting evidence (Barnes, 2018). Data collection for this adverse outcome has resulted in evidence-based guidelines that nursing can use preoperatively, intraoperatively, and postoperatively to reduce SSIs. Although these SSI prevention guidelines are based on small number of recommendations, opportunity still remains to create reliable designed SSI prevention programs using mined data from the EHR (Barnes, 2018).

Individuals who receive their care from various ambulatory care facility clinicians are vulnerable to errors in care, partly due to lack of communication and lack of individual engagement in shared decision-making (Davis, Collier, Situ, Coe, & Cleary-Fishman, 2017). The Agency for Healthcare Research and Quality (AHRQ) created a toolkit specifically for the ambulatory care setting. Several evidence-based resources were adapted to develop the ambulatory care individual and clinician tools in this toolkit. The toolkit contains a detailed implementation guide, pre-intervention assessment, follow-up appointment aide, clinician checklist, and educational video. The findings of this project provided opportunities to engage individuals and their care partners as active participants in avoiding harm during transitions of care. Portions of this toolkit may be implemented within the EHR, which would provide easier access within daily workflows. Additional work is needed to understand how this toolkit impacts safe transitions of care by examining individual outcomes and additional process improvements (Davis et al., 2017).

One of the most promising technology solutions for CCTM focuses on the adoption of HIEs by providers. HIEs consolidate existing individual records from multiple providers into an integrated view for streamlined access by clinicians, independent of care setting. Availability of the record itself as the main benefit is augmented with avoidance of duplicate testing and improved coordination of care. Recent integration of patient portals within HIEs provides the added value of the individual having access to clinical, insurance, and outcome information from every health care provider/location they visit (Abdelhamid, 2018). Both HIEs and patient portals can be harnessed for more efficient and effective care delivery by nurses involved in CCTM, while also putting the individual at the center of care, which leads to better outcomes. Increased access to the individual's own health information, through person-facing technologies, such as a patient portal, can improve information sharing, assist with managing care, and potentially improve medication adherence (Knight & Shea, 2014).

A. Role of HIT and communication technologies.
   1. HIT.
      a. Serves as an important component in care coordination.
      b. Facilitates person-centered care.
      c. Leverages important information and communications technologies. Provides ubiquitous access to information, evidence-based alerts, and reminders across people, functions, and sites over time.
      d. Closes the gap in care and facilitates evidence-based decision making.
      e. Generates new knowledge through data analytics and machine learning.
      f. Supports the 'triple aim:' to improve health outcomes, lower costs, and enhance the individual experience (Rocks & Cooper-Audain, 2015).
   2. Knowledge of HIT in relation to care coordination.
      a. Supports the use of HIT in all domains of care coordination.
         (1) Health care home.
         (2) Proactive and longitudinal care planning.
         (3) Communication and hand-offs within and between settings of care.
         (4) Transition management.
      b. Allows recognition of the role of HIEs in sharing information.
         (1) Uses HIEs to share information between and among facilities.
         (2) Integrates HIEs into practice, education, and research.

Chapter 12

(3) Recognizes the importance of HIEs to exchange information spanning different organizations across diverse regions of care delivery.
3. The CCTM RN's knowledge of HIT in relation to the individual/person/caregiver allows:
   a. Understanding of the role of PHRs in consumer engagement, coordination of information from multiple providers, enhance communication between providers and individuals, availability of individual information, safety, and quality.
   b. Recognition of the importance of mobile technology platforms, such as iPads, tablets, notebooks, smartwatches, and smartphones.
   c. Recognition of the use of body-worn sensors and PROs for early detection of high risk individuals requiring additional care during CCTM.
   d. Practice using mobile technology for on-demand access to information, serving multiple users at once (nurse, physician, nurse practitioner, physician assistant, individual, caregiver, consumer).
4. CCTM RN use of the Internet.
   a. Supports practice using the Internet as a source for access to evidence-based content.
   b. Allows articulation of criteria used to assess sources of information found on the Internet.
   c. Leads to practices using a structure and process for evaluating sources of content on the Internet prior to integration with CCTM functions.
   d. Recognizes the role of the Internet in supporting coordination of care from one setting to another.

II. **Competency 2: Explain Why Information and Technology Skills Are Essential for Safe Individual Care**
(Cronenwett et al., 2007)

Learning Outcome Statement
- Demonstrate understanding of the different HIT solutions and their value in enhancing CCTM.
- Understand the role of clinical decision-support tools in CCTM, recognizing that they are to be utilized to support decision-making in concert with critical thinking and clinical judgment rather than dictate practice.
- Understand the role of analytics in mining individual data to describe care delivered thereby enabling improvements in care and through analysis of large datasets, the ability to predict outcomes.
- Identify functions related to CCTM that can be supported with HIT (e.g., problem list communication, clinical decision support, and care plan management).
- Understand the role of electronic quality reporting in measuring outcomes and improving performance.
- Recognize the importance of using nationally recognized, standardized terminologies to support cross-setting communication and transition across all domains of the person-centered medical home.
- Demonstrate ability to translate the information needs of caregivers to those designing the actual systems to capture and communicate individual care data.
- Understand the role of various HIT solutions, such as EHRs, PHRs, the Internet, smartphones, body-worn sensors, and HIEs into CCTM using the CCTM RN Model as the foundation.
- Identify safety functions related to CCTM that can be supported with HIT (e.g., alerts for out-of-range findings, suggestion of potential problems based on documentation, and access to evidence-based guidelines in real time during CCTM).

Learning Objectives
- Describe ways in which various forms of HIT support CCTM in accordance with the CCTM RN standardized practices that support safety and quality using the CCTM RN Model.
- Demonstrate the role various HIT solutions, such as EHRs, PHRs, the Internet, smartphones, body-worn sensors, and HIEs, have in enhancing CCTM.
- Describe the application of professional practice standards to the use of HIT within the CCTM RN role.
- Describe the importance of technology-enabled workflow in enhancing CCTM.
- Demonstrate the skills needed to use HIT to support CCTM within the scope of the CCTM RN role.
- Contrast benefits and limitations of different communication technologies and their impact on safety and quality.
- Describe the benefits and limitations of selected safety-enhancing technologies (e.g., barcodes, computer provider order entry, medication pumps, and automatic alerts/alarms), when

coordinating care and transitioning individuals from one level of care to another (Cronenwett et al., 2007, 2009).

EHRs have greatly improved individual safety through increasing insight into clinical processes and documentation (Sittig & Singh, 2017). The information contained within EHRs and other forms of HIT provide information to caregivers that is necessary to diagnose health problems, treat effectively, reduce documentation errors and inefficiencies/misunderstandings in care delivery, and lower costs. For decades, nurses at all levels have contributed as leaders in the development, use, and examination of effective technology solutions used at the bedside (Murphy, 2013). For instance, nurses have lead HIT solutions designed to provide clinical decision support technology tools and to guide them through many documentation processes as the individual transitions from one setting of care to another (Murphy, 2013).

HIT supports clinical decision at an individual level through alerts, reminders, and evidence-based guidelines to enhance CCTM. In addition, HIT supports decision making at an aggregate level through analysis of individual outcomes using data mining techniques. For example, data analysis techniques such as exploratory data analysis and data visualization have been used with public health nursing data sets to improve home visiting services (Monsen, Brandt et al., 2017). Essentially, HIT-enabled clinical decision support helps prevent adverse events, improve the quality of care, and increase satisfaction with care (HealthIT.gov, n.d.).

The use of multiple sources of HIT solutions (e.g., use of EHR systems, remote care management and monitoring, linkages to web-based services and information, computer-driven algorithms, tracking clinical and nonclinical metrics, dynamic and remote health assessments, and provider communication and coordination of care), when well integrated, enhance the value of population health management and care coordination. Integration is key to achieving this goal. HIEs currently under development with support from the Health Information Technology for Economic and Clinical Health (HITECH) Act (U.S. Department of Health and Human Services [DHHS], 2010) will increasingly become information sources for data collection and analysis.

A. The role of HIT in ensuring individual safety spans multiple domains of care delivery, all of which impact CCTM, including the following areas:
   1. Support of multiple uses of data contained within HIT systems during CCTM for early identification and prevention of events such as missed-care.
   2. Use of real-time clinical data in EHRs, which is more actionable than claims or billing data, which was used for individual safety improvement efforts in the past (Russo, Sittig, Murphy, & Singh, 2016)
   3. Capture of data to help nurses in monitoring safety while also providing the necessary information to move towards quality management across populations of individuals.
   4. Evaluation of population health outcomes to ensure individuals receive appropriate and timely preventive and chronic care.
   5. Collaboration across team members who are frequently in different settings of care. This enables virtual coordination preventing gaps in care delivery.
   6. Early detection of a change in medical condition after the individual leaves the clinical setting (through use of body-worn sensors in the individual's home).

The growth of HIT use by clinicians, individuals, and consumers generated the need to ensure that electronic systems are fostering safety, particularly EHRs. Safety and Assurance Factors for EHR Resilience (SAFER) guides became available in 2014, allowing organizations to evaluate their EHR for optimal use and safety. The guides cover nine areas and several impact CCTM practice including CPOE, communication, test reports, and monitoring (Whitt, Eden, Merrill, & Hughes, 2017).

B. One of the key areas of HIT focuses on enabling and improving decision-support, for both individuals and populations. The exponential growth of scientific evidence driving nursing practice makes it challenging for nurses to keep up with the changes. HIT can assist in this process by bringing necessary information to the nurse in forms that will enhance decision-making processes. As an example, EHRs can alert a clinician that a lab result is abnormal, while also presenting additional data pertinent to the lab result (such as medications and diagnostic test results), in combination with scientific evidence that supports suggested interventions. Data captured as a byproduct of care delivery, can be leveraged for aggregated data analysis. Data from several individuals are aggregated and used to provide information to support care for individuals. HIT provides comparable, reliable, and relevant data for cost, utilization, and outcome studies; for guideline development; for quality management; and for identification of best practices (Mobley, 2019). An automated decision-support system provides the nurse with a tool that enhances

the nurse's ability to make effective and timely decisions in semi-structured and uncertain situations.
1. The structure of any decision-support system applies algorithms to individual data sending a notification to elicit a recommended action. These actions often guide the clinician based upon clinical guidelines or regulatory requirements (Ortiz, Maia, Ortiz, Peres, & Sousa, 2017). Components of the automated decision-support system include:
   a. Some type of user interface that facilitates or triggers inquiries.
   b. A knowledge base (database) containing expert information organized to promote decision-making.
   c. An inference engine with analytic models that can generate alternative solutions.
   d. A standardized terminology infrastructure that enables data structure and organization to allow data to be shared across health systems.
2. An example of how a decision-support system might operate in a clinical setting is the scheduling of immunizations.
   a. The standardized terminology infrastructure enables organized data to represent of rules and guidelines.
   b. The system would ask for input of the child's date of birth, weight, immunization history, and other pertinent facts.
   c. The database would use the information provided to compare with accepted practice standards contained in the knowledge base.
   d. The algorithm in the inference engine would then be used to provide a recommendation for the next immunization to be scheduled.
C. The advancement of HIT solutions has increased the number of data sources that can be combined to produce completely new insights into nursing practice and outcomes. The insights range from descriptive, showing what happened in the past; to predictive, using historical patterns to predict what might happen in the future. Predictive analytics merges and analyzes multiple sources of data using multiple methods such as pattern recognition (heart rate always increases 8 hours prior to an infection) and statistics (the probability of an infection occurring is high), to provide prognostic output that can be used for decision-making, disease surveillance, and population health management (Cichosz, Johansen, & Hejlesen, 2015).

Data analytics has been used for surveillance using health-related data (typically symptom clusters) that precede a given diagnosis and signal a sufficient probability of a number of cases or a potential population outbreak of a disease (Fogli & Guida, 2013). These collected data, typically from emergency departments, can be used for early identification of a public health crisis or a bioterrorism-related event, thereby enabling a rapid response (Thomas, Yoon, Collins, Davison, & MacKenzie, 2018).

D. Use of evidence-based care guidelines. Evidence-based practice promotes high-value health care, which enhances the quality and reliability of health care to improve health outcomes, and reduce variations in the cost of individual care (Melnyk, Gallagher-Ford, Long, & Fineout-Overholt, 2014). Evidence-based practice is crucial for nurses in their quest for practice knowledge. It is through this implementation nursing will close the gap between theory and practice (Mackey & Bassendowski, 2017). Evidence-based practice is solidly grounded in research and is the combination of three concepts: best research, clinical expertise, and individual preferences (Brower, 2017).
The goal of evidence-based practice for nurses is to:
1. Determine the best care options.
2. Answer clinical questions.
3. Identify areas for care improvement. Care planning and care coordination rely upon identifying best practice models from the literature that derive recommendations from large population studies.

An example of an evidence-based decision support in care coordination is the Project BOOST (Society for Hospital Medicine, n.d.), designed to provide safe transitions in care and prevent unnecessary rehospitalization. Evidence-based nursing sources include computerized literature databases, such as the Cumulative Index of Nursing and Allied Health Literature (CINAHL) and the National Library of Medicine's Medline, and online, published, systematic evidence reviews such as The Cochrane Collaboration, the AHRQ, Zynx Health for interprofessional plans of care, and CINAHL's Clinical Innovations Database.

E. Essential Elements for Improving the Discharge Transition showing integration with HIT includes:

Chapter 12

1. Institutional support for, and prioritization of, this initiative expressed as a meaningful investment in time, equipment, informatics, and personnel in the effort.
2. An interprofessional team or steering committee that is focused on improving the quality of care transitions in the institution. Effective care transitions involve provider and interprofessional team communication between levels of care, practices, and organizations (Rattray et al., 2017).
3. Engagement of individuals and families and recognition of the central role they play in executing the post-hospital care plan.
4. Data collection and reliable metrics that, at a minimum, reflect any relevant CMS (2014) core measures and the relevant Physician Quality Reporting Initiative measures. These data should be transformed into reports that inform the team and front-line workers of progress and problem areas to address.
5. Specific aims, or goals, that are time defined, measurable, and achievable.
6. Standardized discharge pathways that highlight key medications and any medication changes, important follow-up and self-management instructions, and any pending tests.
7. To develop an 'intelligent health care system;' a learning organization that promotes a culture of knowledge and empowerment among its members.
8. An essential component to safe and effective discharge transitions involves the development and dissemination for the longitudinal care plan. Through use of EHRs and HIE's, the care plan, once developed, can be shared across the continuum of care for all stakeholders, irrespective of location, to use in care of the individual. Evidenced-based content, patient-reported outcomes (PROs), order sets, diagnoses, problems, and expected outcomes, become part of the longitudinal care plan.

III. **Competency 3: Integration of the Meaningful Measures Framework Within Use of HIT to Identify the Highest Priorities for Quality Measurement and Improvement in CCTM**

Learning Outcome Statement
- Understand use of the Meaningful Measures Framework to identify the quality issues that are the highest priority in improving the health and health care of individuals and communities.
- Recognize use of the Meaningful Measures Framework to identify those core issues that are most critical to CCTM, such as tracking measurable outcomes and impact.
- Understanding of different HIT solutions and their value in supporting innovative approaches to improve quality, safety, accessibility, and affordability.
- Understand models for population health management and care coordination and associated data elements needed for assessment, planning, intervention, and evaluation of care outcomes.

Learning Objectives
- Describe how HIT can help nurses improve health at a national level through CCTM.
- Identify data elements that are needed to measure individual and population health processes and outcomes.
- Describe the key elements of an evidence-based methodology for improving the discharge transition.

The use of HIT is essential for performance improvement, safety, and high quality outcomes. Care can be better coordinated, and is safer, more efficient, and of higher quality, when data necessary for quality measurement are captured as a byproduct of care delivery (Kennedy, Murphy, & Roberts, 2013). HIT plays an essential role to enable person-centered data capture that is shareable and comparable across care settings to facilitate effective and efficient individual and population level positive health outcomes (Knight & Shea, 2014).

Launched in 2018, the CMS Meaningful Measures Framework focuses the nation on quality measurement of the highest core issues most valuable to high quality care and better outcomes. In addition, MyHealthEData initiative was launched to strengthen interoperability or the sharing of health care data between providers and to easier access for consumers (CMS, 2018). These collective initiatives are centered on using a new approach where every clinician focuses on the development of meaningful quality measures using the following core principles:
- Are person-centered and meaningful to individuals, clinicians, and providers.
- Align across programs and settings.
- Address high-impact measure areas that safeguard public health.
- Are outcome-based where possible.
- Address needs for population-based payment.
- Create significant opportunity for improvement.
- Minimize level of burden for providers.

Chapter 12

A. Promoting effective communication and coordination of care is one of the Meaningful Measures Framework pillars. Both effective communication and coordination of care are dependent on the HIT to facilitate communication and the transfer of information, in a way that measurable outcomes and impact can be tracked.
   1. Coordination of care is the integration of care across the continuum of the individual's health care conditions, needs, and experiences and includes data sharing across multiple settings for:
      a. Individuals.
      b. Families.
      c. Caregivers.
      d. Health care teams.
   2. Primary care and family practice providers are the pivotal members of the health care team.
      a. Sharing information within and outside of the practice.
      b. Integrating specialty care.
      c. Transferring information across and up and down all the settings of care.
B. In primary care, there are six principle tasks for effective communication in care coordination.
   1. Maintaining individual continuity with a primary care clinician team.
   2. Documenting and compiling individual information generated within and outside the primary care office.
   3. Using information to manage and coordinate care delivered in primary care practice.
      a. Access and assess individual data.
      b. Manage and coordinate care.
      c. Population-based tracking for individual panel.
      d. Identify means to include patient-generated health data (PGHD).
   4. Referring and consulting (initiation, communication, and ongoing tracking).
   5. Sharing care with clinicians across practices and settings.
   6. Providing care and/or exchanging information for transitions and emergency care.
C. Data elements required for primary care and population health management include, but are not limited to:
   1. Assessment.
   2. Planning.
   3. Intervention.
   4. Evaluation of care outcomes.
D. Assessment, process, and outcome indicators need to be developed and embedded in nursing documentation screens, coded in standardized terminology (ICN or Systematized Nomenclature of Medicine – Clinical Terms [SNOMED – CT®]) so CCTM RN interventions can be tracked and contributions to outcome can be understood.
   1. A task force to identify and define nurse-sensitive indicators (NSI) specific to the ambulatory care setting. The development of the NSI's are in collaboration with the AAACN. Collaborative Alliance for Nursing Outcomes (CALNOC), and National Database Nursing Quality Indicators (NDNQI). This collaboration created the *Ambulatory Care Nurse-Sensitive Indicator Industry Report: Meaningful Measurement of Nursing in the Ambulatory Patient Care Environment*. NSI help facilitate and articulate value of nursing practice in the ambulatory care setting that are specific to individual outcomes.
   2. The ANA announced continued support for use of standardized nursing terminologies to promote and facilitate data exchange. When exchanging data with another setting for problems and care plans, SNOMED – CT and Logical Observation Identifiers Names and Codes (LOINC®) should be used for exchange (ANA, 2018).
   3. Nurses have a fundamental leadership role in health care to contribute to the triple aim of improving the individual care experience, improving the health of populations, and reducing the cost of health care (Berwick et al., 2008; Institute for Healthcare Improvement, 2018).
   4. Informatics competencies can be leveraged as powerful tools supporting the ability to gather the evidence to understand intervention effectiveness to improve health outcomes. Data has become increasingly accessible as more organizations implement electronic health records and link these electronic systems across care settings. This creates not only the opportunity to understand care delivery for entire populations, but also provides the opportunity for nurses to demonstrate the value their interventions bring in health care delivery systems.
   5. Understanding how to measure the nursing processes and contribution of nursing interventions to individual outcomes is an important competency.
   6. In addition to informing nursing practice, this information is vital for consumers and payers of health care.

Chapter 12

Table 12-2.
CCTM Dimension Indicators

CCTM Dimensions	Measure Sets
Support for Self-Management	1. Pain 2. Hypertension 3. Body Mass Index 4. Depression 5. Community Falls 6. Diabetes mellitus HbA1C Monitoring 7. Advance Care Planning 8. Opioid Misuse 9. Emergency Throughput 10. Staffing 11. Volumes 12. Staff Demographics Structure: • Staffing • Volume • Role Demographics Process: • Risk Assessment and Follow-Up Plans • Reassessment Outcomes: • Admission • Readmission • Diabetes mellitus HbA1C Control
Education and Engagement of Individual and Family	
Cross-Setting Communication and Transition	
Coaching and Counseling of Individual and Family	
Nursing Process: Assessment, Plan, Intervention, Evaluation	
Teamwork and Collaboration	
Person-Centered Planning	
Population Health Management	
Advocacy	

Source: © Haas et al., 2019. D. Brown & R. Start. Reprinted with permission.

7. Measures must evaluate the structure of our delivery system, the processes for care delivery, the health outcomes achieved, and the individual's experience (NQF, 2018).
8. Comparisons across organizations and individual populations help us understand the effectiveness of delivery systems. The development of standardized measures that are sensitive to nursing practice is an important component of nursing leadership, and for ambulatory care nursing, at the beginning of the development journey.
9. Ambulatory care measure development has been a strategic priority for AAACN and CALNOC. CALNOC, a nurse led non-profit organization, has been developing and providing benchmark opportunities for hospitals since 1996.
10. AAACN convened an NSI task force in 2013 to build the expertise for ambulatory care nurse-sensitive measure development with CALNOC nurse leaders sharing their expertise.
11. In 2015, the two organizations began a formal collaboration to develop NSIs. AAACN published the *Ambulatory Care Nurse-Sensitive Indicator Industry Report* (Start, Matlock, & Mastal, 2016) to share the current state of the science to help in prioritization of measure development.
12. As a result of these efforts, ambulatory care nurse-sensitive measures have been developed that address the structure, process, and outcomes of interventions sensitive to nursing practice (Mastal et al., 2016; Matlock et al., 2016; Start, Matlock, Brown, Aronow, & Soban, 2018)
    a. Technical expert panels composed of nurses from organizations across the country convened to provide voice and direction to the development of measures that were feasible to capture in our EHRs and meaningful to practice.
    b. In 2016, measure sets were defined for ambulatory care surgery centers and procedure centers that included the structure of staffing and the outcomes of care (Brown & Aronow, 2016).
    c. In 2017, measures were expanded to primary and specialty care settings for measure sets that evaluated the

process of assessment and follow up planning for pain management, hypertension, community fall risk, depression, and body mass index.
d. The next generation of measures address the more complex work of care coordination, transition management, and virtual care through telehealth.
e. Please see Table 12-2, which provides a sample of currently tested and available indicators for each CCTM dimension.

Table 12-1.
Professional Informatics Practice: Knowledge, Skills, and Attitudes for Competency

COMPETENCY 1: Use of Health Information Technology that Is Aligned with the CCTM® RN Model			
Knowledge	**Skills**	**Attitudes**	**Sources**
Describe ways in which various forms of HIT support CCTM in accordance with the CCTM RN Model.	Demonstrate accountability by practicing using HIT within CCTM. Describe methods for using HIT including EHRs, HIEs, PHRs, mobile technology, and the Internet in professional practice. Communicate the role of HIT to other professionals, individuals, consumers, and stakeholders in health care.	Value systems thinking and use of HIT to improve coordination of care. Value the professional role of the RN in HIT; use to improve coordination of care. Recognize the potential for improvement in HIT using the CCTM RN Model as input.	Androwich & Kraft, 2013 Melby, Brattheim, & Hellesø, 2015
Demonstrate the role that various HIT solutions, such as EHRs, PHRs, the Internet, smartphones, and HIEs have in enhancing CCTM.	Identify ways in which HIT can enhance CCTM. Evaluate use of HIT and impact on care coordination. Demonstrate ability to translate the information needs of caregivers to those designing the actual systems to capture and communicate individual care data.	Appreciate ways in which HIT can support professional practices. Respect the intersection of nursing practice and HIT in care coordination. Appreciate the ways HIT can be designed to improve care coordination.	Bates, 2015 Demiris & Kneale, 2015 Melby, Brattheim, & Hellesø, 2015
Describe the application of professional practice standards to use of HIT within the CCTM RN role in ambulatory care.	Demonstrate accountability by practicing within own scope of competence and training. Recognize and implement nursing best practices in use of HIT to support CCTM.	Value legal, ethical, and professional standards of practice. Value the professional role of the RN and recognize differences in scope of practice of RNs, licensed practical nurses/licensed vocational nurses, and the role of unlicensed assistive personnel. Recognize the potential for improved practices through continuing education.	Cronenwett et al., 2007 Salmond & Echevarria, 2017
Recognize the importance of HIT skills in enhancing practice.	Demonstrate skills in using HIT to support CCTM within the scope of the CCTM RN role.	Value functionality contained within all forms of HIT to enhance nursing practice.	Bauer & Bodenheimer, 2017 Dowding et al., 2018

continued on next page

Table 12-1. (continued)
Professional Informatics Practice: Knowledge, Skills, and Attitudes for Competency

COMPETENCY 1: Use of Health Information Technology that Is Aligned with the CCTM® RN Model			
Knowledge	**Skills**	**Attitudes**	**Sources**
Analyze systems theory and design as applied to health informatics.	Use performance-improvement tools (e.g. Lean, Six Sigma, Plan-Do-Study-Act) in system analysis and design to assess use of technology to improve care. Use project management methods in relation to implementation of new technologies. Model behaviors that support theories and methods of change management.	Value systems thinking and use of technology to improve patient safety and quality. Appreciate the Systems Development Lifecycle in the design of information systems.	Cronenwett et al., 2007 Monsen, Brandt et al., 2017
"Evaluate the strengths and weaknesses of information systems in practice" (p. 15).	"Participate in the selection, design, implementation, and evaluation of information systems" (p. 15). Consistently "communicate the integral role of information technology in nurses' work" (p. 15). "Model behaviors that support implementation and an appropriate use of EHRs" (p. 15). "Assist team members in adopting IT by piloting and evaluating proposed information systems" (p. 15).	"Recognize nursing's important role in selecting, designing, implementing, and evaluating health information systems for practice environments" (p. 15). "Appreciate the need for an interprofessional team to make final decisions related to selection and use of new information systems" (p. 15). "Value the use of information technologies in practice" (p. 15).	American Association of Colleges of Nursing (AACN), 2012
COMPETENCY 2: Explain Why Information and Technology Skills are Essential for Safe Individual Care			
Knowledge	**Skills**	**Attitudes**	**Sources**
Demonstrate understanding of the different HIT solutions and value in enhancing CCTM.	Contrast benefits and limitations of common IT strategies used in the delivery of individual care. Evaluate the strengths and weaknesses of information systems used in individual care. Participate in the selection, design, implementation, and appropriate use of EHRs. Assist team members to adopt IT by piloting and evaluating proposed technologies.	Communicate the value and integral role of information technology in nurses' work.	Cronenwett et al., 2007 McGinnis, Powers, & Grossmann, 2011 AACN, 2012

continued on next page

**Table 12-1. (continued)
Professional Informatics Practice: Knowledge, Skills, and Attitudes for Competency**

COMPETENCY 2: Explain Why Information and Technology Skills are Essential for Safe Individual Care			
Knowledge	**Skills**	**Attitudes**	**Sources**
Understand the role of clinical decision-support tools in CCTM, recognizing they are to be utilized to support decision-making rather than to dictate practice.	Work to develop and maintain an extensive knowledge base to support design and use of HIT to enhance clinical decision-making. Use decision-support tools but apply clinical judgment and critical thinking. Avoid over-reliance on decision support tools. Demonstrate skills in searching, retrieving, and managing data to make decisions at the point of care and an aggregate level across populations to make decisions.	Respect the individual's right to participate in care planning and make his or her own decision about course of action. Recognize the final decision maker is usually the individual/caregiver while remaining sensitive to situations in which the nurse needs to act on the individual's behalf to assure his or her safety. Appreciate the value of decision-support tools to enhance the nurse's knowledge base and as a check list to avoid clinical oversights.	Cronenwett et al., 2007
Understand the major components of automated decision-support tools.	Recognize requirements for decision support including the use of knowledge bases, analytical tools, and user interfaces. Articulate system requirements using nursing practice as the foundation.	Appreciate how HIT could work to support practice, such as reminders related to immunizations, access to evidence-based protocols, and suggestions related to treatment.	Androwich & Kraft, 2013
Understand the benefits and limitations of selected safety-enhancing technologies.	Describe the role of HIT in promoting safety. Recognize HIT limitations in safety while articulating the role of nursing judgment when using HIT. Identify metrics to measure HIT impact on safety.	Appreciate the role of pre-/post-measurement in using HIT to improve safety. Appreciate the role of nursing practice and workflow as a critical lever in improving safety.	Cronenwett et al., 2007 Yanamadala, Morrison, Curtin, McDonald, & Hernandez-Boussard, 2016.
Evaluate benefits and limitations of common information systems strategies to improve safety and quality.	Participate in the design of clinical decision support systems (e.g., alerts and reminders in EHRs).	"Patient safety and quality of care are seriously compromised by flawed EHR system design or functionality or improper used. Failure to address information integrity issues in EHR systems will lead to spiraling, rather than declining, healthcare costs and medical errors as a result of the proliferation of new types of patient safety hazards" (para. 3).	AACN, 2012 Bowman, 2013

continued on next page

**Table 12-1. (continued)
Professional Informatics Practice: Knowledge, Skills, and Attitudes for Competency**

COMPETENCY 2: Explain Why Information and Technology Skills are Essential for Safe Individual Care			
Knowledge	**Skills**	**Attitudes**	**Sources**
"Know the current regulatory requirements for information systems use" (p. 15).	"Use federal and other regulations related to information systems in selecting and implementing information systems in practice" (p. 15).	"Appreciate the role that federal regulation plays in developing and implementing information systems that will improve patient care and create more effective delivery systems" (p. 15). Understand Federal Health IT Strategic Plan 2015-2020.	AACN, 2012 HealthIT.gov, 2015
"Evaluate benefits and limitations of different health information technologies and their impact on safety and quality" (p. 16).	"Promote access to patient care information for all who provide care" (p. 16). "Serve as a resource for documentation of nursing care at basic and advanced levels" (p. 16). "Develop safeguards for protected health information" (p. 16). "Comply with HIPAA regulations in the use of EHRs and other sources of patient information" (p. 16). "Champion communication technologies that support clinical decision-making, error prevention, care coordination, interprofessional collaboration, and protection of patient privacy" (p. 16).	"Appreciate the importance of valid, reliable, and significant data to improve quality and provide efficient care" (p. 15).	AACN, 2012
Identify components of the National Quality Strategy – six aims.	Articulate the six aims of the National Quality Strategy and use of HIT. Identify methods for HIT design to support the National Quality Strategy related to care coordination and person-centered care. Engage in public policy decision making to enhance the National Quality Strategy.	Value the importance of improving health for populations of individuals. Value the important role of public policy in nursing practice.	Agency for Healthcare Research and Quality, 2017 American Recovery and Reinvestment Act of 2009 Centers for Medicare & Medicaid Services, 2014 National Quality Forum, 2006 Samal et al., 2012

continued on next page

**Table 12-1. (continued)
Professional Informatics Practice: Knowledge, Skills, and Attitudes for Competency**

COMPETENCY 3: Integration of National Quality Strategy Requirements within Use of HIT to Improve Care Coordination and Transition Management			
Knowledge	**Skills**	**Attitudes**	**Sources**
Analyze data sets to identify nursing care impact on outcomes.	Demonstrate efficient use of standardized terminologies and HIT applications to technology to perform role. Use standards as defined in the 'meaningful use' rule as a guide for top-priority conditions for analysis of quality. "Use the existing coding and billing system to appropriately reflect the level and type of service delivered in practice" (p. 16). "Model behaviors that support implementation and appropriate use of data accessed through databases, electronic health records, dashboards, remote monitoring devices, telemedicine, and other technologies" (p. 16).	"Appreciate the importance of valid, reliable, and significant data to improve quality and provide efficient and effective care" (p. 15-16).	AACN, 2012 Frankel, Haraden, Federico, & Lenoci-Edwards, 2017

Chapter 12

Case Study 12-1.
Health Information Technology in Clinical Primary Care Coordination

Introduction

Health information delivered electronically has the ability to connect and encourage individuals to be active in their own health by providing tools to help them make informed health decisions. Engaging and empowering individuals and families on the use of HIT is transforming the way care is being delivered across care settings. Access to online health information and technologies can empower individuals and caregivers to ask more questions and influence positive effects on lifestyle all to promote better medical outcomes (HealthIT.gov, 2017; Ricciardi, Mostashari, Murphy, Daniel, & Siminerio, 2013). Over the last decade, the increase in mobile applications and self-tracking devices has changed the way individuals search and receive health information. According to Fox (2013), one in three cellphone owners have used their phone to look for health information and 59% of U.S. adults have searched online for information about a health topic within the past year. There is tremendous opportunity to engage individuals, families, and care providers with web-based and mobile technologies.

CCTM RN Outreach

Patty S. is a 58-year-old who has been living with type 2 diabetes for the last 12 years. Recently, her condition has worsened and she has been prescribed an insulin pump to manage her glucose level. Her primary care provider would like her to track her blood sugars more frequently with a new remote monitoring system the clinic is piloting designed specifically for their high-risk individuals.

While Patty was in the clinic, her primary care provider performed a 'warm-hand-off' to the CCTM® RN. The CCTM RN assesses her immediate needs and schedules time to review the home monitoring device.

Clinical Interactions

During the visit with Patty in the clinic, the CCTM RN assists her with the download and setup of the application (App) on her phone that allows for daily monitoring of glucose. As the CCTM RN reviews this with Patty, she continuously assesses her engagement, computer literacy, and comfort with the process. The app receives information from a sensor on the individual's finger and sends data to her phone display. The CCTM RN demonstrates the entire process to Patty and has her teach it back to demonstrate understanding. It is explained that individual readings are uploaded from her device to a HIPAA compliant, secure, encrypted cloud-based database, which is integrated with the EHR portal. From the portal, the clinic is able to receive and validate individual information and file it into the individual's medical record.

Clinical Implications

Nursing implications for remote monitoring include daily login to the portal to review and download data to the individuals chart and notifying the provider according to insulin protocol criteria. During the initial 30 days, the care coordinator meets with Patty weekly to discuss her overall health, any questions or difficulties she may be experiencing with the pump and remote monitoring process.

Chapter 12

Case Study 12-2.
Health Information Technology in Transitional Acute Care Coordination

Introduction

Secondary to the federal incentive program, EHR adoption rates are exceeding 90% (Henry, Pylypchuk, Searcy, & Patel, 2016). However, despite the advent of widespread and ubiquitous EHRs, exchange of health information between settings has lagged behind (Holmgren & Adler-Milstein, 2017; Perlin, 2016). Health information exchange is necessary for interoperability. The Healthcare Information and Management Systems Society (HIMSS) defines interoperability as "the ability of different information systems, devices, or applications to connect, in a coordinated manner, within and across organizational boundaries to access, exchange, and cooperatively use data amongst stakeholders, with the goal of optimizing the health of individuals and populations" (para. 1).Through interoperability, clinicians from one setting (primary care) can receive information from another setting (acute care), and subsequently interpret and make effective use of the information to provide care.

New technologies, standards development, and strong support from continued policy initiatives provide promise that nurses, from one setting, receiving an individual from another setting, will receive data necessary for continued care for the individual. With interoperability, information about an individual's problem list, medication list, plan of care, and other individual information, can be extracted from an EHR in one location and assimilated into the individual's EHR at another location. The purpose of this use case is to demonstrate how interoperability standards can be used to supply the CCTM® RN with detailed acute discharge information to improve the quality of follow-up care and avoid rehospitalization.

RN CCTM Outreach

Margaret K. is a 65-year-old woman who is being discharged from the hospital with full understanding of her post-discharge instructions. Given her hip replacement, combined with multiple chronic conditions (CHF, type 2 diabetes, Hypertension and Arthritis), she is a high risk for readmission. During her acute care stay, there are changes in her medications combined with instructions on activity, safety precautions, identification of early signs of infection, and other instructions intended to improve outcomes and prevent re-admission. While in the acute care setting, Margaret started to show positive outcomes and demonstrated understanding of the post-discharge instructions. She has been scheduled for a follow-up appointment with her primary care provider and team.

Clinical Interactions

The hospital discharge alert service routes key information about the discharge of Margaret to the CCTM RN in real-time to support the transition of care. This is accomplished through a Health Level Seven International (HL7) message from the inpatient EHR to the primary office EHR. HL7 refers to international standards needed for data transmission between applications across various providers and health care settings and each HL7 message sends information about a particular event, such as an individual discharge (HL7, 2018a). The HL7 message is also routed to the CCTM RN's mobile phone. This attracts the attention of the CCTM RN who then proceeds to gather additional information such as diagnoses, discharge medications, discharge instructions, problem lists, resolved hospital problems, pending results, procedures in the hospital, etc. This discharge summary is sent using a Clinical Document Architecture (CDA) standard. CDA is a popular, flexible markup standard developed by HL7 that defines the structure of certain medical records, such as discharge summaries and progress notes, as a way to better exchange this information between providers and individuals (HL7, 2018b).

With this information, the CCTM RN can review Margaret's case prior to the office visit and because the information was communicated in standard formats, it can be stored in the office EHR, where the CCTM RN reviews and updates the information with Margaret during her visit.

Clinical Implications

CCTM RN implications for access to post-discharge information includes use of a mobile phone to receive an alert that responsibility for a patient is transitioning from an acute to post-acute setting. This is followed with login to an EHR portal to review discharge summary data in preparation for individual care.

Secondary to use of data standards, all clinicians can access the same data from the office, thereby facilitating communication between the CCTM RN, physician, social workers, and other stakeholders in care (including the individual).

Chapter 12

References

Abdelhamid, M. (2018). Greater patient health information control to improve the sustainability of health information exchanges. *Journal of Biomedical Informatics.* 83(1), 150-158.

Agency for Healthcare Research and Quality (AHRQ). (2017). *About the National Quality Strategy (NQS).* Retrieved from https://www.ahrq.gov/workingforquality/about/index.html

American Academy of Ambulatory Care Nursing (AAACN). (2016). *Scope and standards of practice for registered nurses in care coordination and transition management.* Pitman, NJ: Author.

American Association of Colleges of Nursing (AACN). (2012). *Graduate-level QSEN competencies: Knowledge, skills and attitudes.* Retrieved from http://www.aacnnursing.org/Portals/42/AcademicNursing/CurriculumGuidelines/Graduate-QSEN-Competencies.pdf

American Nurses Association (ANA). (2015). *Nursing informatics: Scope and standards of practice* (2nd ed.). Silver Spring, MD: Author.

American Nurses Association (ANA). (2018). *Inclusion of recognized terminologies supporting nursing practice within electronic health records and other health information technology solutions.* Retrieved from https://www.nursingworld.org/practice-policy/nursing-excellence/official-position-statements/id/Inclusion-of-Recognized-Terminologies-Supporting-Nursing-Practice-within-Electronic-Health-Records/

American Recovery and Reinvestment Act of 2009. (P.L. 111-5). 111th Congress of the United States of America.

Androwich, I., & Kraft, M.R. (2013). Informatics. In C.B. Laughlin (Ed.), *Core curriculum for ambulatory care nursing* (3rd ed., pp. 63-75). Pitman, NJ: American Academy of Ambulatory Care Nursing.

Barnes, S. (2018). Surgical site infection prevention in 2018 and beyond. *AORN Journal.* 107(5), 547-550. doi:10.1002/aorn.12144

Bates, D.W. (2015). Health information technology and care coordination: The next big opportunity for informatics? *Yearbook of Medical Informatics, 10*(1), 11-14. doi:10.15265/iy-2015-0020

Bauer, L., & Bodenheimer, T. (2017). Expanded roles of registered nurses in primary care delivery of the future. *Nursing Outlook, 65*(5), 624-632. doi:10.1016/j.outlook.2017.03.011

Baysari, M.T., & Westbrook, J.I. (2015). Mobile applications for patient-centered care coordination: A review of human factors methods applied to their design, development, and evaluation. *Yearbook of Medical Informatics, 10*(1), 47-54.

Berwick, D.M., Nolan, T.W., & Whittington, J. (2008). The triple aim: Care, health, and cost. *Health affairs, 27*(3), 759-769. doi:10.1377/hlthaff.27.3.759

Blake, R., & Shaw, R. (2017). *Technology Informatics Guiding Education Reform: The TIGER initiative.* Retrieved from https://www.himss.org/event/technology-informatics-guiding-education-reform-tiger-initiative

Brennan, P.E., & Bakken, S. (2015). Nursing needs big data and big data needs nursing. *Journal of Nursing Scholarship, 47*(5), 477-484.

Bowman, S. (2013). Impact of electronic health record systems on information integrity: Quality and safety implications. *Perspectives in Health Information Management, 10*(Fall), 1c.

Brower, E.J. (2017). Origins of evidence-based practice and what it means for nurses. *International Journal of Childbirth Education, 32*(2), 14-18.

Brown, D.S., & Aronow, H.U. (2016). Ambulatory care nurse-sensitive indicators series: Reaching for the tipping point in measuring nurse-sensitive quality in the ambulatory surgical and procedure environments. *Nursing Economic$, 34*(3), 147-151.

Centers for Medicare & Medicaid Services (CMS). (2014). *2014 clinical quality measures.* Retrieved from https://www.cms.gov/Regulations-and-Guidance/Legislation/EHRIncentivePrograms/2014_ClinicalQualityMeasures.html

Centers for Medicare & Medicaid Services (CMS). (2018). *Overview of the Centers for Medicare & Medicaid Services Meaningful Measures Framework.* https://www.cms.gov/Medicare/Quality-Initiatives-Patient-Assessment-Instruments/QualityInitiativesGenInfo/Downloads/CMS-Meaningful-Measures_Overview-Fact-Sheet_508_2018-02-28.pdf

Cichosz, S.L., Johansen, M.D., & Hejlesen, O. (2015). Toward big analytics: Review of predictive models in management of diabetes and its complications. *Journal of Diabetes Science and Technology 10*(1), 27-34.

Cipriano, P.F., Bowles, K., Dailey, M., Dykes, P., Lamb, G., & Naylor, M. (2013). The importance of health information technology in care coordination and transitional care. *Nursing Outlook, 61*(6), 475-489.

Cronenwett, L., Sherwood, G., Barnsteiner, J., Disch, J., Johnson, J., Mitchell, P., ... Warren, J. (2007). Quality and safety education for nurses. *Nursing Outlook, 55*(3), 122-131.

Cronenwett, L., Sherwood, G., Pohl, J., Barnsteiner, J., Moore, S., Sullivan, D.T., ... Warren, J. (2009). Quality and safety education for advanced nursing practice. *Nursing Outlook, 57*(6), 338-348.

Davis, K., Collier, S., Situ, J., Coe, M., & Cleary-Fishman, M. (2017). *A Toolkit to engage high-risk patients in safe transitions across ambulatory settings.* Rockville, MD: Agency for Healthcare Research and Quality. Retrieved from https://www.ahrq.gov/sites/default/files/wysiwyg/professionals/quality-patient-safety/hais/tools/ambulatory-surgery/safetransitions/safetrans_toolkit.pdf

Demiris, G., & Kneale, L. (2015). Informatics systems and tools to facilitate patient-centered care coordination. *Yearbook of Medical Informatics, 10*(1), 15-21. doi:10.15265/iy-2015-003

Dowding, D.W., Russell, D., Jonas, K., Onorato, N., Barrón, Y., Merrill, J.A., & Rosati, R.J. (2018). Does level of numeracy and graph literacy impact comprehension of quality targets? Findings from a survey of home care nurses. *AMIA Annual Symposium Proceedings. AMIA Symposium, 2017*, 635-640.

Dowding, D.W., Russell, D., Onorato, N., & Merrill, J.A. (2018). Technology solutions to support care continuity in home care: A focus group study. *Journal for Healthcare Quality, 40*(4), 236-246. doi:10.1097/JHQ.0000000000000104

Fogli, D., & Guida G. (2013) Knowledge-centered design of decision support systems for emergency management. *Decision Support Systems, 55*(1), 336-347.

Fox, S. (2013). *Health and technology in the U.S.* Retrieved from http://www.pewinternet.org/2013/12/04/health-and-technology-in-the-u-s/

Frankel, A., Haraden, C., Federico, F., & Lenoci-Edwards, J. (2017). *A framework for safe, reliable, and effective care.* Retrieved from https://www.medischevervolgopleidingen.nl/sites/default/files/paragraph_files/a_framework_for_safe_reliable_and_effective_care.pdf

Haas, S., Conway-Phillips, R., Swan, B.A., De La Pena, L., Start, R., & Brown, D.S. (2019). Developing a business case for the care coordination and transition management model: Need, methods, and measures. *Nursing Economic$, 37*(3).

Health Information and Management Systems Society (HIMSS). (2018). *Electronic health records.* Retrieved from http://www.himss.org/library/ehr/%3FnavItemNumber%3D13261

Healthcare Information and Management Systems Society (HIMSS). (2019). *What is interoperability?* Retrieved from https://www.himss.org/library/interoperability-standards/what-is-interoperability

HealthIT.gov. (2015). *2015 standards hub.* Retrieved from https://www.healthit.gov/topic/certification/2015-standards-hub

HealthIT.gov. (2017). *Benefits of Health IT.* (2013). Retrieved from https://www.healthit.gov/topic/health-it-basics/benefits-health-it

HealthIT.gov. (n.d.). *Health IT and health information exchange basics.* Retrieved from http://healthit.gov/providers-professionals/learn-ehr-basics

Health Level Seven International (HL7). (2018a). *Frequently asked questions.* Retrieved from http://www.hl7.org/about/FAQs/index.cfm

Health Level Seven International (HL7). (2018b). *Glossary of terms.* Retrieved from http://www.hl7.org/documentcenter/

Chapter 12

public_temp_4EC04C21-1C23-BA17-0C6C07E6D B864836/calendarofevents/FirstTime/Glossary%20of%20terms.pdf

Henry, J., Pylypchuk, Y., Searcy, T., & Patel, V. (2016). *Adoption of electronic health record systems among U.S. non-federal acute care hospitals: 2008-2015*. Retrieved from https://dashboard.healthit.gov/evaluations/data-briefs/non-federal-acute-care-hospital-ehr-adoption-2008-2015.php

Holmgren, A.J., & Adler-Milstein, J. (2017). Health information exchange in US hospitals: The current landscape and a path to improved information sharing. *Journal of Hospital Medicine, 12*(3), 193-198.

Institute of Electrical and Electronics Engineers (IEEE). (1990). *IEEE standard computer dictionary: A compilation of IEEE standard computer glossaries: 610*. New York, NY. 1990.

Institute for Healthcare Improvement. (2018). *Triple aim for populations*. Retrieved from http://www.ihi.org/Topics/TripleAim/Pages/default.aspx

Kennedy, R., Murphy, J., & Roberts, D.W. (2013). An overview of the National Quality Strategy: Where do nurses fit? *The Online Journal of Issues in Nursing, 18*(3), 5.

Knight, E.P., & Shea, K. (2014). A patient-focused framework integrating self-management and informatics. *Journal of Nursing Scholarship, 46*(2), 91-97. doi:10.1111/jnu.12059

Langabeer, J.R., 2nd, & Champagne, T. (2016) Exploring business strategy in health information exchange organizations. *Journal of Healthcare Management, 61*(1), 15-26.

Lu, Y., Zhang, S., Zhang, Z., Xiao, W., & Yu, S. (2017). A framework for learning analytics using commodity wearable devices. *Sensors, 17*(6). doi:10.3390/s17061382

Mackey, A., & Bassendowski, S. (2017). The history of evidence-based practice in nursing education and practice. *Journal of Professional Nursing, 33*(1), 51-55.

Mastal, M., Matlock, A.M., & Start, R. (2016). Ambulatory care nurse-sensitive indicators series: Capturing the role of nursing in ambulatory care – The case for meaningful nurse-sensitive measurement. *Nursing Economic$, 34*(2), 92- 98.

Matlock, A.M., Start, R, Aronow, H., & Brown, D.S. (2016). Ambulatory care nursing-sensitive indicators. *Nursing Management, 47*(6), 16-18.

McGinnis, J.M., Powers, B., & Grossmann, C. (Eds.). (2011). *Digital infrastructure for the learning health system: the foundation for continuous improvement in health and health care: Workshop series summary*. Washington, D.C.: National Academies Press.

McGonigle, D., Hunter, K., & Hebda, T. (2013). How can we promote nursing informatics? *Online Journal of Nursing Informatics, 17*(1). Retrieved from http://ojni.org/issues/?p=2391

Melby, L., Brattheim, B.J., & Hellesø, R. (2015). Patients in transition – Improving hospital-home care collaboration through electronic messaging: Providers' perspectives. *Journal of Clinical Nursing, 24*(23-24), 3389-3399. doi:10.1111/jocn.12991

Melnyk, B.M., Gallagher-Ford, L., Long, L.E., & Fineout-Overholt, E. (2014). The establishment of evidence-based practice competencies for practicing registered nurses and advanced practice nurses in real-world clinical settings: Proficiencies to improve healthcare quality, reliability, patient outcomes, and costs. *Worldviews on Evidence-Based Nursing, 11*(1), 5-15.

Merkow, R.P., Ju, M.H., Chung, J.W., Hall, B.L., Cohen, M.E., Williams, M.V., ... Bilimoria, K.Y. (2015). Underlying reasons associated with hospital readmission following surgery in the United States. *JAMA 313*(5), 483-495.

Mobley, A.M. (2019). Documentation and informatics. In C.B. Laughlin & S.G. Witwer (Eds.), *Core curriculum for ambulatory care nursing* (4th ed., pp. 95-110). Pitman, NJ: American Academy of Ambulatory Care Nursing.

Monsen, K.A., Brandt, J.K., Brueshoff, B.L., Chi, C.L., Mathiason, M.A., Swenson, S.M., & Thorson, D.R. (2017). Social determinants and health disparities associated with outcomes of women of childbearing age who receive public health nurse home visiting services. *Journal of Obstetric, Gynecology, and Neonatal Nursing, 46*(2), 292-303.

Monsen, K.A., Vanderboom, C.E., Olson, K.S., Larson, M.E., & Holland, D.E. (2017). Care coordination from a strengths perspective: A practice-based evidence evaluation of evidence-based practice. *Research and Theory for Nursing Practice, 31*(1), 39-55. doi:10.1891/1541-6577.31.1.39

Murphy, J. (2013). Progress report: Electronic health records and HIT in the United States. *American Nurse Today, 8*(11), 11. Retrieved from https://www.americannursetoday.com/progress-report-electronic-health-records-and-hit-in-the-united-states/

National Quality Forum (NQF). (2006). *National Quality Forum-endorsed definition and framework for measuring care coordination*. Washington, DC: Author.

National Quality Forum (NQF). (2012). *Patient reported outcomes (PROs) workshop #1*. Retrieved from https://www.qualityforum.org/Projects/n-r/Patient-Reported_Outcomes/Workshop_1_Summary_07302012.aspx

National Quality Forum. (NQF). (2013). *Patient reported outcomes (PROs) in performance measurement*. Retrieved from https://www.qualityforum.org/Publications/2012/12/Patient-reported_Outcomes_in_Performance_Measurement.aspx

National Quality Forum (NQF). (2018). *ABCs of measurement*. Retrieved from https://www.qualityforum.org/measuring_performance/abcs_of_measurement.aspx

Ortiz, D.R., Maia, F.O.M., Ortiz, D.C.F., Peres, H.H.C., & Sousa P.A.F. (2017). Computerized clinical decision support system utilization in nursing: A scoping review protocol. *JBI Database of Systematic Reviews and Implementation Reports, 15*(11), 2638-2644.

Perlin, J.B. (2016). Health information technology interoperability and use for better care and evidence. *JAMA. 316*(16), 1667-1668.

Quality and Safety Education for Nurses (QSEN). (2018). *Informatics*. http://qsen.org/competencies/pre-licensure-ksas/#informatics

Raju, D., Su, X., Patrician, P.A., Loan, L.A., & McCarthy, M.S. (2015). Exploring factors associated with pressure ulcers: A data mining approach. *International Journal of Nursing Studies, 52*(1), 102-111.

Rattray N.A., Sico, J.J., Cox, L.M., Russ, A.L., Matthias, M.S., & Frankel, R.M. (2017). Crossing the communication chasm: Challenges and opportunities in transitions of care from the hospital to the primary care clinic. *Joint Commission Journal on Quality and Patient Safety, 43*(3), 127-137.

Ricciardi, L., Mostashari, F., Murphy, J., Daniel, J.G., & Siminerio, E.P. (2013). A national action plan to support consumer engagement via e-health. *Health Affairs, 32*(2), 376-384.

Rocks, D., & Cooper-Audain, E. (2015). Recent research on care coordination. *Home Healthcare Now, 33*(2), 104-109.

Roehrs, A., da Costa, C.A., da Rosa Righi, R., & de Oliveira, K.S.F. (2017). Personal health records: A systematic Literature review. *Journal of Medical Internet Research, 19*(1), e13.

Russo, E., Sittig, D.F., Murphy, D.R., & Singh, H. (2016). Challenges in patient safety improvement research in the era of electronic health records. *Healthcare (Amsterdam, The Netherlands), 4*(4), 285-290.

Salmond, S.W., & Echevarria, M. (2017). Healthcare transformation and changing roles for nursing. *Orthopaedic Nursing, 36*(1), 12-25.

Samal, L., Dykes, P.C., Greenberg, J., Hasan, O., Venkatesh, A.K., Volk, A., & Bates, D.W. (2012). *Environmental analysis of health information technology to support care coordination and care transitions*. Washington, DC: National Quality Forum.

Sittig, D., & Singh, N. (2017). A sociotechnical approach to electronic health record related safety. In A. Sheikh, K.M. Cresswell, A. Wright, & D.W. Bates (Eds.), *Key advances in clinical informatics* (pp. 197-216). Philadelphia, PA: Elsevier.

Society for Hospital Medicine. (2019). *Advancing successful care transitions to improve outcomes*. Retrieved from https://www.hospitalmedicine.org/clinical-topics/care-transitions/

Society for Hospital Medicine (SHM). (n.d.). *SHM's Center for Quality Improvement* [brochure]. Retrieved from https://www.hospitalmedicine.org/globalassests/clinical-topics/clinical-pdf/shm-qi-brochure-2017

Start, R., Matlock, A.M., Brown, D., Aronow, H., & Soban, L. (2018). Realizing momentum and synergy: Benchmarking meaningful ambulatory care nurse-sensitive indicators. *Nursing Economic$, 36*(5), 246-251.

Start, R., Matlock, A.M., & Mastal, P. (2016). *Ambulatory care nurse-sensitive indicator industry report: Meaningful measurement of nursing in the ambulatory patient care environment.* Pitman, NJ: American Academy of Ambulatory Care Nursing.

Thomas, M.J., Yoon, P.W., Collins, J.M., Davison, A.J., & MacKenzie, W.R. (2018). Evaluation of syndromic surveillance systems in 6 US state and local health departments. *Journal of Public Health Management & Practice, 24*(3), 235-240.

U.S. Department of Health and Human Services (DHHS). (2010). *Health Information Technology for Economic and Clinical Health (HITECH) Act.* Washington, DC: Author.

Whitt, K., Eden, L., Merrill, K.C., & Hughes, M. (2017). Nursing student experience regarding safe use of electronic health records: A pilot study of the safety and assurance factors for EHR resilience guides. *CIN: Computers, Informatics, Nursing, 35*(1), 45-53.

Yanamadala, S., Morrison, D., Curtin, C., McDonald, K., & Hernandez-Boussard, T. (2016). Electronic health records and quality of care: An observational study modeling impact on mortality, readmissions, and complications. *Medicine, 95*(19), e3332

Mell, P., & Grance, T. (2011). *The NIST definition of cloud computing, recommendations of the National Institute of Standards and Technology.* Washington, DC: U.S. Department of Commerce.

National Quality Forum (NQF). (2014). *NQF-endorsed measures for care coordination: Phase 3.* Retrieved from http://www.qualityforum.org/Publications/2014/12/NQF-endorsed_Measures_for_Care_Coordination__Phase_3.aspx

O'Carroll, P.W., Yasnoff, W.A., Ward, M.E., Ripp, L.H., & Martin, E.L. (Eds.). (2003). *Public health informatics and information systems.* New York, NY: Springer.

Sackett, D.L., Strauss, S.E., Richardson, W.S., Rosenberg, W., & Haynes, R.B. (2000). *Evidence-based medicine: How to practice and teach EBM* (2nd ed.). Edinburgh, Scotland: Churchill Livingstone.

Sheer, B. (2007). Highlights of the International Council of Nurses 2007 Annual Conference, Yokohama, Japan. Retrieved from http://www.medscape.com/viewarticle/559912

Society for Hospital Medicine (SHM). (n.d.). SHM's Center for Quality Improvement [brochure]. Retrieved from https://www.hospitalmedicine.org/globalassets/clinical-topics/clinical-pdf/shm-qi-brochure-2017

Additional Readings

Agency for Healthcare Research and Quality (AHRQ). (2013). *Findings and lessons from the AHRQ: Ambulatory and safety quality program.* Rockville, MD: Author.

Agency for Healthcare Research and Quality (AHRQ). (2018). *The PSO privacy protection center.* Retrieved from https://www.ahrq.gov/cpi/about/otherwebsites/psoppc.ahrq.gov/index.html

Bahr, S.J., Siclovan, D.M., Opper, K., Beiler, J., Bobay, K.L., & Weiss, M.E. (2017). Interprofessional health team communication about hospital discharge. An implementation science evaluation study. *Journal of Nursing Care Quality, 32*(4), 285-292.

Brower E.J. (2017). Origins of evidence-based practice and what it means for nurses. *International Journal of Childbirth Education, 32*(2), 14-18.

Centers for Medicare & Medicaid Services (2018*). CMS proposes changes to empower patients and reduce administrative burden.* Retrieved from https://www.cms.gov/newsroom/press-releases/cms-proposes-changes-empower-patients-and-reduce-administrative-burden

Committee on Patient Safety and Health Information Technology; Institute of Medicine (IOM). (2011). *Health IT and patient safety: Building safer systems for better care.* Retrieved from https://www.ncbi.nlm.nih.gov/pubmed/24600741

Haas, S., & Androwich, I. (2011). Ambulatory care nursing: Concerns and challenges. In P.S. Cowen & S. Moorhead (Eds.), *Current issues in nursing* (8th ed.). St. Louis, MO: Elsevier.

Harle, C.A., Huerta, T.R., Ford, E.W., Diana, M.L., & Menachemi, N. (2013). Overcoming challenges to achieving meaningful use: Insights from hospitals that successfully received Centers for Medicare & Medicaid Services payments in 2011. *Journal of the American Medical Informatics Association, 20*(2), 233-237.

HealthIT.gov. (n.d.). *Clinical decision support (CDS).* Retrieved from https://www.healthit.gov/topic/safety/clinical-decision-support

Hersch, W. (2009). A stimulus to define informatics and health information technology. *BMC Medical Informatics and Decision Making, 9,* 24.

McGonigle, D., Mastrian, K. (2018). *Nursing informatics and the foundation of knowledge.* Burlington, MA: Jones and Bartlett Learning.

Chapter 13

Instructions for Continuing Nursing Education Contact Hours

Continuing nursing education credit can be earned for completing the learning activity associated with this chapter. Instructions can be found at aaacn.org/CCTMCoreCNE

Telehealth Nursing Practice

Kathryn Koehne, DNP, RN-BC, C-TNP
Suzanne Wells, MSN, RN
Gina Tabone, MSN, RNC-TNP
Jayme M. Speight, MSN, RN-BC

Learning Outcome Statement

After completing this learning activity, the learner will be able to demonstrate the elements of competency in professional telehealth nursing practice that are required for the Care Coordination and Transition Management registered nurse (CCTM® RN).

Learning Objectives

After reading this chapter, the CCTM RN will be able to:
- Integrate knowledge, skills, and attitudes requisite to competency in telehealth nursing with knowledge, skills, and attitudes essential to CCTM competencies.
- Recognize the importance of, and understand, the specialized telehealth skills necessary for safe and effective practice for the CCTM RN.
- Describe principles of successful communication and collaboration unique to telehealth nursing and the provision of care in a virtual or remote encounter.
- Discuss various telehealth technologies and implications in nursing practice.
- Practice safe, timely, and effective CCTM in the ambulatory care setting using telehealth principles, practices, and appropriate telehealth technologies.
- Describe the existing regulatory, ethical, and professional standards associated with telehealth nursing practice in the CCTM RN role.
- Verbalize the importance of continuing education to maintain/enhance knowledge base in telehealth nursing for CCTM.
- List the principles of telehealth triage inherent in the CCTM RN role.
- Collaborate with individual/family/caregiver to facilitate CCTM when using telehealth technology.
- Collaborate with an interprofessional team when using telehealth technology.
- Incorporate appropriate teamwork and delegation within the domain of telehealth nursing.
- Demonstrate the knowledge, skills, and attitudes requisite for telehealth nursing practice for the CCTM RN role (see Tables 13-1 to 13-5).
- Describe how CCTM is impacted and supported by the various telehealth modalities.

AAACN Care Coordination and Transition Management Standards

Standard 1.	Assessment
Standard 2.	Nursing Diagnosis
Standard 3.	Outcomes Identification
Standard 4.	Planning
Standard 5.	Implementation
Standard 5a.	Coordination of Care
Standard 5b.	Health Teaching and Health Promotion
Standard 5c.	Consultation
Standard 6.	Evaluation
Standard 7.	Ethics
Standard 8.	Education
Standard 9.	Research and Evidence Based Practice
Standard 10.	Performance Improvement
Standard 11.	Communication
Standard 12.	Leadership
Standard 13.	Collaboration
Standard 14.	Professional Practice Evaluation
Standard 15.	Resource Utilization, and Standard
Standard 16.	Environment

Source: AAACN, 2016.

Chapter 13

> **Competency Definition**
>
> Telehealth encompasses a broad scope and is defined as the "use of electronic information and telecommunications technologies to support long-distance clinical health care, patient and professional health-related education, public health, and health administration" (Health Resources & Services Administration, 2018, para. 3). Nagel and Penner (2016) described telehealth as the "remote delivery of health care services using technology and digital communications for assessment, information exchange, clinical decision making, interdisciplinary collaboration, and/or providing health care interventions to individuals" (p. 92). "Telehealth nursing is the delivery, management, and coordination of care and services provided via telecommunications technology within the domain of nursing" (Rutenberg & Greenberg, 2012, p. 5).

When the CCTM RN engages in telehealth, all standards are relevant and applicable. Telehealth nursing or *telenursing* is not simply the use of devices and equipment; rather, it is the use of "technology to deliver nursing care and conduct nursing practice" (Schlachta-Fairchild, Elfrink, & Deickman, 2008, p. 3-135).

Telehealth nursing practice uses a variety of telehealth technologies including, but not limited to, telephone, fax, electronic mail, Internet, smartphones, mobile apps, in-home messaging devices, video monitoring, and interactive video. Telehealth nursing interventions are continually evolving to support and coordinate care through virtual information exchange (Greenberg, Espensen, Becker, & Cartwright, 2003). The exchange of information may include advice to manage acute illnesses, wellness promotion, disease or condition management, care coordination during care transitions, and end-of-life support (American Academy of Ambulatory Care Nursing [AAACN], 2018). With greater frequency, nurses are using telehealth technologies to coordinate complex care needs and support individuals and families along the continuum of care.

The CCTM RN engages with individuals during both in-person and remote encounters. A demand for connectedness and access, movement toward value-based reimbursement, and new technologies in care delivery influence individual engagement (Edge, 2016). "When properly implemented, the broad adoption of connected health has the potential to extend care across populations of both acute and chronically ill patients and help achieve the important policy goals of improving access to high-quality and efficient health care" (Kvedar, Caye, & Everett, 2014, p. 194).

The CCTM RN may use various telehealth modalities to address complex needs or provide support during a transition in care. The most basic telehealth device is the telephone which has been used for many decades to manage individuals who do not share the same physical space as the individual who is providing care. More recently, there has been an expansion of telehealth modalities such as health portals, video-conferencing, remote individual monitoring, and mobile health (mhealth), which the CCTM RN may use in the provision of care.

Health Portals

Online or web-based health portals allow individuals to access their personal health record and communicate with the care team in between clinic (on-site) appointments. Individuals may review laboratory test results, immunizations, medications, and allergies; and send messages. These messages are securely routed through the health portal to care team members and may contain a simple inquiry or time-sensitive content such as questions about symptoms, concerns about side effects of medication, or clarification of health information.

Mendu and Waikar (2015) reported that when health records are accessed by means of portals, individual engagement increased for various chronic conditions. The CCTM RN plays an integral role in assisting individuals on how and when to access personal health information through a health portal which has the potential for augmenting care coordination and transition in care management. Rigby and colleagues (2015) explain that an "effective patient portal is not an on-line peephole into the clinical view of the patient but needs to be a portal for two-way and multi-party dialogue" (p. 150). Health portals may offer convenient access, but individuals may find them difficult to navigate and may struggle to understand medical information within the record (Baldwin, Singh, Sittig, & Giardina, 2016). The CCTM RN recognizes there is potential risk and inefficiency in managing care when both visual and verbal cues are absent.

Video Conferencing

The CCTM RN may use live interactive or synchronous video conferencing in a supportive role (telepresenter) or in a primary role. In a supportive role, the CCTM RN is with the individual and "presents" the individual to a provider at a distant location with the use of video conferencing equipment or other specialized devices. In this synchronous or real-time appointment, the CCTM RN assists with the exam by being the "hands" of the clinician and advocates for the individual by assuring privacy and facilitating the interview/dialogue.

In a primary role, the CCTM RN connects directly with the individual and family who are at a distant location (e.g., home or another clinic) using live interactive video to assess, educate, or coach the individual. This modality may be referred to as a *virtual home visit*. Husebo and Storm (2014) report that individuals with a virtual home visit have greater satisfaction with factors such as access and flexibility of the service when compared to recipients who received a traditional homecare visit. It is expected that the use of virtual visits will continue to rise with the increasing demand for this low-cost, convenient, and effective alternative to care administered in other settings (Gordon, Adamson, & DeVries, 2017).

Remote Patient Monitoring

Remote patient monitoring uses digital technologies to collect health data from individuals in one location and electronically transmit that information securely to health care providers in a different location for assessment and recommendations (Center for Connected Health Policy, 2018a). Remote monitoring programs aim to enhance the individual's and care team's monitoring of chronic conditions in order to "anticipate and identify exacerbations, thus avoiding unnecessary emergency room visits, rehospitalizations, surgeries, premature death, and excess costs to the health care system" (Kottek, Stafford, & Spetz, 2017, p. 5). Noah and colleagues (2018) completed a systematic review of the literature and found that remote patient monitoring shows early promise in improving outcomes for individuals with select chronic conditions.

The Veterans Health Administration (VHA) has been an early adopter of home telehealth monitoring. Between July 2003 and December 2007, a national home telehealth program was implemented. This program supports the care for Veterans with chronic conditions in their homes and involves the use of home telehealth and disease-management technologies (Darkins et al., 2008). For fiscal year 2016, the VHA reported that 702,000 veterans (approximately 12%) with 45% of those veterans living in rural communities experienced a telehealth episode of care (Landi, 2017). Although the VA has been developing and implementing telehealth programs for many years, a new ruling will accelerate and expand use among VA providers and veterans.

In 2018, the U.S. Department of Veterans Affairs (VA) announced a new federal rule that allows VA doctors, nurses, and other health care providers to administer care to Veterans using telehealth regardless of where in the United States the provider or veteran is located. With Congressional approval for this legislation, the VA is investing $260 million to further expand telehealth services (Wicklund, 2018). "By enabling veterans nationwide to receive care at home, the rule will especially benefit veterans living in rural areas who would otherwise need to travel a considerable distance or across state lines to receive care" (U.S. Department of Veterans Affairs, 2018, para. 4).

The CCTM RN plays a central role with remote home monitoring. Prior to initiation, the individual and family must receive education and be able to demonstrate understanding, adeptness, and confidence in demonstrating use of home-monitoring equipment. The individual and/or family must be able to understand the requirements and process of transmitting the data. The CCTM RN assesses the individual's learning needs and personalizes education to ensure comprehension. Once the equipment is being utilized in the home, the CCTM RN receives the remote data, assesses the data, and determines whether an intervention is required (Kottek et al., 2017). Further, the CCTM RN offers support and troubleshoots technical issues.

mHealth

Mobile communication-based health care or *mHealth* is defined as "use of portable devices with the capability to create, store, retrieve, and transmit data in real time between end users for the purpose of improving patient safety and quality of care" (Akter & Ray, 2010, p. 75).

Saner and Van der Velde (2016) explain that mobile applications may be either automatic (e.g., passive monitoring of activity using room sensors) or require the individual to take action (e.g., transmitting home-measurement values using conventional telephones or increasingly, and in particular, smartphones). The CCTM RN may receive data from individuals via this route and will need to assess the relevancy and accuracy of the information relayed.

Matthew-Maich and colleagues (2016) completed a literature review and concluded that the use of mHealth interventions has the potential to support successful management of chronic conditions by improving individual self-monitoring and management, building social networks for individuals, informing health care professionals of patients' health status, providing indirect feedback interactions, tailoring care and education to individual needs, and improving communication among health care professionals. Home *telemonitoring* is under the mHealth umbrella and is defined as an automated process for the transmission of data on an individual's health status from home to the respective health care setting. Several studies (Cardozo & Steinberg, 2010; Celler et al., 2017; Graham et al., 2012; Madigan et al., 2013; Paré, Jaana, & Sicotte, 2007) have validated that telemonitoring systems are effective in transition management, improved an individual's outcomes, and reduced readmission rates. Milani and Lavie (2015) report that the "utilization of these technologies has been shown to better engage patients in the care process, leading to improved satisfaction with the health care system, and converts the patient from a passive recipient to an active partner on the health care team" (p. 338).

Mobile Apps

The first mobile device was developed in 1973 by Motorola but was not released for consumer use until 1983 (Hardman & Steinberger-Wilckens, 2014). Over the past three decades the number of mobile devices has gone from zero to 8.6 billion (GSMA Intelligence, 2018). Ninety-five percent of Americans own a cellphone of some kind and use mobile connectivity on a daily basis (Pew Research Center, 2018). The expansion of this technology has impacted the entire world unlike any other single phenomenon. With this unprecedented technological growth, mobile devices have moved into the clinical practice domain.

The rapid integration of mobile devices into clinical practice has, in part, been driven by the rising availability and quality of medical software applications, or apps, which are software programs that have been developed to run on a computer or mobile device for a specific purpose (Ventola, 2014). In 2017, consumers downloaded 178.1 billion mobile apps to their connected devices. It is projected by 2022, an estimated 258.2 billion apps will be downloaded. Grundy, Held, and Bero (2017) explain that mobile health includes diverse stakeholders which include companies, health professionals, and consumers who highly value the collection, analysis, and sharing of user data. To date, there are over 318,000 mHealth apps (Byambasuren, Sanders, Beller, & Glasziou, 2018).

I. **Range of Mobile Apps**
(Boulos, Brewer, Karimkhani, Buller, & Dellavalle, 2014)

A. Apps for health care professionals.
  1. Medication referencing tools.
  2. Clinical decision-support tools.
  3. Communication.
  4. Electronic health record system access.
  5. Individual monitoring.
      a. Remotely monitor the health or location of individuals with chronic diseases or conditions.
B. Specialty or disease-specific apps.
  1. Specialty information.
  2. News and updates in real time.
C. Education.
  1. Portable library.
D. Consumer apps.
  1. Wellness management.
  2. Disease management.
  3. Self-diagnosis.
  4. Medication reminder.
  5. Electronic patient portal.

II. **Benefits of Health Apps**
(Grundy et al., 2017; Ozdalga, Ozdalga, & Ahuja, 2012; Ventola, 2014)

A. Support better clinical decision-making and improved individual outcomes.
B. Evidence-based resources available at the point-of-care.
C. Allow health professionals to make more rapid decisions with a lower error rate, increasing the quality of data management and accessibility, and improving practice efficiency and knowledge.
D. Allow individuals to track and report symptoms.
E. Facilitate disease education, medication information, task notifications, and synchronize records with an online database to better control symptoms.

III. **Concerns with Health Apps**
(Boulos et al., 2014)

A. Lack of health professional involvement in the design of the majority of health apps.
B. Pose a risk to health consumers' privacy; information is sought by third parties.
C. Pose risks related to information leaks, information manipulation, and loss of information.
D. Individuals may use apps to self-diagnose.

IV. **Regulation of Apps**
(U.S. Food & Drug Administration, 2018)

A. In 2013, the U.S. Food and Drug Administration (FDA) released a guide which explains the agency's oversight of mobile medical apps.
B. The FDA applies the same risk-based approach to apps as it does to the safety and effectiveness for other medical devices.

Chapter 13

The CCTM RN should anticipate that telehealth interventions will continually evolve and expand as telehealth technologies advance. The various modalities will offer individuals, families, and the care team new opportunities for safe, effective, person-centered, timely, efficient, and equitable care (Agency for Healthcare Research and Quality [AHRQ], 2016). CCTM will be impacted by current and future innovations.

V. Essential Elements of Telehealth Practice

When engaged in CCTM, the RN will need to be familiar and competent with various telehealth technologies. Greenberg, Rutenberg, and Scheidt (2014) identify five essential elements of telehealth practice, which are:
- Professional Telehealth Practice.
- Telehealth Triage Principles and Practice.
- Effective Communication Using Telehealth Technology.
- Teamwork and Collaboration.
- Technology Expertise.

For safe and effective practice, it is particularly important the CCTM RN understands the potential for triage when interacting with individuals via telehealth technology, and therefore a specialized telehealth triage skill set is required for nurses engaged in CCTM. In this chapter, the five essential elements will be described, along with the requisite knowledge, skills, and attitudes that are needed to attain competence. Although some of these elements are common to nursing in the in-person encounter, information addressed herein incorporates nuances and distinct practice differences necessary for the provision of care using telehealth technology (Greenberg et al., 2014).

VI. Professional Telehealth Practice

Telehealth nursing practice must comply with basic standards put forth by the nursing profession (Rutenberg & Greenberg, 2012). Telehealth, as a modality of delivery of CCTM services, requires knowledge of specific regulatory, ethical, and professional standards as they apply to care delivery.

A. Application of standards to telehealth practices.
1. Regulatory standards.
    a. Adheres to licensure requirements.
    b. Aligns practice with Nurse Practice Act(s) in applicable jurisdiction(s).
    c. Identifies issues related to interstate practice and the Enhanced Nurse Licensure Compact (National Council of State Boards of Nursing, n.d.).
    d. Practices within the guidelines set forth by Health Insurance Portability and Accountability Act (U.S. Department of Health and Human Services, 2013).
    e. Maintains a healthy and ergonomically safe work environment (Occupational Safety and Health Administration, n.d.).
2. Professional standards.
    a. Aligns practice with *Scope and Standards of Practice for Professional Telehealth Nursing* (AAACN, 2018).
    b. Assimilates nursing process in all telehealth encounters.
    c. Recognizes telehealth nursing as a highly collaborative practice; however, functions autonomously and maintains accountability for own actions and associated individual's outcomes.
    d. Documents telehealth encounters thoroughly, accurately, and promptly (AAACN, 2018).
3. Ethical standards.
    a. Complies with American Nurses Association (ANA) Code of Ethics (2015).
    b. Recognizes person's right to self-determination, but in all cases, acts in the best interest of the person to ensure safety (ANA, 2015).
    c. Exercises moral courage to support core values and ethical obligations (Lachman, 2010).
    d. Provides care to all who are in need, regardless of their cultural, social, or economic standing (ANA, 2010).
    e. Engages in ongoing professional development in telehealth.
    f. Recognizes the rapidly evolving state of telehealth nursing.
    g. Remains current in the use of relevant telehealth technology.
    h. Engages in continuing education to maintain comprehensive clinical knowledge base.
    i. Actively seeks to supplement existing knowledge deficits.

VII. Telehealth Principles and Practice

CCTM RNs who provide care using telehealth technology must be poised and prepared to triage symptoms and prioritize care needs (Greenberg et al., 2014). Moreover, CCTM RNs also need to be able to assess knowledge deficits and triage learning needs. Because triage involves identifying and managing incipient and ongoing issues, the nurse must possess a significant depth and breadth

of knowledge to determine the nature and urgency of the problem(s) and refer the individual to the appropriate level of care, provide education and counseling, and offer support as necessary (see Table 13-2).
A. Application of the nursing process in telehealth triage (Rutenberg & Greenberg, 2012).
   1. Performs an adequate assessment including relevant subjective and objective data.
   2. Formulates diagnostic statement to include the nature and urgency of the problem and any potential confounding factors.
   3. Identifies desired outcomes as a basis for development of plan of care to ensure individual safety.
   4. Collaboratively develops an individualized plan of care to assure achievement of desired outcomes.
   5. Implements plan/intervention with attention to continuity of care.
   6. Evaluates effectiveness of triage intervention.
B. Principles of telehealth triage in the CCTM RN role (Rutenberg & Greenberg, 2012).
   1. Interacts directly with the individual to perform accurate assessment of symptoms and/or knowledge and understanding of diagnosis or condition.
   2. Considers the possibility of, and actively looks for, unexpected problems and rules out the worst possible clinical presentation.
   3. Errs on side of caution to ensure safety.
   4. Respects the individual's perception but does not accept the self-diagnosis or caregiver's diagnosis without further assessment.
   5. Avoids jumping to a conclusion about the nature of the individual's problem.
   6. Avoids making assumptions about the individual's level of knowledge and skill in managing a health condition or symptoms.
   7. Exercises critical thinking and judgment in use of support tools.
   8. Provides support and collaboration as needed by the individual.
C. Pediatric considerations.
   1. Applies growth and developmental principles when assessing symptomatology and identifying intended individual outcomes.
   2. Recognizes the child's response to illness through subtle signs based on developmental stages such as:
      a. Children often compensate for illness longer than adults but will deteriorate rapidly once compensatory measures are exhausted.
   3. Incorporates pediatric considerations in telehealth encounters.
      a. Carefully listens to parents or primary caregiver of the child because they know the child best. When caregivers are concerned, this is a red flag.
      b. Involves both the child and caregiver to gather health information for better assessment of illness/injury.
      c. Considers developmental stages when using the nursing process. Is careful to use vocabulary and questioning that is aligned with the individual's level of understanding.

VIII. **Effective Communication Using Telehealth Technology**

The CCTM RN must be able to "communicate effectively using a variety of formats, tools, and technologies to build professional relationships and to deliver care across the continuum" (AAACN, 2016, p. 26). When using telehealth technology, communication strategies must be implemented to accurately and effectively elicit and provide information to individuals, families, nurses, and other team members.

Telehealth interactions may be *synchronous* or *asynchronous*. Synchronous, or real-time telehealth systems, support live interactions between an individual and a health care team member, using audio and video telehealth technology (Center for Connected Health Policy, 2018a). For an example, a synchronous visit may serve as an alternative to an in-person encounter. Wilson and Maeder (2015) describe asynchronous, or store-and-forward communication, as systems that "decouple the components of the interaction so that they can occur at different times at the convenience of the participating parties" (p. 214). Asynchronous telehealth captures relevant data and/or digital samples (e.g., still images, video, audio, text files) in one location and subsequently transmits these files for interpretation at a remote site by health professionals (Deshpande et al., 2009). This store-and-forward model allows for multiple interactions but does not rely on a physical examination or face-to-face contact. Regardless, of the interaction model that is used, the CCTM RN must recognize that the skills necessary for effective communication must be adapted when the nurse is not in the physical presence of the person, his or her family/caregiver, or other members of the health care team (see Table 13-3) (Rutenberg & Greenberg, 2012).
A. Effective non-in-person (virtual) communication. "Effective communication is communication that

is comprehended by both participants; it is usually bidirectional between participants, and enables both participants to clarify the intended message" (Schyve, 2007, p. 360). To effectively communicate via a telehealth encounter, the CCTM RN:
1. Introduces self and role.
2. Expresses empathy.
3. Invites the individual to share perspective and preferences.
4. Uses visualization as a technique to gain a clear picture of the problem and confirms understanding by verifying impression with individual.
5. Confirms comfort with the information/direction given and the plan of care.
6. Interprets (e.g., rephrases) information when necessary to increase understanding.
7. Clearly and promptly documents telehealth interactions so they are accessible to members of the health care team (Greenberg et al., 2014).

B. Communication barriers.
"When effective communication is absent, the provision of health care ends – or proceeds only with errors, poor quality, and risks to patient safety" (Schyve, 2007, p. 360).
1. Language barriers.
The United States Census Bureau (2015) reported that the nation's population is becoming more diverse and identifies that there are at least 350 languages spoken in U.S. homes. Although 90% of the population speaks English, 9% (25.9 million) is Limited English Proficient (Migration Policy Institute, 2016). The CCTM RN employs the following strategies to overcome language barriers (Squires, 2018):
   a. Enlists the services of a medical interpreter when necessary.
   b. Utilizes an approved language line when necessary for language interpretation.
   c. Implements live video remote interpretation when available.
   d. Uses HIPAA-compliant translation apps and devices.
2. Hearing impairment.
According to the National Institute on Deafness and Other Communication Disorders (2016), 10% of the population has some degree of hearing loss which ranges from mild (difficulty hearing or understanding soft sounds) to profound (inability to hear loud sounds).
In virtual encounters, a hearing impairment may pose even a greater challenge than in-person interactions; when both visual and auditory cues are absent, communication effectiveness may be significantly impacted. The CCTM RN may use the following to communicate with an individual who has impaired hearing:
   a. Speak naturally and at a moderate speed directly into the phone mouthpiece.
   b. Reduce background noise; choose quiet setting.
   c. Use health portals as appropriate for relaying information.
   d. Interact with Relay Operator for the Hearing Impaired.
   e. Understand individual phraseology when using TTY or TDD technology.
3. Visual impairment.
The National Institutes of Health (2016) estimates that 1 million Americans are legally blind and 3.2 million have visual impairment (20/40 vision with correction). Telehealth technologies may be an option if the individual has difficulty accessing an in-person visit due to transportation difficulties. The individual may interact with the care team via telephone with a landline or mobile phone by using a voice-activated phone, braille phone, or a phone with enlarged numbers. Communicating through health portals or videoconferencing may offer an opportunity for the individual and CCTM RN to communicate. Various assistive technologies are available to accommodate individuals with visual impairment. The CCTM RN can support the individual by recommending or coordinating use of the following:
   a. Braille keyboard.
   b. Keyboard with large print.
   c. Screen magnifiers for low-vision computer users.
   d. Screen readers for blind individuals.
   e. Voice recognition software.
   Gell, Rosenger, Demiris, LaCroix, and Patel (2015) have identified that vision impairment is associated with lower likelihood of technology use. Despite the availability of assistive technologies, individuals with visual impairment experience barriers including "policies that do not explicitly support accessible design, webpage design and limitations for interpretation by assistive devices,

and lack of financial resources to acquire appropriate assistive technology" (p. 418). It is important that the CCTM RN assess technology use with an individual with a vision impairment and individualizes care as needed to decrease barriers and promote quality communication.
C. Use plain language in interactions.
1. Understand that many individuals may not have the capacity to obtain, process, and understand basic health information and services needed to make appropriate health decisions.
   a. Ninety million Americans have difficulty understanding and acting on health information (The Joint Commission, 2017).
2. Confirm individual understanding of medical conditions, treatments, or other courses of action by using simple and concise language with individuals and applying certain communication methods, such as the "teach-back'" technique (AHRQ, 2015).
3. Explore reasons for non-adherence with medication, missed appointments, and lack of follow-through with tests and referrals as these may be indicators of low health literacy (Safeer & Keenan, 2005).
4. Understand that individuals with low health literacy may be less likely to use health information technology tools (e.g., personalized fitness trackers, apps, health portals) or perceive them as easy or useful (Mackert, Mabry-Flyn, Champlin, Donovan, & Pounders, 2016).
D. Pediatric considerations.
1. When assessing symptoms in the pediatric population, consider limitations with young children and non-verbal children who cannot verbalize or express what is wrong.
2. Using third parties such as caregivers and parents of minor individuals to relay information can cause miscommunications.
3. At times, the nurse may need to address parental concerns that may or may not be related to the actual illness or injury being addressed. The use of compassion and empathy with every question establishes rapport and may uncover concerns that have not yet been addressed and may need to be evaluated.

IX. Teamwork and Collaboration

While utilizing telehealth technology, the CCTM RN must actively foster open communication, facilitate mutual respect, engage in shared decision-making, participate in team learning, delegate as appropriate, and work to achieve optimal care coordination and transition management (Cronenwett et al., 2007). Rouleau and colleagues (2017) performed an extensive review and found that intra- and interprofessional collaboration was positively impacted by the use of information and communication technologies. Effective teamwork and collaboration requires knowledge of interprofessional roles and practices (see Table 13-4).
A. Collaborates with person/family/caregiver to facilitate CCTM when using telehealth technology.
1. Recognizes and respects person/family/caregiver role in decision-making.
2. Identifies, acknowledges, and addresses the individual's agenda (e.g., request or desired outcome) in the telehealth encounter.
B. Facilitates interprofessional collaboration when using telehealth technology.
1. Possesses knowledge of interprofessional roles and practices.
2. Recognizes and avoids risks associated with transferring care responsibilities to another professional (handoff) during transitions in care, especially in the telehealth setting.
3. Applies principles of successful communication and collaboration unique to telehealth nursing during interprofessional interactions (Rouleau et al., 2017).
C. Facilitates appropriate teamwork and delegation within the domain of telehealth nursing.
1. Delegates as appropriate and necessary to enhance efficiency within telehealth encounters.
2. Delegates to licensed practical nurses and unlicensed assistive personnel as appropriate to their level of education, experience, scope of practice, and licensure.
3. Adheres to the five rights of delegation when providing care utilizing telehealth technology.
D. Invites individuals and families to participate in relevant discussions regarding care delivery.

X. Technology Expertise

The CCTM RN must be able to appropriately, safely, and efficiently use telehealth technology to meet the needs of the individual, family, or population. The telehealth technology used by the

CCTM RN will differ across settings. In some situations, permission for various equipment will need to be obtained from the individual or family. The CCTM RN is responsible to attain and maintain competence with the use of the devices or equipment (see Table 13-5).

A. Proficiency in use of telehealth technology used in their setting.
   1. Possesses basic understanding of technology and functionality.
   2. Troubleshoots and consults with technical support staff for technical problems.
   3. Understands documentation and storage of data.
   4. Discusses contingency plan in the event of technology breakdown (downtime process).
B. Maintains individual safety and confidentiality when using telehealth technology.
   1. Confirms with whom they are interacting when using telehealth technology.
   2. Maintains individual privacy while using telehealth technology.
   3. Uses certified practices and systems for secure management of data.
C. Participates in discussions and initiatives related to the implementation of telehealth and electronic technologies.
   1. Advocates for the interests of individuals and families as end users for various health applications.
   2. Ensures that safety, efficiency, and scope of practice issues are taken into consideration when introducing new technologies.
D. Empowers individuals to use advancing technologies to track and manage their health (Mackert et al., 2016).
   1. Avoids making assumptions related individual's ability to engage in technology (e.g., health portal, telephone follow-up).
   2. Explores the individual's resources in using technology for telehealth services.
      a. A division exists between those who have access to, and use information technology, and those who do not. It is known as the *digital divide* (Connolly & Crosby, 2014).
         (1) Absence of devices.
         (2) Lack of access to high-speed Internet.
         (3) Lack of mobile broadband.
         (4) Lack of knowledge of how to operate devices or apps.
   3. Identifies telehealth resources available for individuals.
   4. Advocates for the expansion of telehealth technologies to meet the needs of the underserved (e.g., rural communities).
E. Pediatric considerations.
   1. Attention should be given to potential issues with legal guardianship, individual privacy, legal responsibility, and informed consent at the initiation of a telehealth encounter (Espensen, 2009).
      a. Uses caution about how much and what type of information is given to non-custodial caregivers.
      b. Verifies that there is written authorization/consent given for non-custodial caregivers to obtain treatment and information sharing before proceeding with the telehealth encounter.

Table 13-1.
Professional Telehealth Practice: Knowledge, Skills, and Attitudes for Competency

Knowledge	Skills	Attitudes	Sources
Understand the existing legal, ethical, and professional standards associated with telehealth nursing. Recognize the importance of continuing education to maintain/enhance knowledge base in telehealth nursing.	Demonstrate accountability by practicing within own scope of competence and training. Assure safety in compliance with professional standards and scope of practice laws and regulations. Recognize and implement telehealth best practices in care coordination and transition management.	Value legal, ethical, and professional standards of practice. Value the professional role of the RN and recognize differences in scope of practice of RNs, licensed practical nurses/licensed vocational nurses (LPN/LVNs), and the role of unlicensed assistive personnel (UAP). Recognize the potential for improved practices through continuing education.	Cronenwett et al., 2007
Understand the concept of accountability and responsibility for telehealth nursing practice and for the outcome of that practice.	Uphold and practice within legal, ethical, and professional standards of telehealth nursing practice. Adhere to existing individual privacy, confidentiality, and security laws related to individual information, especially as it pertains to practice using telehealth technology. Appropriately delegate functions to LPNs, LVNs, and UAP. Adhere to individual privacy, confidentiality, and security principles related to sharing/display/storage of individual records and information.	Accept responsibility for own behavior. Value legal and ethical principles and individual's right to privacy. Appreciate the importance of remaining current in a rapidly changing practice	AAACN, 2018 International Council of Nurses (ICN), 2007.
Articulate the elements of the nursing process as they apply to telehealth across settings via telehealth technology.	Adhere to the *Scope and Standards of Practice for Professional Telehealth Nursing*. Participate in lifelong learning specific to telehealth nursing, seeking new education and training opportunities as new practice opportunities become available.	Value and participate in lifelong learning.	AAACN, 2018

continued on next page

Table 13-1. (continued)
Professional Telehealth Practice: Knowledge, Skills, and Attitudes for Competency

Knowledge	Skills	Attitudes	Sources
Understand legal and ethical principles related to sharing individual information.	Apply the nursing process in all telehealth encounters. When care is provided across state lines: • Maintain licensure in states in which he or she is practicing. • Practice within the RN scope of practice in the state in which care is being provided as interpreted by the relevant board(s) of nursing.	Value the individual's rights. Value the nursing process as the basic standard of nursing practice and recognize the importance of utilizing all elements of nursing process in telehealth interactions. Recognize the values the importance of licensure in the practice of nursing across state lines. Appreciate that regulations and standards exist to protect the public, which is a sovereign responsibility of each board of nursing. Commit to providing high-quality, safe, and effective care coordination and transition management.	AAACN, 2018 Rutenberg & Greenberg, 2012
Possess general understanding of different cultural groups. Cognizant that different belief systems exist. Understand components of cultures related to health care practices and illness.	Be respectful of the beliefs of others. Be adaptable to other cultural beliefs and practices. Demonstrate culturally sensitive interview skills. Utilize of interpreter services appropriately.	Maintain flexibility and open-mindedness when caring for persons different than self.	Laughlin, 2018

Source: Cronenwett et al. (2007). *Nursing Outlook, 55*(3), 122-131. Reprinted with permission from Elsevier.

Table 13-2.
Telehealth Triage Principles and Practice: Knowledge, Skills, and Attitudes for Competency

Knowledge	Skills	Attitudes	Sources
Acknowledge the necessity of collaboration in development of a plan of care to achieve desired outcomes.	Elicit care expectations of individual and family. Ensure individual and family have contact numbers to communicate effectively when technology may not be working. Collaborate with the individual/caregiver to develop a plan of care to attain desired outcomes that are realistic and achievable.	Value safety. Respect the individual and caregiver as reliable sources of information. Respect the individual's right to participate in care planning and making his or her own decision about the course of action. Recognize that expectations influence outcomes in management of symptoms. Respect the individual's perspective, valuing individual self-determination.	Cronenwett et al., 2007
Identify strategies for implementing the plan of care as appropriate for the individual and within the clinical context.	Collaborate with the individual/caregiver to identify desired outcomes for the triage encounter. Implement the plan of care in collaboration with the individual/caregiver and other members of the health care team as appropriate.	Recognize the key role of the individual/caregiver in implementation of the plan of care in any telehealth encounter.	Cronenwett et al., 2009
Identify assessment techniques to collect both subjective and objective data using telehealth technologies. Understand the need to be sensitive to auditory, verbal, and emotional cues communicated through speech. Understand the role of outcomes identification in individualizing care using telehealth technology. Is knowledgeable about the process of evaluation of a telehealth encounter to achieve desired outcomes.	Establish a therapeutic relationship with the individual when using technology. Conduct assessments including both subjective and objective data using an array of available resources. Prioritize plan and intervention based on assessment data. Involve other members of the health care team in development of a plan of care as appropriate and necessary. Implement an interprofessional plan of care directly or via geographically remote site person(s) to achieve desired outcomes. Evaluate the individual's progress toward attainment of expected outcomes.	Recognize the duty of nurse to provide safe and effective care. Realize desired outcomes must be individualized and that the individual/caregiver has an important role in their development. Recognize the telehealth encounter doesn't end with implementation of the plan of care, but that the nurse has a responsibility to follow-up, when indicated, to measure attainment of desired outcomes and assure individual safety.	Schlachta-Fairchild et al., 2008 Espensen, 2009

continued on next page

Table 13-2. (continued)
Telehealth Triage Principles and Practice: Knowledge, Skills, and Attitudes for Competency

Knowledge	Skills	Attitudes	Sources
Understand the need to function within a professional code of ethics that ensures individual rights. Understand that implementation in the telehealth setting by necessity must include other individuals since the telehealth nurse is unable to provide physical care or services directly to the individual.	Work toward identifying and honoring the individual's wishes. Employ creative strategies when the individual's desires conflict with health and safety.	Recognize the highly collaborative nature of telehealth nursing. Understand that a plan of care must be personalized to each individual and might be impacted by the motivation of the individual and available resources. Understand the need to balance individual self-determination with assuring safety. Be sensitive to the fact telehealth nursing is highly collaborative. Recognize the final decision-maker in a telehealth encounter is usually the individual/caregiver while remaining sensitive to situations in which the nurse needs to act on the individual's behalf to assure his or her safety. Employ strategies to reduce risk in the performance of triage using telehealth technology.	AAACN, 2018
Demonstrate comprehensive knowledge of the interpersonal, clinical, and technical skills needed to perform triage in non-face-to-face settings. Comprehend the complexity of individual assessment utilizing telehealth technology. Develop nursing diagnostic statements based on assessment. Possess a wide and diverse clinical knowledge base. Acquire knowledge of individual and community resources as well as organizational policies relevant to development of an individualized plan of care.	Assess presence and extent of symptoms. Develop assessment techniques that compensate for the nurse's inability to see or touch the individual. Formulate diagnostic statements that address individual's presenting problems and include the nature and urgency of the individual's problem and related needs. Address the individual's ability to carry out the plan of care and other factors that might impact continuity of care. Assure continuity of care in implementation of the plan of care. Facilitate actions to assure individual safety.	Recognize the ability of the individual/caregiver to provide health data utilizing their visual, tactile, auditory, and olfactory senses with individualized coaching. Recognize the duty of nurse to provide safe and effective care. Maintain sensitivity to the complexity of the health care system and the individual's likely need for support and coaching in navigating the system. Value the role of the team in providing care to an individual and recognize the important contributions of the individual/family, telehealth nurse, and other members of the health care team as well as appropriate community resources. Value lifelong learning and understand that individuals may present with a wide variety of clinical and social problems the nurse must recognize and address.	Rutenberg & Greenberg, 2012

continued on next page

Table 13-2. (continued)
Telehealth Triage Principles and Practice: Knowledge, Skills, and Attitudes for Competency

Knowledge	Skills	Attitudes	Sources
Understand the role of clinical decision-support tools in triage, recognizing they are to be utilized to support decision-making rather than to dictate decision-making. Effectively manage individuals and decrease inappropriate use of health care resources by utilizing clinical decision-support tools and properly directing the individual to an appropriate level of care. Recognize clinical pitfalls in the practice of telehealth triage. Explain the minimum skill set for provision of triage services in the non-face-to-face setting.	Document a complete, accurate, and prompt account of the interaction. Follow-up when appropriate and necessary based on assessment of the likelihood the individual will be able to carry out the plan of care and the risk associated with failure to do so.	Value the role of critical thinking and clinical judgment in the provision of care during a triage encounter. Appreciate the value of decision-support tools to enhance the nurse's knowledge base and as a checklist to avoid clinical oversights. Value the unique nature of triage outside of the face-to-face setting and understand that in the absence of face-to-face assessment and a known medical diagnosis, it requires a somewhat different, often more conservative approach to individual management.	Rutenberg & Greenberg, 2012
Describe the process of a systematic assessment.	Work to develop and maintain an extensive knowledge base to support clinical decision-making in triage encounters. Consistently utilize decision-support tools during triage, but apply clinical judgment and critical thinking. Avoid overreliance on decision-support tools. Practice in a manner that assures individual safety. Perform an adequate assessment with all symptom-based encounters, regardless of the nature of the individual or complaint, or the technology used. Consistently err on the side of caution. Avoid accepting self-diagnosis without adequate investigation. Avoid stereotyping the individual.	Understand individuals are potentially in crisis and their concerns must be identified and addressed in a professional and empathetic manner. Recognize the importance of the role of the RN in telehealth encounters. Approach each encounter with caution and recognize the inherent risk in the provision of care using telehealth technology. Value individual health and safety.	Rutenberg & Greenberg, 2012

continued on next page

Table 13-2. (continued)
Telehealth Triage Principles and Practice: Knowledge, Skills, and Attitudes for Competency

Knowledge	Skills	Attitudes	Sources
	Interact directly with the individual whenever possible.		
	Recognize the perils associated with fatigue and haste.		
	Use critical thinking to recognize and address all concerns, remaining on the alert for unexpected problems.		
	Anticipate problems to be worst possible until proven otherwise.		
	Advocate for the individual, even when it is difficult to do so.		
	Follow-up when indicated by the nursing care plan.		
	Facilitate continuity of care, recognizing the telehealth encounter is often not the endpoint of care, but rather the beginning.		
Pediatric Considerations			
Recognize the child's response to illness through subtle signs based on developmental stages. For example, children often compensate for illness longer than adults but will deteriorate rapidly once compensatory measures are exhausted.	Apply growth and developmental principles when assessing symptomatology and identifying intended individual outcomes.	Appreciate that the management of children requires a family-centered approach.	Rutenberg & Greenberg, 2012
	Listen carefully to parents or primary caregiver of the child because they know the child best. When caregivers are concerned, this is a red flag for the RN.		
	When possible, use both the child and caregiver to gather health information for better assessment of illness/injury.		
	Use vocabulary and questioning that is aligned with the individual's level of understanding.		

Sources: Cronenwett et al. (2007). *Nursing Outlook, 55*(3), 122-131. Reprinted with permission from Elsevier. Cronenwett et al. (2019). *Nursing Outlook, 57*(6), 338-348. Reprinted with permission from Elsevier and the author.

Chapter 13

Table 13-3.
Effective Communication: Knowledge, Skills, and Attitudes for Competency

Knowledge	Skills	Attitudes	Sources
Examine how the safety, quality, and cost effectiveness of health care can be improved through the active involvement of the individual/family.	Elicit and validate values, preferences, and expressed needs.	Respect preferences, values, and needs. Value various forms of communication and accept that others may have differing ways of communicating.	Cronenwett et al., 2007
Analyze differences in communication styles, preferences among individuals, nurses, and other members of the health care team.		Value interprofessional collaboration and communication.	Cronenwett et al., 2009
Recognize subtle changes in interpersonal communication patterns of individual and providers that may indicate potential problems or important changes in status that require attention. Recognize need to create a therapeutic relationship with the individual/family.	Adapt communication style to the goals of the individual and the technology used. Create therapeutic environment using telehealth technologies. Use a variety of formats, tools, and technologies to build professional relationships and to coordinate care. Communicate individual's values, preferences, and expressed needs as appropriate to other members of the health care team.	Recognize own responsibility for contributing to effective communication. Acknowledge role of continuous quality improvement.	ICN, 2007
Identify a variety of communication strategies using technology, including the effective use of both verbal and nonverbal communication. Coordinate care within and across settings via telehealth technology.	Evaluate personal skills and styles of communication via technology to identify areas needing improvement or education. Share communication experiences with peers and ask for feedback and evaluation of effectiveness. Facilitate identification and delivery of services via communication technology.	Understand that effective communication is essential to a telehealth encounter. Understand that effective communication is essential to a telehealth encounter. Value medical record as a communication tool and endeavor to document the encounter in such a way as to be relevant to other members of the team.	AAACN, 2018

continued on next page

**Table 13-3. (continued)
Effective Communication: Knowledge, Skills, and Attitudes for Competency**

Knowledge	Skills	Attitudes	Sources
Recognize the limitations inherent in non-face-to-face communication. Discuss strategies used to "connect" with others when communicating via technology.	Identify self with name and licensure. Engage in active listening. Clarify statements when necessary. Allow individuals to tell their story in their own way, communicating their concerns in a manner most comfortable to and effective for them. Use self-disclosure when appropriate and necessary to connect with the individual/family/caregiver. Encourage the individual to take notes during a telehealth encounter. Document as appropriate and maintain clear records of communications.	Recognize self-disclosure as a strategy which can either enhance or interrupt connection with the individual/family caregiver and realize it must be used judiciously when it is believed that it will enhance the nurse's ability to meet the individual's needs without instead shifting the focus from the individual/family/caregiver to the RN. Understand effective communication is essential to a telehealth encounter.	Rutenberg & Greenberg, 2012
Recognize information needs of patients, providers, and other members of the health care team. Recognize which elements of communication tools improve telehealth interactions and promote positive results.	Verify caller/contact identity and relationship to the individual and identify need or desired outcome of the communication. Adapt communication style as needed to fit the technology used (e.g., tone of voice, facial expression, clear written word, appropriate literacy level). Participate in evaluation of communication tools and encounter forms.	Recognize own responsibility for contributing to effective communication.	Rutenberg & Greenberg, 2012

continued on next page

Table 13-3. (continued)
Effective Communication: Knowledge, Skills, and Attitudes for Competency

Knowledge	Skills	Attitudes	Sources
Pediatric Considerations			
Explain that interactions pertaining to a child require a whole-situation approach which requires developmental considerations as well as parental capabilities that will influence communication strategies.	Consider limitations with young children and non-verbal children who cannot verbalize or express what is wrong. Maintain awareness that the use of third parties such as caregivers and parents of minor individuals to relay information may cause miscommunications. Address parental concerns that may or may not be related to the actual illness or injury being addressed. Use compassion and empathy with every question to establish rapport and uncover concerns that have not yet been addressed and need to be evaluated.		

Sources: Cronenwett et al. (2007). *Nursing Outlook, 55*(3), 122-131. Reprinted with permission from Elsevier. Cronenwett et al. (2019). *Nursing Outlook, 57*(6), 338-348. Reprinted with permission from Elsevier and the author.

Table 13-4.
Teamwork and Collaboration: Knowledge, Skills, and Attitudes for Competency

Knowledge	Skills	Attitudes	Sources
Describe how telehealth technologies enhance teamwork and collaboration across the care continuum. Identify potential and actual barriers and facilitators in the use of telehealth technologies and what it brings to effective team functioning. Discuss the impact of effective team functioning on safety and quality of care. Describe scope of practice and roles of interprofessional and nursing telehealth care team members.	Contribute own expertise and perspective in coordination of care. Implement telehealth technologies that allow the care team to connect with each other and individuals and their families to facilitate transitions in care and coordinate care at a distance. Engage in cross continuum care conferences, educational in-services, and other interprofessional meetings. Engage in communication practices that facilitate cohesion and minimize risks associated with hand-offs among providers and across transitions in care when using telehealth technologies. Consult with interprofessional team members to ensure efficacy and reliability of telehealth technology. Function(s) competently within own scope of practice as a member of the telehealth care team. Integrate the contributions of others in assisting individual/family to achieve health goals. Demonstrate self-awareness of strengths and limitations as a team.	Appreciate that individuals and families are an integral part of the care team and that their preferences, needs, and values will guide clinical decision-making in telehealth encounters. Value telehealth technology as an effective modality for care team members to coordinate and facilitate care across the continuum with individuals and families. Acknowledge that telehealth technologies build relationships between care team members at distant locations. Value the perspectives and expertise of all health team members. Recognize a shared responsibility for effective team functioning in non-in-person encounters. Value own role in identifying risks and preventing errors in delivering care via the utilization of telehealth and electronic technologies. Appreciate the attributes and abilities of care team members that are effective in meeting the needs of individuals and families in the telehealth setting. Prioritize relationship-building among care team members especially when there is separation by distance and work in different settings. Recognize that interprofessional collaboration improves individual outcomes and quality of care in all settings – including telehealth.	AHRQ, 2016 Cronenwett et al., 2007 Naylor, 2011

continued on next page

Table 13-4. (continued)
Teamwork and Collaboration: Knowledge, Skills, and Attitudes for Competency

Knowledge	Skills	Attitudes	Sources
Analyze strategies associated with technology that influence the ability to initiate and sustain effective partnerships with members of nursing and interprofessional teams. Recognize the risks associated with transferring individual care responsibilities to another professional ("hand-over") during transitions in care, especially in the telehealth setting.	Lead or participate in the design and implementation of telehealth systems that support effective teamwork. Act with integrity, consistency, and respect for differing views when coordinating care using telehealth technology.	"Value(s) the influence of system solutions in achieving team functioning in the telehealth setting" (p. 342). "Respect(s) the centrality of the individual/family as core members of any health care team, especially in the telehealth environment" (p. 341). Appreciate the risks associated with hand-offs among providers and across transitions in care, especially in the telehealth setting.	Cronenwett et al., 2009
Recognize the need for teamwork and collaboration to coordinate care within the telehealth domain.	Assure the individual and the care team are aware of potential/actual safety issues. Document the process and outcome of care within the individual's health record in which other care team members have access to ensure continuity of care.		Schlachta-Fairchild et al., 2008
	Demonstrate principles of delegation of duties to team members. Ensure identities/roles of practitioners and clients when coordinating care using telehealth technology. Implement and communicate an interprofessional plan of care to promote positive outcomes via telehealth technology.	Recognize the importance of teamwork and collaboration in the telehealth setting.	AAACN, 2018

Sources: Cronenwett et al. (2007). *Nursing Outlook, 55*(3), 122-131. Reprinted with permission from Elsevier. Cronenwett et al. (2019). *Nursing Outlook, 57*(6), 338-348. Reprinted with permission from Elsevier and the author.

Table 13-5.
Technology Expertise: Knowledge, Skills, and Attitudes for Competency

Knowledge	Skills	Attitudes	Sources
Develop process and outcome measures that allow for the implementation and continual improvement of the use of telehealth technologies in care coordination and transition management. Identify knowledge and skills required to provide care and to communicate via specific telehealth technologies. Analyze features of technology that support or pose barriers to coordinating care and managing transitions. Explore innovative telehealth technology options to expand care delivery options. Appraise technological options to determine appropriate tools for effective and efficient care delivery in care coordination and transition management. Identify potential privacy risks with the use of telehealth technology.	Demonstrate efficient use of technology devices to perform role. Apply appropriate telehealth technology to support CCTM. Champion communication technologies that support care coordination. Assure safety of self and others when using telehealth technology.	Value innovative technologies that support care coordination and transition management. Appreciate the need for continuing education. Prioritize safety, privacy, and confidentiality when implementing telehealth and electronic technology in care delivery. Advocate for the introduction of new and innovative technologies to enhance and support care delivery.	Cronenwett et al., 2007 Hall & McGraw, 2014
Explain the impact of consumerism in care delivery. Identify federal and state regulations applicable to telehealth care delivery. Discuss functions and features related to the technology and tools being utilized. Identify safety features and requirements of devices and equipment utilized in a telehealth encounter. Describe care delivery that is safe, efficient, and within scope for the employee's role.	Use technology appropriately and safely to coordinate care for individuals. Provide and/or coordinate education for individuals and families when utilizing technological devices and equipment. Establish a collegial relationship with key technical support person(s) to ensure technical problems/questions can be addressed efficiently. Examine strategies for improving systems to support team functioning.	Prioritize person-centered care by exploring individual and family preferences. Accept personal responsibility for performance. Acknowledge accountability for competency in the use of telehealth technology and the practices that support the utilization of the tools.	AAACN, 2018

continued on next page

Table 13-5. (continued)
Technology Expertise: Knowledge, Skills, and Attitudes for Competency

Knowledge	Skills	Attitudes	Sources
Recognize the need for organizational policies or standard operating procedures to support/guide the use of telehealth technology in practice: • Locate existing standards and maintain • Participate in development of standards • Modify standards as needed to reflect current state	Maintain safe and proper use of devices and equipment. Participate in training related to telehealth technology. Anticipate potential technical problems by having back-up plan or alternative action ready. Utilize technology according to organizational or agency policy. Participate in the selection, design, implementation, and evaluation of technology. Maintain competence in technology use.		

Source: Cronenwett et al. (2007). *Nursing Outlook, 55*(3), 122-131. Reprinted with permission from Elsevier.

Chapter 13

Case Study 13-1. Videoconferencing

Existing literature suggests that the use of telehealth technology for appointments can increase access to care and is valued by individuals, families and providers (Reider-Demer, Raja, Martin, Schwinger, & Babayan, 2017). Telehealth video conferencing is a viable alternative to traditional health care delivery, enabling providers and consultants across distances to provide care in a cost-effective and convenient way (Armstrong, Semple, & Coyte, 2014). Synchronous or real-time video conferencing is not just an option for physicians or advanced practice providers; nurses use telemedicine for triage and transitional care (Glavind, Bjørk, & Lindquist, 2014). Telehealth enables nurses to evaluate individuals' current situation, manage symptoms, review medications, and determine the appropriate level of care.

Introduction

- Forty-five-year-old healthy man presented with a 1-week history of a drooping eyelid (ptosis).
- Magnetic resonance imaging identified a right carotid artery dissection.
- Transitioned home on aspirin therapy and pain medication for complaints of a "vice-like" headache.

Clinical Interaction

- A telemedicine video conferencing appointment was scheduled with an RN 2 days after the transition home. The RN reviewed medications and confirmed upcoming appointments. The nurse assessed the individual, who reported a "worsening" headache.
- The RN collaborates with the nurse practitioner who recommends an urgent in-person appointment. The re-scan is negative. Treatment management is changed and follow-up is scheduled.

Clinical Implications

- Telemedicine visit is scheduled sooner than a traditional follow-up appointment and results in earlier identification of problems.
- RN in the ambulatory care setting provides consistency in care during a vulnerable time.
- Individuals and families do not have to leave home or travel distance; increase in satisfaction and decrease in cost of care.
- Telemedicine appointment is effective in eliminating health disparity caused by distance.
- Families do not have to rearrange schedule to accommodate an in-person appointment.

This case was contributed by Melissa Reider-Demer, DNP, MN, CPNP who serves individuals and families in the Department of Neurology, University of California Los Angeles.

Case Study 13-2.
Electronic Patient Portals

A patient portal is a secure online website that gives individuals convenient access to personal health information from anywhere with an Internet connection. Using a secure username and password, health information such as recent appointments, discharge summaries, list of medications, immunizations, allergies, and lab results can be viewed (HealthIT.gov, 2017). Individuals may also engage in additional health portal activities such as send secure messages to the care team, request medication refills, schedule an appointment, or access educational resources.

Introduction

- Twenty-eight-year-old female transmits a secure message through the health portal requesting a change in her prescription.
- The medication that is identified is sertraline and she states that she is taking 50 mg and would like to take more.
- Message states, "I was told to follow-up if I didn't feel better." The message was brief and there was no additional information.

Clinical Interaction

- The RN reviews the message that was sent by the individual and reviews the problem list, medication list, and recent appointments in the health record.
- Individual was hospitalized for an injury sustained from a bike accident 1 month ago. Although her injuries resolved and she was able to return to her usual routine, she was experiencing low energy, inability to sleep, and poor appetite.
- Individual had appointment with her primary care provider 10 days ago.
- The individual's PHQ-9 score was 18, indicating moderate depression.
- Sertraline 50 mg was initiated and individual was encouraged to schedule a counseling appointment.
- The RN recognizes that interacting, assessing symptoms, and making recommendations through a health portal may not be effective, efficient, and may potentially be risky.
- The RN locates the individual's mobile phone number in her medical record and calls the individual.

Clinical Implications

- While health portals facilitate communication with an individual's care team, symptom information requires an assessment.
- In a health portal interaction, the RN cannot see or hear the individual which prevents the ability to obtain an accurate description of the situation.
- A recent diagnosis of depression and request for an increase in medication is a serious and potentially life-threatening request.
- A follow-up contact to a clinic after a diagnosis of depression has been made requires a thorough assessment and exploration of the individual's follow-through.
- The RN should assess the status of the individual and then ask if the counseling appointment was scheduled; discuss if the medication is being taken as directed; and explore other supports in the individual's life (e.g., family, friends, pets, etc.).
- The RN must consider worst possible in this situation and discuss suicidal ideation by exploring thoughts of self-harm or presence of a suicide plan.

Case Study 13-3.
Remote Patient Monitoring

Remote patient monitoring uses digital technologies to collect health data from individuals in one location and electronically transmit that information securely to health care providers in a different location for assessment and recommendations (Center for Connected Health Policy, 2018).

Introduction
- Sixty-eight-year-old male with diagnosis of congestive heart failure (CHF), chronic obstructive pulmonary disease (COPD), osteoarthritis, and mild anxiety.
- Has experienced multiple admissions for exacerbation of symptoms.
- Resides 75 miles from hospital in a rural community – limited transportation.
- Recent hospitalization; status stabilized and prescribed new medications.
- Prior to leaving the hospital, the RN provided the individual with wireless devices for remote telemontioring and automated ("smart pill") medication box; education completed.

Clinical Interaction
- The individual sends in daily or scheduled measurement of weight, blood pressure, heart rate, and single lead ECG rhythm to the RN.
- Data transmitted through telephone line or broadband connection. Two-way audio/video allows nurses, providers, and individuals to communicate.
- The RN reviews data reported by monitoring devices and contacts the individual if the data indicate the treatment plan needs to be adjusted.
- Based on predefined threshold values, an alert may be generated when a physiological measurement is out of the acceptable range, and notifies the RN to intervene with individuals.
- The automated pill box indicates whether medication is being taken as ordered.

Clinical Implications
- Remote patient monitoring is an option for managing chronic illnesses and assisting during transitions in care.
- The CCTM® RN must ensure the individual has proficiency and confidence with the equipment to obtain and transmit accurate health data.
- Individuals with CHF are an appropriate population to monitor remotely since there is a readmission rate of 25% at 30 days and nearly 50% at 6 months (Hale, Jethwani, Kandola, Saldana, & Kvedar, 2016).
- The medication dispensing device was designed to simplify the complex task of medication management with the aim of reducing medication errors and improving communication with providers (Reeder, Demiris, & Marek, 2013).

Chapter 13

References

Agency for Healthcare Research and Quality (AHRQ). (2015). *Health literacy universal precautions toolkit* (2nd ed.). Retrieved from https://www.ahrq.gov/professionals/quality-patient-safety/quality-resources/tools/literacy-toolkit/healthlittoolkit2-tool5.html

Agency for Healthcare Research and Quality (AHRQ). (2016). *Organizing measures by quality domain.* Retrieved from https://www.ahrq.gov/professionals/quality-patient-safety/talkingquality/create/organize/qualitydomain.html

Akter, S., & Ray, P. (2010). mHealth – An ultimate platform to serve the unserved. *Yearbook of Medical Informatics, 2010,* 94-100. doi:10.1055/s-0038-1638697

American Academy of Ambulatory Care Nursing (AAACN). (2016). *Scope and standards of practice for registered nurses in care coordination and transition management.* Pitman, NJ: Author.

American Academy of Ambulatory Care Nursing (AAACN). (2018). *Scope and standards of practice for professional telehealth nursing* (6th ed.). T. Anglea, C. Murray, M. Mastal, & S. Clelland (Eds.). Pitman, NJ: Author.

American Nurses Association (ANA). (2010). *Nursing's social policy statement: The essence of the profession* (3rd ed.). Silver Spring, MD: Author.

American Nurses Association (ANA). (2015). *Code of ethics for nurses.* Silver Spring, MD: Author.

Armstrong, K.A., Semple, J.L., & Coyte, P.C. (2014). Replacing ambulatory surgical follow-up visits with mobile app home monitoring: Modeling cost-effective scenarios. *Journal of Medical Internet Research, 16*(9), e213. doi:10.2196/jmir.3528

Baldwin, J.L., Singh, H., Sittig, D.F., & Giardina, T.D. (2016). Patient portals and health apps: Pitfalls, promises, and what one might learn from the other symptoms. *Health Care: The Journal of Delivery Science and Innovation, 5*(3), 81-85.

Boulos, M.N.K., Brewer, A.C., Karimkhani, C., Buller, D.B., & Dellavalle, R.P. (2014). Mobile medical and health apps: State of the art, concerns, regulatory control and certification. *Online Journal of Public Health Informatics, 5*(3), 229. doi:10.5210/ojphi.v5i3.4814

Byambasuren, O., Sanders, S., Beller, E., & Glasziou, P.G. (2018). Prescribable mHealth apps identified from an overview of systematic reviews. *npj Digital Medicine, 1,* 1-12. Retrieved from https://www.nature.com/articles/s41746-018-0021-9

Cardozo, L., & Steinberg, J. (2010). Telemedicine for recently discharged older patients. *Telemedicine and e-Health, 16(1),* 49-55. doi:10.1089/tmj.2009.0058.

Celler, B., Varnfield, M., Nepal, S., Sparks, R., Li, J., & Jayasena, R. (2017). Impact of at-home telemonitoring on health services expenditure and hospital admissions in patients with chronic conditions: Before and after control intervention analysis. *Journal of Medical Internet Research, 5*(3), e29.

Center for Connected Health Policy. (2018a). *Remote patient monitoring.* Retrieved from http://www.cchpca.org/remote-patient-monitoring-rpm

Center for Connected Health Policy. (2018b). *What is telehealth?* Retrieved from http://www.cchpca.org/about/about-telehealth

Connolly, K.K., & Crosby, M.E. (2014). Examining e-Health literacy and the digital divide in an underserved population in Hawai'i. *Hawai'i Journal of Medicine & Public Health, 73*(2), 44-48.

Cronenwett, L., Sherwood, G., Barnsteiner, J., Disch, J., Johnson, J., Mitchell, P., ... Warren, J. (2007). Quality and safety education for nurses. *Nursing Outlook, 55*(4), 122-131. doi:1016/j.outlook.2007.02.006

Cronenwett, L., Sherwood, G., Pohl, J., Barnsteiner, J., Moore, S., Sullivan, D.T., ... Warren, J. (2009). Quality and safety education for advanced nursing practice. *Nursing Outlook, 57*(6), 338-348.

Darkins, A., Ryan, P. Kobb, R., Foster, L. Edmonson, E. Wakefield, B., & Lancaster, A.E. (2008). Care coordination/home telehealth: The systematic implementation of health informatics, home telehealth, and disease management to support the care of veteran patients with chronic conditions. *Telemedicine and eHEALTH,14*(10), 1118-1126. doi:10.1089/tmj.2008.0021 1118-1127

Deshpande, A., Khoja, S., Lorca, J., McKibbon, A., Rizo, C., Husereau, D., & Jadad, A.R. (2009). Asynchronous telehealth: A scoping review of analytic studies. *Open Medicine, 3*(2), e69-e91.

Espensen, M. (Ed.). (2009). *Telehealth nursing practice essentials.* Pitman, NJ: American Academy of Ambulatory Care Nursing.

Edge, P. (2016). Using health information technology to improve patient engagement. *HIT Perspectives.* Retrieved from https://www.pocp.com/hit-perspectives-health-information-technology/

Gell, N.M., Rosenberg, D.E., Demiris, G., LaCroix, A.Z., & Patel, K.V. (2015). Patterns of technology use among older adults with and without disabilities. *The Gerontologist, 55*(3), 412-421. doi:10.1093/geront/gnt166

Glavind, K., Bjørk, J., Lindquist, A.S. (2014). A retrospective study on telephone follow-up of anterior colporrhaphy by a specialized nurse. *The International Urogynecology Journal, 25*(12),1693-1697.

Gordon, A.S., Adamson, W.C., & DeVries, A.R. (2017). Virtual visits for acute, nonurgent care: A claims analysis of episode-level utilization. *Journal of Medical Internet Research, 19*(2), e35. doi:10.2196/jmir.6783

Graham, J., Tomcavage, J., Salek, D., Sciandra, J., Davis, D.E., & Stewart, W.F. (2012). Post-discharge monitoring using interactive voice response system reduces 30-day readmission rates in a case-managed Medicare population. *Medical Care, 50*(1), 50-57.

Greenberg, M.E., Espensen, M., Becker, C., & Cartwright, J. (2003). Telehealth nursing practice special interest group adopts teleterms. *ViewPoint, 25*(1), 8-10.

Greenberg, M.E., Rutenberg, C. & Scheidt, K.B. (2014). Telehealth nursing practice. In S.A. Haas, B.A. Swan, & T.S. Haynes (Eds.), *Care coordination and transition management* (175-188). Pitman, NJ: American Academy of Ambulatory Care Nursing.

Grundy, Q., Held, F., & Bero, L. (2017). A social network analysis of the financial links backing health and fitness apps. *American Journal of Public Health, 107*(11), 1783-1788. doi:10.2105/AJPH.2017.303995

GSMA Intelligence. (2018). *Definitive data and analysis for the mobile industry.* Retrieved from https://www.gsmaintelligence.com/

Hale, T.M., Jethwani, K., M.S., Sadana, F., & Kvedar, J.C. (2016). A remote medication monitoring system for chronic heart failure patients to reduce readmissions: A two-arm randomized pilot study. *Journal of Medical Internet Research, 18*(5), e91. doi:10.2196/jmir.5256

Hall, J.L., & McGraw, D. (2014). For telehealth to succeed, privacy and security risks must be identified and addressed. *Health Affairs (Millwood), 33*(2), 216-221. doi:10.1377/hlthaff.2013.0997

Hardman, S., & Steinberger-Wilckens, R. (2014). Mobile phone infrastructure development: Lessons for the development of a hydrogen infrastructure. *Science Direct, 39*(16), 8185-8193. doi:10.1016/j.ijhydene.2014.03.156

HealthIT.gov. (2017). *What is a patient portal?* Retrieved from https://www.healthit.gov/faq/what-patient-portal

Health Resources & Services Administration. (2018). *Telehealth programs.* Retrieved from https://www.hrsa.gov/rural-health/telehealth/index.html

Husebo, A.M.L., & Storm, M. (2014). Virtual visits in home health care for older adults. *The Scientific World Journal, 2014,* 1-11, doi:10.1155/2014/689873

International Council of Nurses (ICN). (2007). *International competencies for telenursing.* Geneva, Switzerland: Author.

Kottek, A., Stafford, Z., & Spetz, J. (2017). *Remote monitoring technologies in long-term care: Implications for care team organization and training.* Retrieved from https://healthworkforce.ucsf.edu/sites/healthworkforce.ucsf.edu/files/REPORT_FINAL_RemoteMonitoring.pdf

Kvedar, J., Caye, M.J,. & Everett, W. (2014). Connected health: A review of technologies and strategies to improve patient care with telemedicine and telehealth. *Health Affairs, 33*(2), 194-199. doi:10.1377/hlthaff.2013.0992

Lachman, V.D. (2010). Strategies necessary for moral courage. *OJIN: The Online Journal of Issues in Nursing 15*(3). doi:10.3912/OJIN.Vol15No03Man03

Landi, H. (2017). VA issues proposed rule to allow home-based telemedicine for veterans. *Health Informatics.* Retrieved from https://www.healthcare-informatics.com/news-item/telemedicine/va-issues-proposed-rule-allow-home-based-telemedicine-veterans

Laughlin, C.B. (2018). *Core curriculum for ambulatory care nursing* (4th ed.). Pitman, NJ: American Academy of Ambulatory Care Nursing.

Mackert, M., Mabry-Flynn, A., Champlin, S., Donovan, E.E., & Pounders, K. (2016). Health literacy and health information technology adoption: The potential for a new digital divide. *Journal of Medical Internet Research, 18*(10), e264. doi:10.2196/jmir.6349

Madigan, E., Schmotzer, B.J., Struk, C.J., DiCarlo, C.M., Kikano, G., Piña, I.L., & Boxer, R.S. (2013). Home health care with telemonitoring improves health status for older adults with heart failure. *Home Health Care Services Quarterly, 32*(1), 57-74. http://doi.org/10.1080/01621424.2012.755144

Matthew-Maich, N., Harris, L., Ploeg, J., Markle-Reid, M., Valaitis, R., Ibrahim, S., ... Isaacs, S. (2016). Designing, implementing, and evaluating mobile health technologies for managing chronic conditions in older adults: A scoping review. *JMIR mHealth and uHealth, 4*(2), e29. doi:10.2196/mhealth.5127

Mendu, M.L., & Waikar, S.S. (2015). Electronic health record patient portals in CKD and hypertension management: Meaningfully used? *Clinical Journal of the American Society of Nephrology, 10*(11), 1897-1899. doi:10.2215/CJN.10070915

Migration Policy Institute. (2016). *Language diversity and English proficiency in the United States.* Retrieved from https://www.migrationpolicy.org/article/language-diversity-and-english-proficiency-united-states

Milani, R.V., & Lavie C.J. (2015). Health care 2020: Reengineering health care delivery to combat chronic disease. *American Journal of Medicine, 128*(4), 337- 343. doi:10.1016/j.amjmed.2014.10.047

Nagel. D.A., & Penner, J.L. (2016). Conceptualizing telehealth in nursing practice: Advancing a conceptual model to fill a virtual gap. *Journal of Holistic Nursing, 34*(1), 91-104. doi:10.1177/0898010115580236

National Council of State Boards of Nursing. (n.d.). *Licensure compacts.* Retrieved from https://www.ncsbn.org/compacts.htm

National Institute on Deafness and Other Communication Disorders. (2016). *Quick statistics about hearing.* Retrieved from https://www.nidcd.nih.gov/health/statistics/quick-statistics-hearing

National Institutes of Health. (2016). *Visual impairment, blindness cases in U.S. expected to double by 2050.* Retrieved from https://www.nih.gov/news-events/news-releases/visual-impairment-blindness-cases-us-expected-double-2050

Naylor, M.D. (2011). Viewpoint: Interprofessional collaboration and the future of health care. *American Nurse Today, 6*(6). Retrieved from https://www.americannursetoday.com/viewpoint-interprofessional-collaboration-and-the-future-of-health-care/

Noah, B., Keller, M.S., Mosadeghi, S., Stein, L., Johl, S., Delshad, S., ... Spiegel, B.M. (2018). Impact of remote patient monitoring on clinical outcomes: An updated meta-analysis of randomized controlled trials. *npj Digital Medicine.* Retrieved from https://www.nature.com/articles/s41746-018-0027-3

Occupational Safety and Health Administration. (n.d.). *Computer workstations eTool.* Retrieved from https://www.osha.gov/SLTC/etools/computerworkstations/comnents.html

Ozdalga, E., Ozdalga, A., & Ahuja, N. (2012). The smartphone in medicine: A review of current and potential use among physicians and students. *Journal of Medical Internet Research, 14*(5), e128. doi:10.2196/jmir.1994

Paré, G., Jaana, M., & Sicotte, C. (2007). Systematic review of home telemonitoring for chronic diseases: The evidence base. *Journal of the American Medical Informatics Association, 14*(3), 269-277. doi:10.1197/jamia.M2270

Pew Research Center. (2018). *Mobile fact sheet.* Retrieved from http://www.pewinternet.org/fact-sheet/mobile/

Reeder, B., Demiris, G., & Marek, K.D. (2013). Older adults' satisfaction with a medication dispensing device in home care. *Informatics for Health & Social Care, 38*(3), 211-222. doi:10.3109/17538157.2012.741084

Reider-Demer, M., Raja, P., Martin, N. Schwinger, M., & Babayan, D. (2017). Prospective and retrospective study of videoconference telemedicine follow-up after elective neurosurgery: Results of a pilot program. *Neurosurgical Review, 41*(2), 497-501. doi:10.1007/s10143-017-0878-0

Rigby, M., Georgiou, A., Hyppönen, H., Ammenwerth, E., de Keizer, N., Magrabi, F., & Scott, P. (2015). Patient portals as a means of information and communication technology support to patient-centric care coordination – the missing evidence and the challenges of evaluation: A joint contribution of IMIA WG EVAL and EFMI WG EVAL. *Yearbook of Medical Informatics, 10*(1), 148-159. doi:10.15265/IY-2015-007

Rouleau, G., Gagnon, M.P., Côté, J., Payne-Gagnon, J., Hudson, E., & Dubois, C.A. (2017). Impact of information and communication technologies on nursing care: Results of an overview of systematic reviews. *Journal of Medical Internet Research, 19*(4), e122. doi:10.2196/jmir.6686

Rutenberg, C., & Greenberg, M.E. (2012). *The art and science of telephone triage: How to practice nursing over the phone.* Hot Springs, AR: Telephone Triage Consulting, Inc.

Safeer, R.S., & Keenan, J. (2005). Health literacy: The gap between physicians and patients. *American Family Physician, 72*(3), 463-468.

Saner, H., & Van der Velde, E. (2016). eHealth in cardiovascular medicine: A clinical update. *European Journal of Preventive Cardiology, 23*(25), 5-12. doi:10.1177/2047487316670256

Schlachta-Fairchild, L., Elfrink, V., & Deickman, A. (2008). Patient safety, telenursing, and telehealth. In R.G. Hughes (Ed.), *Patient safety and quality: An evidence-based handbook for nurses.* Rockville, MD: Agency for Healthcare Research and Quality.

Schyve, P.M. (2007). Language differences as a barrier to quality and safety in health care: The Joint Commission perspective. *Journal of General Internal Medicine, 22*(Suppl. 2), 360-361. doi:10.1007/s11606-007-0365-3

Squires, A. (2018). Strategies for overcoming language barriers in healthcare. *Nursing Management, 49*(4), 21-26.

The Joint Commission. (2017). *Facts about patient-centered communications.* Retrieved from https://www.jointcommission.org/facts_about_patient-centered_communications/

United States Census Bureau. (2015). *Census Bureau reports at least 350 languages spoken in U.S. homes.* Retrieved from https://www.census.gov/newsroom/press-releases/2015/cb15-185.html

U.S. Department of Health and Human Services. (2013). *Summary of the HIPAA security rule.* Retrieved from https://www.hhs.gov/hipaa/for-professionals/security/laws-regulations/index.html

U.S. Department of Veterans Affairs (VA). (2018). *VA expands telehealth by allowing health care providers to treat patients across state lines.* Retrieved from https://www.va.gov/opa/pressrel/pressrelease.cfm?id=4054

U.S. Food and Drug Administration (FDA). (2018). *Mobile medical applications.* Retrieved from https://www.fda.gov/medicaldevices/digitalhealth/mobilemedicalapplications/default.htm

Ventola, C.L. (2014). Mobile devices and apps for health care professionals: Uses and benefits. *Pharmacy and Therapeutics, 39*(5), 356-364.

Wicklund, E. (2018). VA puts telehealth to work in 'anywhere to anywhere' care initiative. *mHealthIntelligence.* Retrieved from https://mhealthintelligence.com/news/va-puts-telehealth-to-work-in-anywhere-to-anywhere-care-initiative

Wilson, L.S., & Maeder, A.J. (2015). Recent directions in telemedicine: Review of trends in research and practice. *Healthcare Informatics Research, 21*(4), 213-222. doi:10.4258/hir.2015.21.4.213

Glossary

5 A's Behavior Change Model Adapted for Self-Management Support Improvement – An interactive closed-loop model for implementing self-management strategies.

Abandonment – Relationship between individual and health care provider is terminated abruptly and without individual's consent; provider disregards legal and ethical obligations to facilitate continuity of care and to avoid harm caused by prematurely terminating the relationship.

Accessibility of Care – Refers to the ease with which consumers can initiate interaction with a clinician about health problems; includes activities to eliminate barriers raised by geography, financing, culture, race, language, etc.

Accountable Care Organization (ACO) – Groups of doctors, hospitals, and other health care providers who come together voluntarily to provide high-quality, coordinated care for Medicare individuals, avoiding unnecessary or duplicative care.

Accreditation – A process in which an authoritative body formally recognizes an organization or a person is competent to carry out specific tasks.

Accreditation Association for Ambulatory Health Care (AAAHC) – A private, non-profit agency that offers voluntary, peer-based review of the quality of health care services of ambulatory care health organizations, including ambulatory care and office-based surgery centers, managed care organizations, Federally Qualified Community Health Centers, and diagnostic imaging centers, among others.

Active Listening – A way of listening and responding to another person that improves mutual understanding. Active listening skills are conversational techniques that enable better understanding and more productive communication.

Acute Care Nursing – Nursing care of individuals typically in a hospital setting who are receiving treatment for illness, accident, trauma, or surgical procedure, with the goal of promoting, restoring, or maintaining optimal health.

Addiction – A condition in which a person engages in the use of a substance or in a behavior for which the rewarding effects provide a compelling incentive to repeatedly pursue the behavior despite detrimental consequences; and may involve the use of substances such as alcohol, inhalants, opioids, cocaine, nicotine, and others, or behaviors such as gambling.

Advance Care Planning (ACP) – A process of planning for an individual's future through discussion of goals, values, and beliefs, and how they influence end-of-life care preferences and completion of appropriate documents.

Advance Directives – Allow competent adults to make certain kinds of health care decisions in advance of an acute (such as a car accident) or chronic (such as dementia or stroke) incapacity, thus ensuring their wishes are respected even if they are unable to communicate them directly; two types are living wills and durable power of attorney for health care.

Advocacy – Act or process of advocating or supporting (a cause or proposal) on behalf of another.

Agency for Healthcare Research and Quality (AHRQ) – The lead federal agency charged with improving the safety and quality of America's health care system. AHRQ develops the knowledge, tools, and data needed to improve the health care system and help Americans, health care professionals, and policymakers make informed health decisions and health care safer, and improve quality.

Algorithm – A step-by-step procedure that is explicit and in a logical order to achieve a specific result.

Ambulatory Care – Outpatient care in which patients generally stay less than 24 hours and are discharged to their normal residential situation after care.

Ambulatory Care Nursing – A unique domain of specialty nursing practice that focuses on individuals, families, groups, communities, and populations in primary and specialty care, virtual encounters, and non-acute outpatient settings.

Ambulatory Patient Classifications (APCs) – Used by the Centers for Medicare & Medicaid Services for prospective payment in hospital outpatient departments and ambulatory surgery centers; based on procedures and adjusted for severity.

Ambulatory Patient Groups (APGs) – Patient classification system designed to explain amount and type of resource used in ambulatory care visit.

Glossary

American Academy of Ambulatory Care Nursing (AAACN) – The nursing professional organization that promotes leadership, collaboration, and innovation in ventures that advance the delivery of nursing and health care services in ambulatory care settings through professional clinical, educational, research, and health policy initiatives.

Americans with Disabilities Act (ADA) – Provides equal opportunity rights to disabled citizens in employment, access to state and local government agencies, public accommodations, transportation, and telecommunications; defines a disabled person as someone who has a substantial physical or mental impairment that significantly limits a major life activity.

Autonomy – The right to self-determine or freedom to choose one's course of action; support of independent decision-making.

Balanced Scorecard – Graphic or pictorial display of the organization's indicators chosen to support the strategic plan and vision of the organization; allows for examination of relationships among the separate indicators (care, quality, financial, operational, etc.).

Benchmarking – A continuous quality improvement process of comparing processes, strategies, and/or outcomes to those of the toughest competitor, to those considered industry leaders, or to similar activities in the organization, and using the information to change/improve practices, resulting in superior performance as determined by measured outcomes.

Beneficence – An act of charity, mercy, and kindness, with a strong connotation of doing good to others, including moral obligation. All professionals have the foundational moral imperative of doing right. Doing good requires defining what is meant by "good" in the situation. It is a concept in research ethics that states researchers should have the welfare of the research participant as a goal of any clinical trial or other research study. The antonym of this term, maleficence, describes a practice that opposes the welfare of any research participant.

Better Outcomes by Optimizing Safe Transitions (BOOST) – A national initiative led by the Society of Hospital Medicine to improve the care of individuals as they transition from hospital to home. Project BOOST has developed tools to assist in transitions.

Big Data – Refers to datasets that are large in volume, high in velocity, complex, variable, and diverse, requiring advanced techniques and technologies to enable the capture, storage, distribution, management, and analysis of the information.

Bundled Payments – A method in which payments to health care providers are based on the expected costs for a clinically defined episode or bundle of related health care services.

CAGE-AID – A questionnaire that focuses on both drug and alcohol abuse.

Capitation – Method for funding expenses of enrollees in prepaid health plans; pays providers a fixed fee per member regardless of services used. For example, a plan pays a per member per month (PMPM) amount to a physician group to provide primary care services for each enrollee in the plan.

Care Coordination –
1. Agency for Healthcare Research and Quality (AHRQ) definition: "Care coordination is the deliberate organization of patient care activities between two or more participants (including the patient) involved in a patient's care to facilitate the appropriate delivery of health care services. Organizing care involves the marshaling of personnel and other resources needed to carry out all required patient care activities and is often managed by the exchange of information among participants responsible for different aspects of care" (McDonald et al., 2007; McDonald et al., 2011, p. 4).
2. National Quality Forum (NQF) (2010) definition: "Care coordination is defined as an information-rich, patient-centric endeavor that seeks to deliver the right care (and only the right care) to the right patient at the right time… A function that helps ensure that the patient's needs and preferences for health services and information sharing across people, functions, and sites are met over time… Care coordination maximizes the value of services delivered to patients by facilitating beneficial efficient, safe, and high-quality patient experiences and improved health care outcomes" (p. 2).
3. NQF (2016) updated definition: Care coordination is "the deliberate synchronization of activities and information to improve health outcomes by ensuring that care recipients' and families' needs and preferences for health care and community services are met over time" (p. 13).

Glossary

Care Coordination Transition Management Registered Nurse (CCTM® RN) Model – Standardizes work of all Registered Nurses using evidence from nursing and interprofessional literature on care coordination and transition management.

Care Transitions – "The movement patients make between health care practitioners and settings as their condition and care needs change during the course of a chronic or acute illness. For example, in the course of an acute exacerbation of an illness, a patient might receive care from a primary care physician or specialist in an outpatient setting, then transition to a hospital physician and nursing team during an inpatient admission before moving on to yet another care team at a skilled nursing facility. Finally, the patient might return home, where he or she would receive care from a visiting nurse. Each of these shifts from care providers and settings is defined as a care transition" (Coleman & Boult, 2003, p. 556).

Case Management – A collaborative process that assesses, plans, implements, coordinates, monitors, and evaluates the options and services required to meet the client's health and human service needs. It is characterized by advocacy, communication, and resource management, and promotes quality and cost-effective interventions and outcomes (Commission for Case Manager Certification, 2018).

Centers for Disease Control and Prevention (CDC) – The nation's health protection agency, working 24/7 to protect from health and safety threats, both foreign and domestic.

Centers for Medicare & Medicaid Services (CMS) – Formerly Health Care Financing Administration (HCFA); division within the U.S. Department of Health and Human Services that determines the standard rules and reporting mechanisms for health care services.

CMS Meaningful Measures Framework – Quality measurement of the highest core issues most valuable to high quality care and better outcomes.

Certification – Process that uses predetermined standards to validate and recognize an individual's knowledge, skills, and abilities in a defined functional and clinical area of specialty practice approved by the American Nurses Association as an area of specialty practice.

Chronic Pain – Pain that lasts beyond the expected healing time, usually greater than 3 months; can be constant or intermittent, and is often subcategorized as associated with or without a terminal disease.

Clinical Care Classification (CCC) – Formerly Home Health Care Classification (HHCC); Saba's Georgetown System for Patient Problems, Interventions, and Outcomes.

Clinical Data Registries (CDRs) – Databases with medical information about immunizations, screenings, chronic disease prevalence, or disease-specific lab results for a panel of patients/individual patients of a physician, provider, or practice.

Clinical Decision Support System (CDSS) – Provides clinicians with intelligently filtered information at appropriate times to foster better processes, better individual patient care, and better population health.

Clinical Practice Guidelines – Statements that have been systematically developed based on evidence to assist practitioners and individuals in making decisions about appropriate health care for specific clinical circumstances.

Cognitive Impairment – Failing of short- and long-term recall and general thinking logic skills.

Collaboration – Working together toward a common goal; to pursue a common purpose and a sharing of knowledge to resolve problems, decide issues, and set goals within a structure of collegiality.

Commercial Indemnity Plans – A type of insurance contract in which the insurer pays for care received up to a fixed amount per encounter or episode of illness.

Competence – Having the ability to demonstrate the knowledge, technical and critical thinking, and interpersonal skills necessary to perform one's job responsibilities.

Competency – An expected level of performance that integrates knowledge, skills, abilities, and judgment.

Complementary, Alternative, and Integrative Therapies (CAM) – Care that includes nontraditional therapies either in place of or together with conventional medicine.

Glossary

Comprehensive Geriatric Assessment (CGA) – A multidisciplinary diagnostic and treatment process that identifies medical, psychosocial, and functional limitation of a frail older person to develop a coordinated plan to maximize overall health with aging.

Confidentiality – To protect the individual's and family's right to privacy regarding information the nurse or institution holds about the individual.

Confusion – Disorientation, inappropriate behavior or communication, and/or hallucinations.

Co-Payment – Out-of-pocket expense paid by an individual for a specific service defined in the insurance plan each time a health service is used.

Core Competencies for Nursing – A standard set of performance "domains" in which it is necessary to demonstrate proficiency to enter into professional practice.

Cost Benefit Analysis – A formal financial analysis completed by organizations to determine the cost of a program and projected revenues, and to identify and quantify program benefits; includes assumptions about specific expenses and projected revenue. Often part of evaluating the feasibility of a new program or service.

CPT – The Physicians' Current Procedural Terminology, published by the American Medical Association; the internationally recognized coding system for reporting medical services and procedures.

Credentialing – Review and verification of credentials (i.e., education, training, licensure, certification, experience). Most states required a criminal background check prior to granting licensure.

Critical Thinking – A deliberate nonlinear process of collecting, interpreting, analyzing, drawing conclusions about, presenting, and evaluating information that is both factually and belief-based. This is demonstrated in nursing by clinical judgment, which includes ethical, diagnostic, and therapeutic dimensions and research.

Cultural Competence – Requires developing cultural awareness (conscious learning process through which one becomes appreciative and sensitive to the cultures of other people), cultural knowledge (process of understanding the key aspects of a group's culture), cultural skills (ability to collect relevant data regarding health histories and perform culturally specific assessments), and cultural encounters (process that encourages one to engage directly in cross-cultural interactions with people from culturally diverse backgrounds).

Cultural Safety – Providing culturally safe care requires the nurse to be respectful of nationality, culture, age, sex, and political and religious beliefs.

Decision Support System (Clinical Decision Support) – Automated tool that enhances the nurse's ability to make decisions in semi-structured, uncertain situations by bringing necessary information, evidence, expertise, and resources to the point of care.

Deductible – Amount an insured individual is responsible to pay before insurance covers costs. For example, an individual may have to pay a $200 deductible for hospitalization before the remainder of the hospital stay is covered by insurance.

Delegation – The transfer of responsibility for the performance of a task from one person to another.

Dementia – An umbrella term that covers several chronic, progressive brain disorders caused by brain disease or injury; all types of dementia can include symptoms of memory disorders, personality changes, impaired reasoning, and difficulty with language and motor function.

Deontology – Also known as duty-based ethics; based on the belief there are duties to which one must be faithful and which one is obligated to carry out because these duties are owed to all human beings and because of the expectations implied by one's professional role.

Depression (Major) – Possessing five or more symptoms of depression (e.g., insomnia, fatigue, weight loss or gain, low self-esteem, sudden bursts of anger, excessive sleeping).

Diagnosis-Related Groups (DRGs) – A system for classifying hospital inpatients into groups requiring similar quantities of resources according to characteristics, such as diagnosis, age, procedure, complications, and co-morbidities.

Glossary

Distance Learning – Provides access to learning modalities initially designed to reach/include persons in rural/isolated areas, providing educational opportunities/resources.

Domain of Ambulatory Nursing Practice – The overall scope of nursing practice in the ambulatory arena; it includes attributes of the environment in which practice occurs, individual requirements for care, and specific nursing role dimensions.

Drug Abuse Screening Test (DAST) – A 20- or 28-item self-report scale for abuse of drugs other than alcohol.

Education Process – Systematic planned course of action consisting of two major interdependent operations: teaching and learning.

Electronic Health Record (EHR) – A secure, real-time, point-of-care, person-centric information resource for clinicians. Longitudinal electronic record of an individual's health information and can include one or more encounters across multiple health settings.

Electronic Nicotine Delivery System (ENDS) – Also known as e-cigarettes, personal vaporizers, vape pens, e-cigars, e-hookah, or vaping devices that produce an aerosolized mixture containing flavored liquids and nicotine and inhaled by the user.

Emergency Medical Treatment and Active Labor Act (EMTALA) – Federal law passed in 1986 to ensure an individual's access to emergency services regardless of ability to pay.

Emotional Intelligence – Ability to accurately perceive one's own and others' emotions, to understand the signals that emotions send about the relationship, and influence emotional states of the people they lead.

Engagement in Health Care – Actions individuals must take to obtain the greatest benefit from the health care services available to them.

Enhanced Nursing Licensure Compact (eNLC) – Allows nurses (RNs and LPNs/VNs) to have one compact license in the nurse's primary state of residence (home state) and allows practice (physically, telephonically/electronically) in other compact states unless the nurse is under discipline or restricted license.

Environmental Management – The assurance of appropriate management plans to provide a safe, accessible, effective, and functional environment of care.

Equal Employment Opportunity Commission (EEOC) – A federal agency that issues and enforces regulations concerning equal opportunity and non-discrimination in the workplace.

Ethics – A branch of philosophy dealing with values related to human conduct, with respect to the rightness or wrongness of certain actions, and to the goodness and badness of the motives and ends of such actions; a set of moral principles or values, the principles of conduct governing an individual or a group.

Evidence-Based Practice – "The conscientious and judicious use of current best evidence in conjunction with clinical expertise and patient values to guide health care decisions" (Titler, 2008).

Existential Distress – Suffering that arises from a sense of meaningless, hopelessness, fear, and regret in individuals who are knowingly approaching the end of life.

Fee for Service – Reimbursement method in which payment is made for each service or item.

Fidelity – Faithfulness; involves duty owed to patients, families, and colleagues to do what one says.

Fixed Costs – Costs do not change with volume of service units or activity, such as patient visits.

Generalized Anxiety Scale (GAD-7) – A self-reported questionnaire for screening and severity measuring of generalized anxiety disorder (GAD).

Geriatric Resources for Assessment and Care of Elders (GRACE) – A team-developed care plan to improve the quality of geriatric care and optimize health and functional status, decrease excess health care use, and prevent long-term nursing home placement.

Get Up and Go Test – A timed test for measurement of mobility. It includes a number of tasks, such as standing from a seated position, walking, turning, stopping, and sitting down.

Grief – The individualized feelings and responses that a person makes to real, perceived, or anticipated loss.

Glossary

Health Care Financing Administration (HCFA) – See Centers for Medicare & Medicaid Services (CMS).

Health Care Financing Administration (HCFA) Common Procedure Coding System (HCPCS) – A uniform method for health care providers and medical suppliers to report professional services, procedures, and supplies to health care plans.

Health Care Reform – As described by the Patient Protection and Affordable Care Act (PPACA) of 2010, introduces changes related to health insurance coverage, access to services, quality of care, costs of health care, and overall population health.

Health Care Team – Includes the individual, family, and other members of the health care system who are involved in the development and implementation of the care plan.

Health Coaching – A practice that educates individuals while promoting self-management of individualized health goals.

Health Education – Any combination of planned learning experiences based on sound theories that provide individuals, groups, and communities the opportunity to acquire the information and skills needed to make quality health decisions.

Health Informatics – The interprofessional study of the design, development, adoption, and application of IT-based innovations in health care services, delivery, management, and planning.

Health Information Exchange (HIE) – The transmission of health care-related data among facilities, health information organizations (HIOs), and government agencies according to national standards. HIE is an integral component of the health information technology (HIT) infrastructure under development in the United States and the associated National Health Information Network (NHIN).

Health Information Technology (HIT) – The application of computers and technology to the provision of health care in all settings, including all stakeholders involved in health.

Health Insurance Portability and Accountability Act (HIPAA) – Federal law that establishes a "floor" for privacy protection and implementing privacy and security regulations; applies to all health plans, health care clearinghouses, and those health care providers (including nurses) who bill electronically for their services; provides that individuals have a right to control their information and must "authorize" use or disclosure of their health information.

Health Literacy – Capacity to obtain, process, and understand basic information and services needed to make appropriate decisions regarding health.

Health Maintenance Organization (HMO) – A health plan that uses physicians as gatekeepers. In this model, the individual chooses a primary care provider (PCP) who is responsible for all aspects of care management and who must authorize (gatekeeper) or give permission for referral to other providers; an organized system that accepts responsibility to provide or deliver an agreed-upon set of basic and supplemental health maintenance and treatment services to an enrolled group of persons. The group is reimbursed through a predetermined fixed periodic prepayment made by or on behalf of each person or family unit enrolled.

Healthcare Effectiveness and Data Information Set® (HEDIS®) – A set of standardized performance measures designed to assure purchasers and consumers have the information they need to reliably compare the performance of health plans; sponsored and maintained by the National Committee for Quality Assurance (NCQA).

Healthy People 2020 – Federal government's health care improvement priorities managed by federal agencies; provides measurable objectives applicable at national, state, and local levels; increases public awareness and understanding of determinants of health.

Healthy People 2030 - The fifth edition of Healthy People, which is a national effort that sets goals and objectives to improve the health and well-being of people in the United States; aims at new challenges and builds on lessons learned from its first four decades.

Hospice – Comprehensive, noncurative services are provided to a terminally ill individual and his/her family by an interprofessional team (including physicians, nurses, social workers, chaplains, counselors, certified nursing assistants, therapists, and volunteers) wherever the individual is.

Glossary

ICD-10-CM (*International Classification of Diseases*, 10th Edition, Clinical Modification Procedure Coding System) – Classification system that is the international standard for reporting diseases and conditions for all clinical and research purposes.

Independent Practice Association (IPA) – A legal entity whose members are independent physicians who contract with the IPA for the purpose of having the IPA contract with one or more HMOs.

Index of Independence in Activities of Daily Living (IADL) – An instrument used in assessing functional status when measuring a person's ability to perform activities of daily living independently.

Informatics – Use and support the use of information and technology to communicate, manage knowledge, mitigate error, and support decision-making.

Informed Consent – Process by which a person is provided relevant information about a proposed procedure, test, or course of treatment; given an opportunity to ask questions; and asked to voluntarily agree.

Institute of Medicine (IOM) – An independent, nonprofit organization that works to provide unbiased and authoritative advice to decision-makers and the public to improve health.

Interprofessional Team – A group of individuals from different disciplines working and communicating with each other, providing his/her knowledge, skills, and attitudes to augment and support the contributions of others.

Interstate Compacts – See *Enhanced Nursing Licensure Compact (eNLC)*.

I-SMART Goals – Adds "I" for Important to the SMART Goals acronym.

The Joint Commission (TJC) (formerly The Joint Commission on Accreditation of Healthcare Organizations [JCAHO]) – An independent, not-for-profit organization that accredits and certifies 21,000 U.S. health care organizations and programs in a variety of settings, including ambulatory care organizations.

Justice – Fair, equitable distribution of resources.

Logic Model – A tool used to clarify and graphically display; most often used by managers and evaluators of programs to evaluate the effectiveness of a program.

Magnet Recognition Program® – American Nurses Credentialing Center's program to recognize health care organizations that provide the very best in nursing care and uphold the tradition within professional nursing practice.

Managed Care – A system that combines financing and care delivery through comprehensive benefits delivered by selected providers and financial incentives for enrolled members to use these providers; goals of managed care are quality, cost-effectiveness, and accessible health care. It is a coordinated system of health care, which achieves outcomes (reduced utilization and improved population health) through preventive care, case management, and the provision of medically necessary and appropriate care.

Meaningful Use (MU) – In a health information technology (HIT) context, it is the use of electronic health records (EHRs) and related technology within a health care organization.

Medicaid – A plan jointly funded by federal and state governments introduced in 1966 to cover low-income individuals; it is managed by each state.

mHealth – Mobile communication-based health care using portable devices capable of storing, retrieving, and transmitting data in real time between end users for the purpose of improving patient safety and quality of care.

Mini Cog – An assessment tool to determine the mental status of older adults and identify individuals in need of further evaluation by a neurologist.

Mini-Mental State Examination (MMSE) – A brief 30-point questionnaire used to screen for cognitive impairment.

Mobile Application – Most commonly referred to as an app; is a type of application software designed to run on a mobile device, such as a smartphone or tablet computer.

Modified Caregiver Strain Index – A 13-question tool that measures strain related to care provision.

Glossary

Modified LACE – An assessment tool that incorporates **L**ength of stay, **A**cuity of admission, **C**o-morbidity, and **E**mergency department visits to identify individuals with a high-predicted risk for readmission or death.

Montreal Cognitive Assessment (MoCA) – A cognitive screening test designed to assist health professionals in detecting mild cognitive impairment.

Motivational Interviewing (MI) – Method of guiding individuals to explore their own health behaviors and to strengthen their motivation to change; a skillful clinical communication style for eliciting from individuals their own motivations for making behavior changes in the interest of their health.

Mourning – The outward social expression or public display of loss/grief; often dictated by cultural norms, customs, and practices, including religious customs, rituals, and traditions surrounding death; is also influenced by the individual's personality and life experiences; the process of adapting to life after a loss.

MyChart – A tool that provides individuals with secure access to their medical record in an online and app format.

MyHealthEData Initiative – Strengthens interoperability or the sharing of health care data between providers and consumers, and allows consumers to select health care services that best meet their needs, improve their understanding of their overall health, and make more informed decisions about their personal care.

National Committee for Quality Assurance (NCQA) – An independent, nonprofit organization that assesses, evaluates, and publicly reports on the quality of health plans, health care provider groups, and individual physicians.

National Database of Nursing Quality Indicators (NDNQI) – A repository for nursing-sensitive indicators; contains data collected at the nursing unit level to make informed staffing decisions and improve a person's care and outcomes.

National Patient Safety Goals (NPSGs) – The Joint Commission's series of specific actions that accredited organizations are required to meet with the purpose of preventing medical errors and improving processes for patient safety.

Negligence – A duty of care owed to the individual is breached, with a reasonable direct relationship to the patient suffering damages.

Nonmaleficence – Acting in such a way that avoids harm, either intentional harm or harm as an unintended outcome.

Nurse Practice Act (NPA) – The state's duty to protect those who receive nursing care is the basis for a nursing license. Safe, competent nursing practice is grounded in the law as written in the state NPA and state rules/regulations. Together, the NPA and rules/regulations guide and govern nursing practice.

Nurse-Sensitive Indicators (NSIs) – Measures and indicators that reflect the structure, processes and outcomes of nursing care (American Nurses Association, 2004). These measures reflect the impact of nursing care.

Nursing – The protection, promotion, and optimization of health and abilities; prevention of illness and injury; alleviation of suffering through the diagnosis and treatment of human response; and advocacy in the care of individuals, families, communities, and populations.

Nursing Code of Ethics – A guide for carrying out nursing responsibilities in a manner consistent with quality in nursing care; an expression of nursing's own understanding of its commitment to society; the ethical obligations and duties of every individual who enters the nursing profession.

Nursing Diagnosis – A clinical judgment about individual, family, or community experiences/responses to actual or potential health problems/life processes. NANDA-I nursing diagnoses are the most evidence-based and comprehensive.

Nursing Informatics – A specialty that integrates nursing science, computer science, and information science to manage and communicate data, information, and knowledge in nursing practice.

Nursing Informatics Competency – Adequate knowledge, skills, and abilities to perform specific informatics tasks.

Nursing Interventions Classification (NIC) – Taxonomy for classifying nursing interventions; used in all settings where care is delivered to document nursing interventions; developed by a team at University of Iowa, led by McCloskey and Bulechek.

Glossary

Nursing Minimum Data Set (NMDS) – A concept developed to ensure all data important to nursing were collected in a standardized manner in every encounter, across all settings; includes 16 data elements; not widely implemented in practice.

Nursing Outcomes Classification (NOC) – A system to evaluate the effects of nursing care as part of the nursing process that assists the nurse to document a person's status before and after nursing interventions are deployed.

Nursing Plan of Care – A nursing care plan outlines the nursing care to be provided to an individual/family/community. It is a set of actions the nurse will implement to resolve/support nursing diagnoses identified by nursing assessment; guides in the ongoing provision of nursing care and assists in the evaluation of that care.

Nursing Process – The essential core of practice for the registered nurse to deliver holistic, person-focused care.

Nursing-Sensitive Outcomes – Changes in the actual or potential health status, behavior, or perceptions of individuals, families, or populations that can be attributed to nursing interventions provided.

Nursing Services – Organized services delivered to groups of individuals by nursing staff; includes nursing care, as well as services to support or facilitate direct care, such as referral and coordination of care.

Occupational Safety and Health Administration (OSHA) – Branch of the U.S. Department of Labor responsible for enforcing laws and regulations on workplace safety.

Opioids – The term used to refer to "opiates" (drugs derived from naturally opium, such as morphine and codeine) and "opioids" (chemically manufactured drugs resembling opiates, such as methadone, fentanyl, oxycodone, hydrocodone, hydromorphone, and synthetic heroin).

Orientation – A program that introduces a new employee to an organization's mission, values, and culture, in addition to providing a structure to learning job skills expected of his/her role. The orientation program reviews organizational policies, as well as work setting expectations, policies, and work unit norms.

Out-of-Pocket Expense – Refers to the portion of health care cost for which the individual is responsible.

Ozbolt's Patient Care Data Set (PCDS) – Taxonomy used by nurses to document care in all settings, but primarily developed for the acute care setting; is composed of nursing diagnoses, patient care actions, and nursing outcomes.

Pain – An unpleasant sensory and emotional experience associated with actual or potential tissue damage, or described in terms of such damage.

Palliative Care – Both a philosophy of care and an organized, highly structured system for delivery of care; its goal is to prevent and relieve suffering and to support the best possible quality of life for individuals and their families, regardless of the stage of the disease or the need for other therapies.

Patient – Individuals, families, caregivers/support systems, groups, and populations that approach the health care system either in face-to-face encounters, by telephone, or in other types of virtual encounters.

Patient Activation Measure® (PAM®) – An assessment that gauges the knowledge, skills, and confidence essential to managing one's own health and health care.

Patient Advocacy – The support and empowerment of individuals to make informed decisions, navigate the health care system to access appropriate care, and build strong partnerships with providers, while working towards system improvement to support patient-centered care.

Patient- and Family-Centered Care – An approach to the planning, delivery, and evaluation of health care that is grounded in mutually beneficial partnerships among health care providers, individuals, and families.

Patient-Centered Care – Recognizing the individual or designee as the source of control and full partner in providing compassionate and coordinated care based on respect for the individual's preferences, values, and needs.

Patient-Centered Medical Home (PCMH) – A care delivery model that facilitates partnerships between individual patients, their health care team, and when appropriate, the patient's family; attributes include patient centeredness, continuous improvement, and care that is comprehensive, coordinated, and accessible.

Glossary

Patient Education – Process of assisting people to learn health-related behaviors (knowledge, skills, attitudes, and values) so they can incorporate them into their everyday lives with the goal of optimal health and independence in self-care.

Patient Health Questionnaire (PHQ-2 or 9) – A multipurpose instrument used to assess signs and symptoms of depression.

Patient Protection and Affordable Care Act (PPACA) – U.S. law passed in 2010 to reform health care; focused on health promotion, disease prevention, and increased access through insurance reform.

Pay for Performance – Government and other third-party payer programs to incentivize adherence to suggested evidence-based guidelines that lead to improved patient outcomes.

Peer Review – Process of reviewing and assessing the clinical competence and conduct of health professionals on an ongoing basis; an integral part of quality assessment and improvement processes.

Performance Improvement – Systematic analysis of the structure, processes, and outcomes within systems to improve the delivery of care.

Personal Health Portal – An electronic portal that individuals can access directly to maintain and manage their own health information.

Physician Hospital Organization (PHO) – Entity formed by a hospital and attending medical staff to contract with managed care plans. This type of entity is rapidly being replaced by the ACO.

Point of Service (POS) – A plan that defines service providers in the service area outside of the usual preferred provider network.

Polypharmacy – Involves clients with one condition or more who are using multiple medications, some of which are not clinically indicated.

Population Health – Encompasses the ability to assess the health needs of a specific population, implement and evaluate interventions to improve the health of that population, and provide care for individuals in the context of the culture, health status, and health needs of the populations of which that individual is a member.

Population Health Management – Generally refers to programs and delivery of services targeted to a defined population that uses a variety of individual, organizational, and societal interventions, and is measured by specific health care-related metrics to improve health outcomes.

Practice-Based Population Health (PBPH) – An approach to care that uses information on a group of individuals within a primary care practice or group of practices to improve the care and clinical outcomes of individuals within that practice.

Pre-Visit Chart Review – Collaborate review of an individual's chart 24 to 48 hours before visit.

Precertification – Process of obtaining authorization or certification from a health plan for hospital admissions, referrals, procedures, or tests.

Preferred Provider Organization (PPO) – Program in which contracts exist between providers and health care plans. Providers agree to provide care for negotiated set rates. Set prices are usually less than current prevailing rates. The plan provides financial incentives for individuals to utilize in-network providers through decreased out-of-pocket expense.

Prescription Drug Monitoring Program (PDMP) – Electronic database that tracks information related to prescription drugs and includes individual, drug and dose prescribed, prescriber, and dispensing pharmacy.

Presence – Effective listening; occurs at five different levels: hearing, understanding, retaining information, analyzing and evaluating information, and helping/active empathizing.

Primary Care – The provision of integrated, accessible health care services by clinicians who are accountable for addressing a large majority of personal health care needs, developing a sustained partnership with individuals, and practicing in the context of family and community.

Primary Care Provider (PCP) – The health care provider who oversees the medical care of an individual or family, when well or ill, such as a physician, nurse practitioner, or physician assistant.

Glossary

Primary Prevention – Includes health promotion (HP) interventions and specific protections (SP); may be directed at individuals, groups, or populations; targeted at well populations or those already ill (e.g., HP = nutrition education; SP = use of seatbelts, avoidance of allergens, or importance of immunizations).

Productivity – Measure of the efficiency with which labor and materials are converted into service or care; volume of output related to amount of resources consumed/used to produce a specified output/service.

Quality Improvement – A systematic and continuous action leading to measurable improvement in health care services and the health status of targeted groups of individuals.

Quality Improvement Using Evidence-Based Practice – Evaluation of practice evidence and research using data to monitor the outcomes of care processes and improvement methods to design and test changes to continuously improve the quality and safety of health care systems.

Re-Engineered Discharge (Project RED) – A training program that is a person-centered, standardized approach to discharge planning designed to help hospitals re-engineer their discharge process.

Remote Patient Monitoring – Using digital technologies to collect health data from individuals in one location and electronically transitioning that information securely to health care providers in a different location for assessment and recommendations.

Report Cards – Identify performance measures that include quality indicators (immunization, Pap smear, and mammogram rates), utilization indicators (membership, access, finances, hospital, and emergency department admission), and satisfaction levels; consumers use report card data to compare the performance of different organizations against a predetermined standard/best practice.

Research Utilization – A process of using research findings as a basis for practice; typically based on a single study.

Resource-Based Relative Value Scale (RBRVS) – A classification system that attempts to assign the resource requirements within a defined setting based on weights, according to relative cost of each service.

Revenue – Total amount of income received or that is entitled to be received based on services rendered or goods provided.

Risk Management – An organization-wide program to identify risks, control occurrences, prevent damage, and control legal liability; a process whereby risks to an institution are evaluated and controlled.

Risk Stratification – The process of separating patient populations into high-risk, low-risk, and the ever-important rising-risk groups. Having a platform to stratify individuals according to risk is key to the success of any population health management initiative. Proactively identify and outreach to at-risk individuals to develop person-centered care planning.

Root Cause Analysis (RCA) – A systematic process for identifying "root causes" of problems or events and an approach for responding to them. It is based on the basic idea that effective management requires more than merely "putting out fires" for problems that develop, but finding a way to prevent them.

Secondary Prevention – Involves early diagnosis and prompt treatment to avoid disability (e.g., screening, biopsies, medication, surgery).

Self-Care – Individuals learn to care for themselves and participate in collaborative goal setting and decision-making.

Self-Efficacy – A person's confidence in his/her ability to carry out behaviors necessary to achieve the desired goal.

Self-Management Support – The systematic provision of education and supportive interventions by health care staff to increase a person's skills and confidence in managing their health problems, including regular assessment of progress and problems, goal setting, and problem-solving support.

Situation, Background, Assessment and Recommendation (SBAR) Tool – A handoff technique used to facilitate prompt and appropriate communication between members of the health care team about a person's condition. ISBAR – as above, with "I" representing "Identification."

SMART Goals – SMART is a mnemonic, giving criteria to guide in the setting of objectives: **S**pecific, **M**easurable, **A**ttainable, **R**ealistic, and **T**imely.

Glossary

SNOMED-CT® – Systematic Nomenclature for Medicine-Reference Terminology (College of American Pathologists); comprehensive, multi-axial nomenclature classification system created for the indexing of the entire medical and health care vocabulary.

Social Determinants of Health (SDOH) – Conditions where people live, learn, work, and play that affect a wide range of risks and health outcomes.

Standard – An authoritative statement developed and disseminated by a professional organization or governmental or regulatory agency by which the quality of practice, services, research, or education can be judged.

Standard of Practice – Authoritative statements that delineate responsibilities and competencies for which nurses are responsible.

State Practice Acts – A combination of laws and regulations that define and regulate the practice of medicine, nursing, and other health professions.

Strategic Planning – The continuous process of systematically evaluating the nature of the organization, defining its long-term objectives, identifying quantifiable goals, developing strategies to reach these objectives and goals, and allocating resources to carry out these strategies.

Supervision – The direction and oversight of the performance of others.

Systems Level Advocacy in Nursing – Refers to nurses' actions that promote health broadly at a systems level by remaining focused on the context of the health care delivery system and policy making at the organization, local, state, and national levels.

"Teach Back" – A way of checking understanding by asking individuals to state in their own words what they need to know or do about their health. It is a way to confirm that you have explained things in a manner the person understands.

Team Building and Collaboration – To build, support, and participate effectively within nursing and interprofessional teams, fostering open communication, mutual respect, and shared decision-making to achieve quality patient care during care transitions.

TeamSTEPPS™ (Team Strategies and Tools to Enhance Performance and Patient Safety) – An evidence-based teamwork system aimed at optimizing a person's outcomes through improving communication and teamwork skills among team members across the health care delivery system.

Teamwork and Collaboration – Effectively functioning within nursing and interprofessional teams, fostering open communication, mutual respect, and shared decision-making to achieve quality patient care.

Teamwork in Health Care – A dynamic process involving two or more health professionals with complementary backgrounds and skills, sharing common health goals and exercising concerted physical and mental effort in assessing, planning, or evaluating a person's care.

Telehealth – The delivery, management, and coordination of health services that integrate electronic information and telecommunication technologies to increase access, improve outcomes, and contain or reduce costs of health care.

Telehealth Nursing – The delivery, management, and coordination of care and services provided via telecommunications technology within the domain of nursing; encompassing practices that incorporate a vast array of telecommunications technologies (telephone, fax, electronic mail, Internet, video monitoring, and interactive video) to remove time and distance barriers for the delivery of nursing care.

Telehealth Nursing Practice – The delivery, management, and coordination of care and services provided via telecommunications technology within the domain of nursing.

Telemedicine – The delivery of health care services between two locations by all health care professionals using information and communication technologies for the exchange of valid information for diagnosis, treatment and prevention of disease and injuries, research and evaluation, and the continuing education of health care providers to advance the health of individuals and their communities.

Telemonitoring – Monitoring of physiologic parameters over distance utilizing telehealth technology.

Glossary

Telephone Nursing – All care and services within the scope of nursing practice that are delivered over the telephone; component of telehealth nursing practice restricted to the telephone.

Telephone Triage – An interactive process between the nurse and individual that occurs over the telephone; involves identifying the nature and urgency of client health care needs and determining the appropriate disposition; a component of telephone nursing practice that focuses on assessment and prioritization and referral to the appropriate level of care.

Tertiary Prevention – Aims to achieve the highest level of function, minimize complications, and reduce disability. Examples of tertiary prevention measures include occupational and physical therapy after a stroke, wearing proper shoes with diabetic neuropathy, and assigning appropriate diet post-surgery to promote healing.

Transition Management – The ongoing support of individuals and their families over time as they navigate care and relationships among more than one provider and/or more than one health care setting and/or more than one health care service. The need for transition management is not determined by age, time, place, or health care condition, but rather by individuals' and/or families' needs for support for ongoing, longitudinal evidence-based, individualized plans of care and follow-up plans of care within the context of health care delivery (Haas, Swan, & Haynes, 2018).

Transitional Care –
1. "A broad range of time-limited services designed to ensure health care continuity, avoid preventable poor outcomes among at-risk populations, and promote the safe and timely transfer of patients from one level of care to another or from one type of setting to another" (Naylor, Aiken, Kurtzman, Olds, & Hirschman, 2011, p. 747).
2. "A set of actions designed to ensure the coordination and continuity of health care as patients transfer between different locations or different levels of care within the same location. Representative locations include (but are not limited to) hospitals, sub-acute and post-acute nursing facilities, the patient's home, primary and specialty care offices, and long-term care facilities" (Coleman & Boult, 2003, p. 556).

Translational Research – Involves the use of theory to guide development, implementation, diffusion, and evaluation of effectiveness and sustainability of evidence-based practice.

Transtheoretical Model – Describes behavioral change, which takes into account the individual's desire to change. Created and tested by DiClemente and Prochaska.

TriCare – A federal program providing coverage to families of active duty military personnel, military retirees, spouses, and dependents (replaced CHAMPUS [Civilian Health and Medical Program of the United States]).

U.S. Preventive Services Task Force (USPSTF) – Nongovernmental expert panel of primary care, evidence-based medicine experts who review current preventive services and make practice recommendations.

Usual, Customary, and Reasonable (UCR) – A method used to determine if a fee is usual, customary, and reasonable; customary is based on a percentile of aggregated fees charged in the geographic area for the same service; usually refers to fees normally charged by a physician or health care provider for a service.

Utilitarianism – Also known as consequence-based ethics; the theory that seeks to choose the thing that will offer the most good to the greatest number of people, increase pleasure, and avoid pain.

Utilization Management – A set of techniques used by or on behalf of purchasers of health care benefits to manage health care costs by influencing patient care decision-making through case-by-case assessments of the appropriateness of care prior to its provision as defined by the Institute of Medicine (IOM) (American physical Therapy Association [APTA], 2017).

Variable Costs – Costs that vary with changes in volumes of service units, such as person visits.

Veracity – Truth telling.

Video Conferencing – Live, visual connection between two or more people residing in separate locations for the purpose of communication.

Wearable Technology – Electronics that can be worn on the body, either as an accessory or as part of material used in clothing, and often includes tracking information related to health and fitness.

Zarit Burden Interview – A 22-item caregiver self-reported questionnaire that identifies the stresses experienced by caregivers.

Glossary

References

American Nurses Association (ANA). (2004). *Nursing: Scope & standards of practice.* Silver Spring, MD: Nursesbooks.org.

American Physical Therapy Association (APTA). (2017). *What is utilization management.* Retrieved from http://www.apta.org/WhatIsUM/

Coleman, E.A., & Boult, C. (2003). Improving the quality of transitional care for persons with complex care needs. *Journal of the American Geriatric Society, 51*(4), 556-557.

Commission for Case Manager Certification. (2018). *Definition and philosophy of case management.* Retrieved from https://ccmcertification.org/about-ccmc/about-case-management/definition-and-philosophy-case-management

Haas, S.A., Swan, B.A., & Haynes, T.S. (2018). *Care coordination and transition management core curriculum* (2nd ed.). Pitman, NJ: American Academy of Ambulatory Care Nursing.

McDonald, K., Sundaram, V., Bravata, D., Lewis, R., Lin, N., Kraft, S.A. ... Owens, D.K. (2007). Care coordination. In K. Shojania, K. McDonald, R. Wachter, & D. Owens (Eds.), *Closing the quality gap: A critical analysis of quality improvement strategies* [AHRQ Publication No. 04(07)0051-7]. Rockville, MD: Agency for Healthcare Research and Quality.

McDonald, K.M., Schultz, E.S., Albin, L., Pineda, N., Lonhart, J., Sundaram, V., ... Malcolm, E. (2011). *Care coordination measures atlas* [AHRQ Publication No.11-0023-EF]. Rockville, MD: Agency for Healthcare Research and Quality.

National Quality Forum (NQF). (2010). *Preferred practices and performance measures for measuring and reporting care coordination: A consensus report.* Washington, DC: Author.

National Quality Forum (NQF). (2016). *Looking back to plan ahead* [NQF Care Coordination Standing Committee Quarterly Off-Cycle Webinar]. Washington, DC: Author. Naylor

Naylor, M.D., Aiken, L.H., Kurtzman, E.T., Olds, D.M., & Hirschman, K.M. (2011). The care span: The importance of transitional care in achieving health reform. *Health Affairs, 30*(4), 766-754.

Titler, M.G. (2008). The evidence for evidence-based practice implementation. In R.G. Hughes (Ed.), *Patient safety and quality: An evidence-based handbook for nurses* [Vol. 1, Chapter 7]. (AHRQ Publication No. 08-0043). Rockville, MD: Agency for Healthcare Research and Quality. Retrieved from http://archive.ahrq.gov/professionals/clinicians-providers/resources/nursing/resources/nurseshdbk/nurseshdbk.pdf

Resources

Resources (Discussed in Text)	Description	Resource/Website
Better Outcomes by Optimizing Safe Transitions (BOOST)	A national initiative led by the Society of Hospital Medicine to improve the care of patients as they transition from hospital to home. Project BOOST has developed tools to assist in transitions.	**Society of Hospital Medicine** http://www.hospitalmedicine.org
CAGE and CAGE-AID	A questionnaire that focuses on alcohol and/or drug and alcohol abuse.	**The Michigan Quality Improvement Consortium** http://www.mqic.org/pdf/CAGE_CAGE_AID_QUESTIONNAIRES.pdf **Washington State Agency Medical Directors' Group** http://www.agencymeddirectors.wa.gov/Files/cageover.pdf
Comprehensive Geriatric Assessment (CGA)	A multidimensional, multiprofessional diagnostic process used to determine medical, functional, and psychosocial problems and capabilities in an elderly patient who may be at risk for functional decline.	**U.S. National Library of Medicine National Institutes of Health** https://www.ncbi.nlm.nih.gov/pmc/articles/PMC4282277/
Drug Abuse Screening Test (DAST)	20- or 28-item self-report scale for abuse of drugs other than alcohol.	**CounsellingResources.com** http://counsellingresource.com/lib/quizzes/drug-testing/drug-abuse/ **The Drug Abuse Screening Test (DAST)** http://www.drtepp.com/pdf/substance_abuse.pdf
Generalized Anxiety Scale (GAD-7)	A self-reported questionnaire for screening and severity measuring of generalized anxiety disorder (GAD).	**Patient Health Questionnaire (PHQ) Screeners** http://www.phqscreeners.com/sites/g/files/g10016261/f/201412/GAD-7_English.pdf
Geriatric Resources for Assessment and Care of Elders (GRACE)	A team-developed care plan to improve the quality of geriatric care and optimize health and functional status, decrease excess health care use, and prevent long-term nursing home placement.	*Journal of the American Geriatrics Society* http://onlinelibrary.wiley.com/doi/10.1111/j.1532-5415.2006.00791.x/abstract
Get Up and Go Test	A timed test for measurement of mobility. It includes a number of tasks, such as standing from a seating position, walking, turning, stopping, and sitting down.	**Oncology Nursing Society and Centers for Disease Control and Prevention** https://www.ons.org/sites/default/files/TUG_Test-a.pdf
Index of Independence in Activities of Daily Living (IADL)	An instrument used in assessing functional status when measuring a patient's ability to perform activities of daily living independently.	**The Hartford Institute for Geriatric Nursing, New York University Rory Meyers College of Nursing** https://consultgeri.org/try-this/general-assessment/issue-2.pdf

continued on next page

Resources

Resources (Discussed in Text)	Description	Resource/Website
Mini Cog	An assessment tool to determine the mental status of older adults and identify patients in need of further evaluation by a neurologist.	**International Journal of Geriatric Psychiatry** http://www.ncbi.nlm.nih.gov/pubmed/11113982 **Mini Cog©** https://mini-cog.com
Mini-Mental State Examination (MMSE)	A brief 30-point questionnaire used to screen for cognitive impairment.	**PAR®** http://www.minimental.com/
Modified Caregiver Strain Index (MCSI)	A 13-question tool that measures strain related to care provision.	**ConsultGeriRN.org** https://consultgeri.org/try-this/general-assessment/issue-14
Modified LACE	An assessment tool that incorporates **L**ength of stay, **A**cuity of admission, **C**o-morbidity, **E**mergency department visits to identify patients with a high predicted risk for re-admission or death.	**Hospital Quality Institute** https://view.officeapps.live.com/op/view.aspx?src=http%3A%2F%2Fwww.hqinstitute.org%2Fsites%2Fmain%2Ffiles%2Ffile-attachments%2F1_modified_lace_tool.docx
Montreal Cognitive Assessment (MoCA)	A cognitive screening test designed to assist health professionals for detection of mild cognitive impairment.	**Z. Nasreddine, MD** http://www.mocatest.org/
Patient Activation Measure® (PAM®)	An assessment that gauges the knowledge, skills, and confidence essential to managing one's own health and health care.	**Insignia Health** http://www.insigniahealth.com/solutions/patient-activation-measure **Health Services Research** http://www.ncbi.nlm.nih.gov/pmc/articles/PMC1361231/
Patient Health Questionnaire (PHQ-2 or 9)	A multi-purpose instrument used to assess signs and symptoms of depression.	**American Psychological Association** https://www.apa.org/pi/about/publications/caregivers/practice-settings/assessment/tools/patient-health.aspx **Pfizer** http://phqscreeners.com/
Re-Engineered Discharge (Project RED)	A training program that is a patient-centered, standardized approach to discharge planning designed to help hospitals re-engineer their discharge process.	**Project RED (Re-Engineered Discharge)** http://www.bu.edu/fammed/projectred/
YZarit Burden Interview	A 22-item caregiver self-reported questionnaire that identifies the stresses experienced by caregivers.	**American Psychological Association** https://www.apa.org/pi/about/publications/caregivers/practice-settings/assessment/tools/zarit.aspx

Applications (Apps)

Applications (apps) for mobile devices serve to engage the individual and/or family/caregiver through active involvement in managing health parameters, such as diet, exercise, and some blood monitoring. Apps should be used with caution and with the discretion of the health care team so the person is informed of the benefits and risks (Groshek, Oldenburg, Sarasohn-Kahn, & Sitler, 2015). Governmental and professional organization apps are usually dependable, but some apps provided by commercial vendors may not be. Rigorous evaluation, validation, and the development of best-practice standards for medical apps are needed to ensure quality and safety when used (Ventola, 2014).

Compiled by Cheryl Lovlien, MS, RN-BC; Denise Rismeyer, MSN, RN, RN-BC; and Jayme M. Speight, MSN, RN-BC.

Mobile Apps for Patient Use

Simply Sayin' – Medical Jargon for Families (IOS)
Uses pictures, sounds, and terms to assist with understanding medical jargon for a child or caregiver.

Up-to-Date for Patients and Caregivers
Access information for patients, including pictures, graphs, and charts.

HeartMapp (Android)
Intended to assist patients with heart failure in managing symptoms and medications.

mySugr Diabetes Training
Makes type 2 diabetes learning fun and easy to comprehend.

Mango Health (IOS)
Medicine reminder app. Reminds patient to take pills, tracks refills, and identifies food and drug interactions.

MyRA
Rheumatoid arthritis tracker, picks, communications.

Fooducate
Diabetes nutrition and diet tracker. Identifies food content of groceries purchased and alternatives for people with diabetes.

iBGstar Diabetes Manager
Records, tracks, and manages diabetes data. Integrates with iBGStar blood glucose monitors.

HealthTap
Gives tips and answers related to health concerns and other topics.

Diabetes App
Blood sugar, glucose, and carb counter.

Pillboxie
Helps the person remember to take medications.

goMeals
Identifies nutrition from meals and restaurants.

WebMD for iPad
Health information and tools to check symptoms. Provides first aid information.

Asthma Tracker for Adolescents (American Academy of Pediatrics)
Patient education section is prepopulated with pediatric-relevant educational content, instructions, and videos.

The Amazings
Gameplay to help kids recognize and avoid asthma triggers, such as pollen, cigarette smoke, and pollution, and to stay vigilant about their health. Target audience is children with asthma aged 7 to 12 years.

Wizdy Pets
Health-oriented gaming start-up promoting patient self-management through engaging mobile games.

KidsDoc (American Academy of Pediatrics)
Helps parents know when to have their child seen by a doctor.

Mobile Apps for Nurse/Provider Use

The following are mobile apps that may be of interest for nurses seeking information to share with individuals and families/caregivers. This list is not all inclusive but noted from the article by Aditi Pai (2013).

Nursing Central
Knowledge app for nurses to find answers to questions about diseases, labs, and procedures.

NurseTabs
Fundamentals: Step-by-step procedures for 120+ skills.

NurseTabs – MedSurg
Offers the ability to search across diseases and disorders to have medical information easily available.

Shots by STFM
A digital reference on immunizations.

Lab Notes
A nurse's guide to laboratory and diagnostic tests with patient education. Provides information related to laboratory values and radiology imaging, with patient education and imaging.

References

Groshek, M.R., Oldenburg, J., Sarasohn-Kahn, J., & Sitler, B. (2015). *mHealth App essentials: Patient engagement, considerations, and implementation.* Retrieved from http://www.himss.org/mhealth-app-essentials-patient-engagement-considerations-and-implementation

Pai, A. (2013). *Apple's top 118 apps for doctors, nurses, patients.* Retrieved from http://www.mobihealthnews.com/23740/apples-top-118-apps-for-doctors-nurses-and-patients/page/0/9

Ventola, C.L. (2014). Mobile devices and apps for health care professionals: Uses and benefits. *Pharmacy & Therapeutics, 39*(5), 356-364. Retrieved from https://www.ncbi.nlm.nih.gov/pmc/articles/PMC4029126/

Index

A

AAACN (American Academy of Ambulatory Care Nursing), **316**
AAAHC (Accreditation Association for Ambulatory Health Care), **315**
AAP (American Academy of Pediatrics) Asthma Tracker for Adolescents, 60, 331
Abandonment, **315**
Abilities, assessment of, 52–53
ACA (Affordable Care Act, 2010), 4, 6, 160, 200, **324**
Accessibility
  of care, **315**
  of health information, 180, 182
Accountable Care Organization (ACO), 6, 213, **315**
Accreditation, **315**
Accreditation Association for Ambulatory Health Care (AAAHC), **315**
Accuracy of health information, 180
"Acknowledgment of connection," 83
ACP (advance care planning), 83–84, 87–88, **315**
Acronyms in education of individuals and families, 55
ACSC (ambulatory care sensitive conditions), 8
Actionability of health information, 180
Action plan in self-management model, 79f, 82, 127–128
Action stage of change, 76
Active listening, **315**
Acute care
  defined, **315**
  transition between ambulatory and, 235–261
    application of evidence-based tools to, 243
    case studies on, 248–261
    competency in, 235–236
    defining, 237
    engagement of individual, family, and interprofessional team in, 242–243
    evidence-based models for, 239–242
    evidence-based practice in, 247t
    knowledge, skills, and attitudes for, 244t–247t
    opportunities for, 237–239
    person-centered care in, 244t
    safety in, 245t
    standards guiding, 236–237
    teamwork and collaboration in, 245t–246t
  transition from extended care to, 239
  transition to long-term care from, 238–239
ADA (Americans with Disabilities Act), **316**
Addiction, **315**
  to opioids, 59
Adolescent(s)
  Asthma Tracker for, 60, 331
  confidentiality for, 37
  education of, 55
  health literacy of, 31–32
Advance care planning (ACP), 83–84, 87–88, **315**
Advance directives, **315**
Advise in self-management model, 79f, 80f, 82
Advocacy, 19–46
  antecedents of, 20
  and behavioral/mental health, 32–36
  in care of children, 36–38
  case studies on, 45–46
  in CCTM Model, 27–28
  competency in, 19
  core attributes of, 20
  defined, **315, 323**
  and ethics, 21–23
  future considerations related to, 42
  and health literacy, 30–32
  knowledge, skills, and attitudes for, 43t–44t
  and leadership, 41–42
  at macrosocial level, 20, 21, 21f
  at microsocial level, 20–21, 21f
  in nursing practice, 19, 20–21, 21f
  in organizational policy development, 38–39
  outcomes evaluation of, 20–21, 21f
  professional organization, 45
  in public policy development and health care reform, 39–41
  social determinants of health and, 28–30
  and standards of practice, 23–27
  systems level, 19, **326**
Affordable Care Act (ACA, 2010), 4, 6, 160, 200, **324**
Agency for Healthcare Research and Quality (AHRQ), 2, 31, 103, 268, **315**
Agree in self-management model, 79f, 80f, 82
Alarm algorithms, 266
Alcohol abuse, CAGE questionnaire on, 92
Algorithm, **315**
Alzheimer's disease, 35
The Amazings, 60, 331
Ambulatory care
  defined, **315**
  transition between acute and, 235–261
    application of evidence-based tools to, 243
    case studies on, 248–261
    competency in, 235–236
    defining, 237
    engagement of individual, family, and interprofessional team in, 242–243
    evidence-based models for, 239–242
    evidence-based practice in, 247t
    knowledge, skills, and attitudes for, 244t–247t
    opportunities for, 237–239

Note: Page numbers followed by t and f indicate tables and figures, respectively; those in **boldface** refer to glossary entries

Index

person-centered care in, 244t
safety in, 245t
standards guiding, 236–237
teamwork and collaboration in, 245t–246t
Ambulatory Care Nurse Sensitive Indicator Report, 38–39
Ambulatory care nursing, **315**
Ambulatory care sensitive conditions (ACSC), 8
Ambulatory Patient Classifications (APCs), **315**
Ambulatory Patient Groups (APGs), **315**
American Academy of Ambulatory Care Nursing (AAACN), 316
American Academy of Pediatrics (AAP) Asthma Tracker for Adolescents, 60, 331
American Organization of Nurse Executives (AONE), 197
American Recovery and Reinvestment Act (2009), 160
Americans with Disabilities Act (ADA), 316
Analytics in population health management, 210–211
Analytic skills, knowledge, skills, and attitudes for, 106t–107t
Annual wellness visits (AWV), geriatric, 100
Anonymity, removing mask of, 83
Anticipatory guidance counseling, 55
AONE (American Organization of Nurse Executives), 197
APCs (Ambulatory Patient Classifications), **315**
APGs (Ambulatory Patient Groups), **315**
Applications (apps), 58, 59–60, 289, 290–291, **321,** 331
Arrange in self-management model, 79f, 81f, 82
'Ask Me 3,' 55
Assessment
advocacy in, 23, 27
comprehensive needs, 92–94
family-centered nursing, 143
functional, 92
knowledge, skills, and attitudes for, 106t–107t
nursing informatics and indicators in, 273–275
in nursing process, 139
pediatric, 94
in plan of care, 98
in population health care coordination process, 208, 209f
in self-management model, 79f, 82
Assist in self-management model, 79f, 81f, 82
Asthma Tracker for Adolescents, 60, 331
Asynchronous interactions in telehealth nursing, 292
Autonomy, **316**
AWV (annual wellness visits), geriatric, 100

B

Baby Boomers, 53
Balanced Scorecard, **316**
Behavioral change, management of responses to, 128
Behavioral health, advocacy and, 32–36
Behavioral health services for veterans, 46
Benchmarking, **316**
Beneficence, **316**
Better Outcomes for Older Adults through Safe Transitions (Project BOOST)
and communication, 183
defined, 316
description and contact information for, 329
General Assessment of Preparedness of, 252t–253t, 259t–260t
Patient PASS of, 254t, 261t
and population health management, 204
Risk Assessment 8 P Screening tool of, 210, 249t–251t, 256t–258t
transition model of, 240
Universal Discharge Checklist of, 179, 252t–253t, 259t–260t
Big data
defined, **316**
in nursing informatics, 267–268
in population health management, 204–205, 215
Bridge Model, 183
Bright Futures, 94, 209
Bundled payments, 213, **316**

C

CAGE-AID questionnaire, 92, 316, 329
CAGE questionnaire, 92, 329
CAM (complementary, alternative, and integrative therapies), 317
Cancer screenings, 208
Capitation, **316**
Care
gaps in, 95
true negotiation of, 83
Care coordination
application of evidence-based tools for, 243
background of, 175–176
case studies on, 248–261
communication and, 178
defined, 2–3, 176, 236, **316**
engagement of individual, family, and interprofessional team during, 242–243
evidence-based models for, 239–242
knowledge, skills, and attitude for, 244t–247t
nursing informatics and, 273
opportunities for, 237–239
patient-centered, 236

Index

in population health management, 208–209, 209f, 216
standards guiding, 236–237
standards of practice for advocacy in, 24
and teamwork, 161
Care Coordination and Transition Management (CCTM)
    between acute care and ambulatory care, 235–261
        application of evidence-based tools to, 243
        case studies on, 248–261
        competency in, 235–236
        defining, 237
        engagement of individual, family, and interprofessional team in, 242–243
        evidence-based models for, 239–242
        evidence-based practice in, 247t
        knowledge, skills, and attitudes for, 244t–247t
        opportunities for, 237–239
        person-centered care in, 244t
        safety in, 245t
        standards guiding, 236–237
        teamwork and collaboration in, 245t–246t
    defined, 3–4
    developing competencies for, 8–10
    identifying dimensions of, 9, 10f
    leadership in, 41–42
    verifying dimensions and competencies for, 10, 13t
Care Coordination and Transition Management registered nurse (CCTM RN) Model, 1–16
    advocacy and nursing practice in, 27–28
    and Affordable Care Act, 4, 6
    background and significance of, 4–6
    contents of, 11–12
    core curriculum as foundation for, 2
    defined, **317**
    definitions related to, 2–4
    existing care models vs., 4
    history of, 1–2
    Logic Model for, 10–11, 14t–16t
    mechanics of, 11
    methodology for, 8–10, 10f, 13f
    and Patient-Aligned Care Teams (PACT) Model, 7–8
    purpose of, 1
    rationale and need for, 4–5
Care Coordination and Transition Management (CCTM) Toolkit, 1
Care Coordination Task Force (CCTF), 41
Caregiver, in population health management, 207
Caregiver burden, assessment of, 124
Caregiver Strain Index, Modified, 93
Care plan(s), 98–100
    barriers to participating in, 76
    defined, **323**

identifying best family members to support patient in, 77–78
interprofessional, 163
longitudinal nursing informatics and, 272
in population health management, 210
nursing process and, 144, 152–153
person-centered. See Person-centered care planning
Care team, 76
Care transition(s)
    application of evidence-based tools for, 243
    background of, 235–236
    communication during, 175–193
        and care coordination, 178
        and care transition models, 183–184
        case studies on, 191–193
        challenges of, 178
        competency in, 175
        and continuity of care, 178–179, 182
        defined, 178
        examples of, 176
        failures of, 181–182
        and fragmentation of care, 177
        importance of, 177
        interpersonal, 178
        interventions to ensure, 182
        involving chronic care, 192
        involving emergency care, 192–193
        knowledge, skills and attitudes for, 185t–190t
        and medical errors, 177
        methods of, 179–180
        pediatric considerations with, 178, 181, 182
        pediatric to adult, 184
        principles of, 180–181
    defined, 3, 176, 235, 237, **317**
    engagement of individual, family, and interprofessional team during, 242–243
    evidence-based models for, 239–242
    huddles in, 172
    managing complex cases in, 173
    models for, 183–184
    opportunities for, 237–239
    in population identification, 204
Care Transitions Intervention (CTI), 183, 241
Case management
    vs. CCTM RN Model, 4
    defined, **317**
CCC (Clinical Care Classification), **317**
CCCTM (Certified in Care Coordination and Transition Management) certification, 1

Note: Page numbers followed by t and f indicate tables and figures, respectively; those in **boldface** refer to glossary entries

Index

CCCTM (Certified in Care Coordination and Transition Management) competencies, 1–2
CCD (Continuity of Care Document), 210
CCM (Chronic Care Model), 9, 10f, 200–201, 202f
CCTF (Care Coordination Task Force), 41
CCTM. See Care Coordination and Transition Management (CCTM)
CCTM RN Model. See Care Coordination and Transition Management registered nurse (CCTM RN) Model
CCTP (Community-based Care Transitions Program), 240
CDRs (clinical data registries)
 defined, **317**
 in population identification, 203
CDSS (clinical decision support systems), 144, 317
CDT (Clock Drawing Test), 92
Centers for Disease Control (CDC), 103, 317
Centers for Medicare and Medicaid Services (CMS)
 defined, **317**
 Meaningful Measures Framework of, 272–275, 274t, **317**
 in population health management, 213
Certification, **317**
Certified in Care Coordination and Transition Management (CCCTM) certification, 1
Certified in Care Coordination and Transition Management (CCCTM) competencies, 1–2
CGA (Comprehensive Geriatric Assessment), 93–94, **318**, 329
Change
 readiness to, 76, 127
 stages of, 98
"Change talk," 98
Chart review, pre-encounter, 94–95, **324**
Children
 assessment of, 94
 behavioral and mental health services for, 32, 35–36
 care of
  advocacy in, 36–38
  health literacy and, 31–32
 communication and care coordination involving, 178, 181, 182
 concussion management in, 37
 confidentiality with, 37
 distracted driving and, 37–38
 education of, 55
 electronic nicotine delivery systems for, 38
 gun safety for, 37
 immunization of, 37
 impact of social determinants on health of, 29
 passenger safety of, 37
 person-centered care planning for, 115–116
 physical education of, 37
 poverty of, 37
 refugee, 38
 response to trauma by, 29, 36
 in telehealth nursing, 292, 294, 295, 301t
 transition to young adult care of, 184, 239
Choices for Care, **84**
Chronic care, cross setting communication involving, 191
Chronic Care Model (CCM), 9, 10f, 200–201, 202f
Chronic disease
 nursing process and management of, 143–144
 risk stratification tool for, 95, 96t
 support knowledge and understanding of, 122–124
Chronic pain
 advocacy for, 34–35
 defined, **317**
 education of individuals and families on management of, 59, 70–71
Clinical alerts in population health management, 210
Clinical Care Classification (CCC), **317**
Clinical data registries (CDRs)
 defined, **317**
 in population identification, 203
Clinical decision support
 health information technology in, 270
 in population identification, 204
Clinical decision support systems (CDSS), 144, **317**
Clinical indicators in population health management, 212
Clinical notes, 58
Clinical operations, big data and, 205
Clinical practice committees (CPCs), 38
Clinical Practice domain, standards of practice for advocacy in, 23–25
Clinical practice guidelines, 317
Clinical reasoning, 137
Clock Drawing Test (CDT), 92
Cloud computing, 266
CMS (Centers for Medicare and Medicaid Services)
 defined, 317
 Meaningful Measures Framework of, 272–275, 274t, 317
 in population health management, 213
Coaching and counseling, 75–88
 on advance care planning, 83–84, 87–88
 case studies on, 87–88
 competency in, 76
 defined, **320**
 developing relationship with individuals and families in, 76–77
 encouraging individuals and families to be active members of team in, 77
 equipping individual and family in, 78–82, 79f–

Index

   81f
   evaluation and outcomes in, 85
   knowledge, skills, and attitudes for, 86t
   maintaining relationship with individuals and families in, 82–83
   on palliative care, 84–85
   for self-management support, 129
   strategies in identifying best family member to support patient in, 77–78
Coalitions, 39
Code of Ethics for Nurses with Interpretive Statements (ANA), 22
Cognitive barriers to self-management, 125
Cognitive impairment, **317**
Cognitive learning theory, 50
Coleman Transitions Intervention Model, 241
Collaboration
   background of, 160–161
   in cross-setting communications and transitions, 186t–187t
   defined, 160, **317, 326**
   in education of individuals and families, 56
   interprofessional approach to, 162–163
   in interprofessional practice, 101
   in population health management, 199t, 220t–223t
   and professional practice standards, 161–162
   standards of practice for advocacy in, 26
   vs. teamwork, 159–160
   in telehealth nursing, 294, 305t–306t
   in transition between acute and ambulatory care, 237, 245t–246t
Commercial indemnity plans, **317**
Communication
   advocacy in, 26
   during care transitions (cross setting), 175–193
      between acute and ambulatory care, 236
      and care coordination, 178
      and care transition models, 183–184
      case studies on, 191–193
      challenges of, 178
      competency in, 175
      and continuity of care, 178–179, 182
      examples of, 176
      failures of, 181–182
      and fragmentation of care, 177
      importance of, 177
      interventions to ensure, 182
      involving chronic care, 192
      involving emergency care, 192–193
      knowledge, skills and attitudes for, 185t–190t
      methods of, 179–180
      pediatric considerations with, 178, 181, 182
      pediatric to adult, 184
      principles of, 180–181
      defined, 178
      with family/caregiver and friends, 58
      with health care professionals, 58–59
      interpersonal, 178
      interprofessional, 112t–113t
      nursing informatics and, 273
      in plan of care, 99, 103
      and teamwork, 161, 165–166, 170t, 207
      with telehealth technology, 292–294, 302t–304t
Communication Catalyst Program, 180
Communication skills, knowledge, skills, and attitudes for, 107t–108t
Communication technologies
   in nursing informatics, 268–269
   for self-management support, 129
Community-based Care Transitions Program (CCTP), 240
Community dimensions of practice skills, knowledge, skills, and attitudes for, 108t–109t
Community health worker in population health management, 207
Community outreach, advocacy related to, 29
Competence, defined, 2, **317**
Competency(ies)
   cultural, 108t
   defined, 2, **317**
   development for CCTM of, 8–9
   interprofessional, 101
   verifying, 10, 13t
Complementary, alternative, and integrative therapies (CAM), **317**
Comprehensive Geriatric Assessment (CGA), 93–94, **318**, 329
Comprehensive needs assessment, 92–94
Computerized Patient Record System (CPRS), 8
Computerized provider order entries, 178
Concussion management in children, 37
Confidentiality
   for adolescents and young adults, 37
   and advocacy, 23
   defined, **318**
Confusion, **318**
Connection, acknowledgment of, 83
Consent, informed, **321**
Consultation and teamwork, 162
Contemplation stage of change, 76
Continuity of care
   communication and, 178–179, 182
   defined, 178
Continuity of Care Document (CCD), 210
The Conversation Project, 84
Coordination of care. See Care coordination
   Co-payment, **318**

Note: Page numbers followed by t and f indicate tables and figures, respectively; those in **boldface** refer to glossary entries

Index

Coping
  barriers to, 76
  in plan of care, 99
Core competences for nursing, **318**
Core curriculum as foundation for CCTM Model, 2
Cost(s), variable, **327**
Cost benefit analysis, **318**
Counseling. See Coaching and counseling
  CPCs (clinical practice committees), 38
CPRS (Computerized Patient Record System), 8
CPT (Current Procedural Terminology), **318**
Credentialing, **318**
Critical thinking, 137–138, **318**
Cross setting communication. See Communication, during care transitions (cross setting)
CTI (Care Transitions Intervention), 183, 241
Cultural barriers to self-management, 125
Cultural competency, 108t, **318**
Culturally competent resources, 76
Cultural safety, **318**
Culture and education of individuals and families, 52–53
Current Procedural Terminology (CPT), **318**

D

Dashboards in population health management, 212
DAST (Drug Abuse Screening Test), **319**, 329
Data, objective vs. subjective, 139
Data analysis and selection in Population Health Care Coordination Process, 208, 209f
Data analytics, 271
Data systems in population identification, 203
Decision-making
  in self-management support, 59, 127
  shared, 163
  by surrogate, 83
Decision support
  evidence-based, 271
  nursing informatics and, 270–271
  nursing process and, 144
Decision support systems
  defined, **318**
  in population health management, 199t, 209–211, 227t–230t
Deductible, **318**
Delegation, **318**
Dementia, 32, 35, **318**
  considerations in plan of care for, 100
  Mini-Cog–Mental Status Assessment of Older Adults for, 92–93
Deontology, **318**
Depression
  advocacy and, 32, 33
  defined, **318**
  Patient Health Questionnaire (PHQ-2 or PHQ-9) for, 92
Device monitoring
  big data and, 205
  wearable devices for, 58, 266
Diabetes
  education of individuals and families on, 69
  self-management support for, 129, 134
  treat-to-target for, 141f
Diabetes App, 60, 221
Diagnosis-related groups (DRGs), 318
Dimensions of CCTM
  defining, 9
  identifying, 9, 10f
  verifying, 10, 13t
Discomfort, self-management support for, 123
Disease, assessing knowledge of, 53
Disease certification programs, population health and, 212
Disease management programs, population health management vs., 200
Disease prevention
  in population health management, 208–209
  primary, **325**
  secondary, **325**
  in self-management support, 124
  tertiary, **327**
Distance learning, **319**
Domain of ambulatory nursing practice, **319**
Do Not Intubate (DNI), 84
Do Not Resuscitate (DNR), 84
DRGs (diagnosis-related groups), **318**
Drug abuse, CAGE questionnaire on, 92
Drug Abuse Screening Test (DAST), **319**, 329
Dyslexia, education of individuals and families with, 50

E

EBP. See Evidence-based practice (EBP)
Economic barriers to self-management, 125
E-consults, 58
Education
  of individuals and families, 49–71
    accessing and evaluating reliable health information for, 57
    acronyms in, 55
    for adolescents, 55
    age differences for, 50, 51t–52t
    anticipatory guidance counseling in, 55
    apps for, 59–60
    assessing knowledge and abilities for, 52–53
    assessing readiness for learning and, 50–52, 51t–52t
    case studies on, 69–71
    for children, 55
    collaboration and teamwork in, 56

Index

    definition for competency in, 49
    on diabetes, 69
    engagement and, 58
    evaluation of learning in, 56–57
    with hearing loss, 50
    individualized, 54
    with intellectual disability, 50–52
    knowledge, skills, and attitudes for, 61t–67t
    with learning disabilities, 50
    methods to provide, 53–55, 68t
    for opioid medications, 59, 70–71
    self-management skills in, 58–59
    "teach-back" method for, 54, 56–57
  interprofessional, 101
  in plan of care, 99
  process of, **319**
  of public, 39–40
  standards of practice for advocacy in, 25
EEOC (Equal Employment Opportunity Commission), 319
Effectiveness measures, 103
Electronic health records (EHRs)
  and cross-setting communication, 178, 179–180
  defined, 266, **319**
  in nursing informatics, 265–266
  and person-centered care, 210
  in population health management, 204, 207, 210, 212
  and safety, 270
  types of, 58
Electronic nicotine delivery systems (ENDS), 38, **319**
Electronic patient portals, 58, 268, 288, 310, **324**
ELNEC (End of Life Nursing Education Consortium), 84
Emergency care, cross setting communication involving, 192–193
Emergency Medical Treatment and Active Labor Act (EMTALA), **319**
Emotional intelligence, **319**
Empathy, 77
Empowerment approach to self-management support, 128
EMTALA (Emergency Medical Treatment and Active Labor Act), 319
End of Life Nursing Education Consortium (ELNEC), 84
ENDS (electronic nicotine delivery systems), 38, **319**
Engagement of individuals and families, 41, 58, **319**
Enhanced Nursing Licensure Compact (eNLC), **319**
Environment
  standards of practice for advocacy in, 27
  and teamwork, 162
Environmental management, **319**
Equal Employment Opportunity Commission (EEOC), **319**
Essential Elements for Improving the Discharge Transition, 271–272
Ethical sensitivity, 21, 22
Ethical standards for telehealth nursing, 291
Ethics
  in CCTM nursing, 21–23
  Code of, 22
  defined, **319**
  for interprofessional practice, 110t
  standards of practice for advocacy in, 25
  and teamwork, 162
Evaluation
  advocacy in, 25, 28
  in nursing process, 142–143
  in population health care coordination process, 208, 209f
  and teamwork, 162
Evidence-based care guidelines, nursing informatics and, 268, 271
Evidence-based care resources, 102
Evidence-based decision support, 271
Evidence-based medicine, big data and, 205
Evidence-based practice (EBP)
  components of, 102
  in cross-setting communications and transitions, 188t–189t
  defined, **319**
  goals of, 271
  nursing process and, 146t
  in population health management, 199t, 223t–224t
  quality improvement using, **325**
  standards of practice for advocacy in, 25–26
  in transition between acute and ambulatory care, 247t
Evidence-based tools for care coordination and transition management, 243
Evidence-based transition models, 239–242
Evidentiary Review, 8
Exercise
  by children, 37
  education of individuals and families on, 58
Existential distress, **319**
Extended care, transition to acute care from, 239

F

Fact-based information, 57
Family, defined, 143
Family care, applying nursing process to, 143

Note: Page numbers followed by t and f indicate tables and figures, respectively; those in **boldface** refer to glossary entries

Index

Family-centered care, 323
Family-centered nursing assessment, 143
Family health, defined, 143
Family process, defined, 143
Fatigue, self-management of, 99, 122–123
Fee for service, **319**
Fentanyl, 35
Fidelity, **319**
Firearm safety, 37
5 A's Behavior Change Model Adapted for Self-Management Support Improvement, 78–82, 79f–81f, 128, **315**
Five Wishes, 84
Fixed costs, **319**
Flinders Program, 129
Focus Group Method, 8–9
Fooducate, 60, 331
For-profit organization, 57
Four Pillars, 241
Fraud analysis, big data and pre-adjudication, 205
Functional status assessment, 92
    in population health management, 211
Fundamental Guidelines for Motivational Interviewing, 77–78
The Future of Nursing (IOM), 160

G

Gaps in care, 95
General Assessment of Preparedness (GAP), 179, 252t–253t, 259t–260t
Generalized Anxiety Scale (GAD-7), **319**, 329
Generation X, 53
Generation Z, 53
Genomic analytics, big data and, 205
Geriatric Assessment, Comprehensive, 93–94, **318**, 329
Geriatric patients
    annual wellness visits for, 100
    considerations in plan of care for, 100
    evaluation for transitions to acute care of, 249t–251t, 256t–258t
Geriatric Resources for Assessment and Care of Elders (GRACE), 183, 242, **319**, 329
Get Up and Go Test, 93, **319**, 329
Goal identification in nursing process, 140–142, 141f
Goal setting
    in plan of care, 98–99
    in self-management support, 126
goMeals, 60, 331
GRACE (Geriatric Resources for Assessment and Care of Elders), 183, 242, 319, 329
Graphs for education of individuals and families, 54
Grief, **319**
Group discussions for education of individuals and families, 55

Guided care, 183
Gun safety, 37

H

HCFA (Health Care Financing Administration) Common Procedure Coding System (HCPCS), **320**
HCPCS (HCFA Common Procedure Coding System), **320**
Health
    assessing knowledge of, 53
    social determinants of
        and advocacy, 28–30
        defined, **326**
        in population health management, 211
Health apps, mobile, 58, 59–60, 289, 290–291
Health behaviors in population health management, 211
Health Belief Model in self-management support, 127
Healthcare Effectiveness and Data Information Set (HEDIS), 103, **320**
Health Care Financing Administration (HCFA) Common Procedure Coding System (HCPCS), **320**
Healthcare Information and Management Systems Society (HIMSS), 200, 265–266
Health care policy development, population health and, 212–213
Health care quality measures, population health and, 212
Health care reform, advocacy and, 39–41, **320**
Health care team, **320**
Health care utilization in population health management, 211
Health coaching. See Coaching and counseling
Health education, **320**
Healthfinder.gov, 208–209
Health informatics, 209, 320. See also Informatics
Health information
    accessing and evaluating reliable, 57
    in cross setting communication, 180–181
Health information exchanges (HIEs)
    defined, **320**
    in nursing informatics, 266, 268, 270
    in population health management, 203, 210
Health information technology (HIT), 265–282
    aligned with CCTM RN Model, 266–269, 276t–277t
    and assessment, process, and outcome indicators, 273–275, 274t
    and big data, 267–268, 271
    and care coordination, 273
    case studies on, 281–282
    in clinical decision making, 270
    in clinical primary care coordination, 281

Index

competency in, 265–267
in cross-setting communications and transitions, 189t–190t
and decision-support, 270–271
defined, 209–210, 265, **320**
for education of individuals and families, 54
and Essential Elements for Improving the Discharge Transition, 271–272
and evidence-based care guidelines, 268, 271
knowledge, skills, and attitudes for, 276t–280t
and Meaningful Measures Framework, 272–275, 274t
nursing, 209–210
and patient-reported outcomes, 265
in population health management, 199t, 209–211, 227t–230t, 270
QSEN competencies for, 267
and quality improvement, 272–275, 274t, 280t
role of, 268–269
and safe individual care, 269–272, 277t–279t
technologies included in, 265–266
and Technology Informatics Guiding Education Reform (TIGER), 267
in transitional acute care coordination, 282
Health Information Technology for Economic and Clinical Health (HITECH) Act (2009), 178, 270
Health Insurance Portability and Accountability Act (HIPAA), 182, **320**
Health literacy, 30–32
and care of children, 31–32
and CCTM RN practice, 31
communication breakdown and, 182
definition and context of, 30, **320**
and education of individuals and families, 52, 53
importance of, 30
and macrosocial level, 30
at microsocial level, 30
nursing call to action for, 32
Health Literacy Task Force, 31, 32
Health Literacy Universal Precautions, 31
Health maintenance organization (HMO), **320**
Health portals, 58, 268, 288, 310, **324**
Health promotion
in nursing process, 142
in population health management, 208–209
in self-management support, 124
standards of practice for advocacy in, 24–25
Health-promotion diagnosis, 140
Health risk assessments in population identification, 203
Health status indicators in population health management, 211–212
HealthTap, 60, 331
Health teaching
in nursing process, 142
standards of practice for advocacy in, 24–25
Healthy People 2020, **320**

Healthy People 2030, **320**
Hearing impairment
education of individuals and families with, 50
telehealth nursing with, 293
HeartMapp, 59–60, 331
HEDIS (Healthcare Effectiveness and Data Information Set), 103, **320**
Heroin, 35
HIEs (health information exchanges)
defined, **320**
in nursing informatics, 266, 268, 270
in population health management, 203, 210
HIMSS (Healthcare Information and Management Systems Society), 200, 265–266
HIPAA (Health Insurance Portability and Accountability Act), 182, **320**
HIT. See Health information technology (HIT)
HITECH (Health Information Technology for Economic and Clinical Health) Act (2009), 178, 270
HMO (health maintenance organization), **320**
Home visit, virtual, 289
Hospice, **320**
Housing support, advocacy related to, 29

I

IADL (Independence in Activities of Daily Living), Katz Index of, 92, **321**, 329
iBGstar Diabetes Manager, 60, 331
ICD-10-CM (International Classification of Diseases, 10th Edition, Clinical Modification Procedure Coding System), **321**
ICN (International Council of Nursing), 273
Immigrant children, 38
Immunizations
childhood, 37
in population health management, 208
IMPACT ICU (Integrating Multidisciplinary Palliative Care into the intensive care unit), 84
Implementation
in nursing process, 142
standards of practice for advocacy in, 24
Incontinence, self-management support for, 123
Independence in Activities of Daily Living (IADL), Katz Index of, 92, **321**, 329
Independent practice association (IPA), 321
Index of Independence in Activities of Daily Living (IADL), 92, **321**, 329
Individual care experience in population health management, 211
Informatics, 265–282
aligned with CCTM RN Model, 266–269, 276t–277t

Note: Page numbers followed by t and f indicate tables and figures, respectively; those in **boldface** refer to glossary entries

Index

and assessment, process, and outcome indicators, 273–275, 274t
and big data, 267–268, 271
case studies on, 281–282
in clinical primary care coordination, 281
and communication, 273
competency in, 265–267
in cross-setting communications and transitions, 189t–190t
and decision-support, 270–271
defined, 209–210, **321**
and Essential Elements for Improving the Discharge Transition, 271–272
and evidence-based care guidelines, 268, 271
health, 209
knowledge, skills, and attitudes for, 276t–280t
and Meaningful Measures Framework, 272–275, 274t
nursing, 209–210
and patient-reported outcomes, 265
in population health management, 199t, 209–211, 227t–230t, 270
QSEN competencies for, 267
and quality improvement, 272–275, 274t, 280t
role of, 268–269
and safe individual care, 269–272, 277t–279t
and Technology Informatics Guiding Education Reform (TIGER), 267
in transitional acute care coordination, 282
Informational continuity, 178
Information technology, 58
for self-management support, 129
Information transfer, 178
Informed consent, **321**
Institute of Medicine (IOM), **321**
Integrating Multidisciplinary Palliative Care into the intensive care unit (IMPACT ICU), 84
Intellectual disability, education of individuals and families with, 50–52
International Classification of Diseases, 10th Edition, Clinical Modification Procedure Coding System (ICD-10-CM), 321
International Council of Nursing (ICN), 273
Internet use, 269
Interoperability, 266
Interpersonal communication, 178
Interpreters, 53
Interprofessional collaborative practice, 101
Interprofessional communication, knowledge, skills, and attitudes for, 112t–113t
Interprofessional competencies in health care, 101
Interprofessional education, 101
Interprofessional Education Collaborative (IPEC)
Core Competencies of, 13t
in person-centered care planning, 100–101
and teamwork, 160
Interprofessionality, defined, 163

Interprofessional practice
roles and responsibilities for, 111t–112t
values/ethics for, 110t
Interprofessional team, 162–163
defined, **321**
in person-centered care planning, 100–102, 110t–114t
in population health management, 207
Interstate compacts, 321
Interventions
advocacy in, 27–28
in population health care coordination process, 208, 209f
Interviewing, motivational, 76–78, 97–98, 128, **322**
Invitational Conference on Ambulatory Care Registered Nurse Performance Measurement, 5
IOM (Institute of Medicine), **321**
IPA (independent practice association), **321**
IPEC (Interprofessional Education Collaborative)
Core Competencies of, 13t
in person-centered care planning, 100–101
and teamwork, 160
ISBAR format, 179
I-SMART goals, 126, **321**
Itching, self-management support for, 123

J

The Joint Commission on Accreditation of Healthcare Organizations (JCAHO), **321**
Justice, **321**

K

Katz Index of Independence in Activities of Daily Living (IADL), 92, **321**, 329
KidsDoc, 60, 331
Knowledge, assessment of, 52–53
Knowledge, Skills, and Attitudes (KSA) tables, 9–10

L

Lab Notes, 60, 331
Language barriers to telehealth communication, 293
Leadership
in CCTM, 41–42
and nursing informatios, 273
social determinants of health and, 30
standards of practice for advocacy in, 26
in transition between acute and ambulatory care, 236–237
Learning
electronic methods of, 52
environment of, 52
evaluation of, 56–57
readiness for, 50–52, 51t–52t

style of, 53
Learning disabilities, education of individuals and families with, 50
Lifestyle adaptations in self-management support, 124–126
Listening, active, **315**
Listening skills, 77, 97
Logic Model, 10–11, 14t–16t, **321**
Longitudinal care plans
    nursing informatics and, 272
    in population health management, 210
Long-term care, transition from acute to, 238–239
Long-term opioid therapy (LTOT), 34–35

M

MACRA (Medicare Access and CHIP Reauthorization Act), 200
Magnet Recognition Program, 38–39, **321**
Maintenance stage of change, 76
Managed care, **321**
Mango Health, 60, 331
MCSI (Modified Caregiver Strain Index), 93, **321,** 330
Meaningful Measures Framework, 272–275, 274t, **317**
Meaningful use (MU), **321**
Measurements in care planning, 102–103
Measures of effectiveness (MOE), 103
Measures of performance (MOP), 103
Medicaid, **321**
Medical errors during care transitions, 177
Medical home, patient-centered, **323**
Medical Home model, 160
Medical Orders for Life-Sustaining Treatment (MOLST), 84
Medicare Access and CHIP Reauthorization Act (MACRA), 200
Medicare reimbursement and quality of care, 236
Medication injuries, communication breakdown and, 181
Medication management in plan of care, 99
Medication nonadherence, 181
Medication use, education of individuals and families on, 58, 59
Memory loss, self-management support for, 123
Mental health
    advocacy and, 32–36
    post-acute transitional care models for, 33
mHealth (mobile communication-based health care), 289–290, 321
MI (motivational interviewing), 76–78, 97–98, 128, **322**
Millennials, 53
Mini-Cog–Mental Status Assessment of Older Adults, 92–93, **321,** 330
Mini-Mental State Examination (MMSE), **321,** 330

MMSE (Mini-Mental State Examination), **321,** 330
Mobile applications (mobile apps), 58, 59–60, 289, 290–291, **321,** 331
Mobile communication-based health care (mHealth), 289–290, **321**
Mobile technology, 266
Mobility, Get Up and Go Test for, 93
MoCA (Montreal Cognitive Assessment), **322,** 330
Modified Caregiver Strain Index (MCSI), 93, **321,** 330
Modified LACE, 204, 322, 330
MOE (measures of effectiveness), 103
MOLST (medical Orders for Life-Sustaining Treatment), 84
Monitoring
    big data and, 205
    in care planning, 102–103
    remote patient
        big data and, 205
        defined, **325**
        in telehealth nursing, 289, 290, 311
    wearable devices for, 58, 266
Montreal Cognitive Assessment (MoCA), **322,** 330
MOP (measures of performance), 103
Moral action, 21
Moral agency, 21
Moral distress, 21–22
Motivational interviewing (MI), 76–78, 97–98, 128, **322**
Motor vehicle accidents
    distracted driving and, 37–38
    involving children, 37
Mourning, **322**
MU (meaningful use), **321**
Multimedia approach for education of individuals and families, 53
MyChart, 180, **322**
MyHealthEData initiative, 272, **322**
MyRA, 60, 331
mySugr Diabetes Training, 60, 331

N

NANDA (North American Nursing Diagnosis Association), 140, 145
National Committee for Quality Assurance (NCQA), 103, **322**
National Database of Nursing Quality Indicators (NDNQI), **322**
National Healthcare Decisions Day, 84
National Patient Safety Goals (NPSGs), **322**
National Quality Forum (NQF) on care coordination, 2–3

Note: Page numbers followed by t and f indicate tables and figures, respectively; those in **boldface** refer to glossary entries

Index

National Standards for Diabetes Self-Management Education and Support, 129
Navigator role vs. CCTM RN Model, 4
NCQA (National Committee for Quality Assurance), 103, **322**
NDNQI (National Database of Nursing Quality Indicators), **322**
Needs assessment, comprehensive, 92–94
Negligence, **322**
NI. See Nursing informatics (NI)
NIC (Nursing Interventions Classification), 142, 145, **322**
NMDS (Nursing Minimum Data Set), 323
NOC (Nursing Outcomes Classification), 140–141, 145, 323
Nonmaleficence, **322**
Nonprofit organization, 57
North American Nursing Diagnosis Association (NANDA), 140, 145
NPA (Nurse Practice Act), **322**
NPSGs (National Patient Safety Goals), **322**
NQF (National Quality Forum) on care coordination, 2–3
Nurse leaders, 41–42
Nurse Practice Act (NPA), **322**
Nurse-sensitive indicators (NSIs), 38–39, 273–275, 274t, **322**
NurseTabs, 60, 331
NurseTabs–MedSurg, 60, 331
Nursing, defined, **322**
Nursing assessment, advocacy in, 23, 27
Nursing Central, 60, 331
Nursing Code of Ethics, **322**
Nursing diagnosis(es)
    defined, **322**
    in nursing process, 139–140
    standards of practice for advocacy in, 23
Nursing informatics (NI), 265–282
    aligned with CCTM RN Model, 267–269, 276t–277t
    and assessment, process, and outcome indicators, 273–275, 274t
    and big data, 267–268, 271
    and care coordination, 273
    case studies on, 281–282
    in clinical decision making, 270
    in clinical primary care coordination, 281
    competency in, 265–267, **322**
    in cross-setting communications and transitions, 189t–190t
    and decision-support, 270–271
    defined, 209–210, 265, **322**
    and Essential Elements for Improving the Discharge Transition, 271–272
    and evidence-based care guidelines, 268, 271
    knowledge, skills, and attitudes for, 276t–280t
    and Meaningful Measures Framework, 272–275, 274t
    and patient-reported outcomes, 265
    in population health management, 199t, 209–211, 227t–230t, 270
    QSEN competencies for, 267
    and quality improvement, 272–275, 274t, 280t
    role of, 268–269
    and safe individual care, 269–272, 277t–279t
    and Technology Informatics Guiding Education Reform (TIGER), 267
    in transitional acute care coordination, 282
Nursing interventions, advocacy in, 27–28
Nursing Interventions Classification (NIC), 142, 145, **322**
Nursing Minimum Data Set (NMDS), 323
Nursing Outcomes Classification (NOC), 140–141, 145, **323**
Nursing plan of care. See Care plan(s)
Nursing practice, advocacy in, 19, 20–21, 21f
    in CCTM Model, 27–28
Nursing process, 137–154
    applied to family care, 143
    case studies on, 152–154
    and chronic disease management, 143–144
    clinical reasoning and thinking in, 137–138
    competency in, 137
    and decision support, 144
    defined, 137, 138, **323**
    evidence-based practice in, 146t
    expanding CCTM RN role and, 144–145
    knowledge, skills, and attitudes for, 146t–151t
    and person-centered care, 138, 147t–151t
    and plan of care, 144, 152–153
    quality improvement in, 146t
    safety in, 147t
    and standardized nursing terminology, 145, 145f
    steps of, 138–143
        assessment as, 139
        evaluation as, 142–143
        implementation as, 142
        nursing diagnosis as, 139–140
        outcomes/goals identification as, 140–142, 141f
        planning as, 142
Nursing-sensitive outcomes, 140–142, 141f, **323**
Nursing services, 323
Nursing terminologies, standardized, 273
Nutrition
    education of individuals and families on, 59
    in plan of care, 99
Nutritional support, advocacy related to, 29
Nutrition assistance programs, 37

O

Objective data, 139
Occupational Safety and Health Administration (OSHA), 323

Index

Oncology nurse navigator (ONN), 4
Opioid(s)
    addiction to, 59
    defined, **323**
    misuse and abuse of, 59
    risks of, 59
    storage and disposal of, 59
    tolerance and withdrawal from, 59
Opioid crisis, 32, 33–35
Opioid medications, education of individuals and families on, 59, 70–71
Organizational performance, standards of practice for advocacy in, 25–27
Organizational policy development, advocacy in, 38–39
Orientation, **323**
OSHA (Occupational Safety and Health Administration), **323**
Outcome(s)
    nursing-sensitive, 140–142, 141f, **323**
    patient-reported, 265
Outcome indicators, nursing informatics and, 273–275
Outcomes identification
    in nursing process, 140–142, 141f
    standards of practice for advocacy in, 23–24
Outcomes measurement in population health management, 211–212
Out-of-pocket expense, **323**
Ozbolt's Patient Care Data Set (PCDS), **323**

P

PACT (Patient-Aligned Care Teams) Model, 7–8
Pain
    chronic
        advocacy for, 34–35
        defined, **317**
        education of individuals and families on management of, 59, 70–71
    defined, **323**
Pain management
    education of individuals and families on, 59, 70–71
    in plan of care, 99
    self-management support for, 123
Palliative care, 84–85, **323**
PAM (Patient Activation Measure), 93, **323**, 330
Partnerships for Patients program, 6
Passenger safety of children, 37
Patient, defined, **323**
Patient Activation Measure (PAM), 93, **323**, 330
Patient advocacy. See Advocacy
Patient-Aligned Care Teams (PACT) Model, 7–8
Patient Care Access System (PCAS), 8
Patient Care Data Set (PCDS), **323**
Patient-centered care, **323**. See also Person-centered care
Patient-centered care coordination, 236
Patient-centered medical home (PCMH), **323**
Patient education, **324**
Patient Health Questionnaire (PHQ-2 or PHQ-9), 92, **324**, 330
Patient panels in population health management, 206, 207
Patient portals, 58, 268, 288, 310, **324**
Patient Preparation to Address Situations (after discharge) Successfully (Patient PASS), 254t, 261t
Patient Protection and Affordable Care Act (2010), 4, 6, 160, 200, **324**
Patient-reported outcomes (PROs), 265
Pay-for-performance (P4P), 213–214, **324**
PBPH (practice-based population health), **324**
PCA (Primary Care Almanac), 8
PCAS (Patient Care Access System), 8
PCDS (Patient Care Data Set), **323**
PCMH (patient-centered medical home), **323**
PCPs (primary care providers)
    behavioral and mental health services by, 33
    defined, **324**
    in population health management, 205–206, 207
PDMPs (prescription drug monitoring programs), 34, **324**
Pediatric patients. See Children
Peer coaching for self-management support, 128–129
Peer discussions for education of individuals and families, 55
Peer review, **324**
Performance improvement
    defined, **324**
    standards of practice for advocacy in, 26
Performance measures, 103
Personal action plan in self-management model, 79f, 82
Personal health portal, 58, 268, 288, 310, 324
Personal health records (PHRs), 266
Personalized health information, 58
Personal medical record, 55, 68t
Personal safety in plan of care, 99
Person attribution in population identification, 202–203
Person-centered care
    defined, **323**
    informatics and, 210
    nursing process and, 138, 147t–151t
    in population health management, 199t, 218t–220t

Note: Page numbers followed by t and f indicate tables and figures, respectively; those in **boldface** refer to glossary entries

Index

in transition between acute and ambulatory care, 244t
Person-centered care planning, 91–117
    case studies on, 115–117
    communicating plan of care in, 103
    competency in, 91
    comprehensive needs assessment in, 92–94
    core concepts for, 91–92
    evidence-based care resources in, 102
    interprofessional team approach in, 100–102
    knowledge, skills, and attitudes for, 104t–114t
    monitoring and measuring of individuals in, 102–103
    motivational interviewing in, 97–98
    pediatric, 115–116
    plan of care in, 98–100
    pre-encounter chart review and visit planning in, 94–95
    quality measures and outcomes in, 103
    risk stratification in, 95–97, 96t
Person profile analytics, big data and, 205
Pharmacist in population health management, 207
PHM. *See* Population health management (PHM)
PHO (physician hospital organization), **324**
PHQ-2 or PHQ-9 (Patient Health Questionnaire), 92, **324**, 330
PHRs (personal health records), 266
Physical activity
    by children, 37
    education of individuals and families on, 58
Physical barriers to self-management, 124
Physical discomfort, self-management support for, 123
Physical education at school, 37
Physician hospital organization (PHO), **324**
Picture-based instructions/illustrations, 53–54
Pillboxie, 60, 221
Planning. *See also* Person-centered care planning
    in nursing process, 142
    in population health care coordination process, 208, 209f
    strategic, **326**
Plan of care, 98–100. *See also* Person-centered care planning
    advocacy in, 24, 27
    defined, **323**
    interprofessional, 163
    nursing process and, 144, 152–153
Policy development
    advocacy in, 38–39
    population health and, 212–213
Policy initiatives for care coordination, 40–41
POLST (Provider Orders for Life-Sustaining Treatment), 84
Polypharmacy, **324**
Population health, 199–200
    defined, **324**
    and policy development, 212–213
    practice-based, **324**
Population Health Care Coordination Process, 208–209, 209f, 216
Population Health Conceptual Framework, 200, 201t
Population health management (PHM), 197–230
    background of, 198–201
    big data in, 204–205, 215
    care coordination in, 208–209, 209f, 216
    case studies on, 215–217
    competency in, 197–198, 198t, 199t
    defined, 199–200, **324**
    evidence-based practice in, 199t, 223t–224t
    informatics and decision-support systems in, 199t, 209–211, 227t–230t, 270
    key characteristics of, 200
    knowledge, skills, and attitudes for, 218t–230t
    measuring outcomes in, 211–212
    models for, 200–201, 201f, 202f
    person/population-centered care in, 199t, 218t–220t
    policies supporting, 200
    and policy development, 212–213
    population identification in, 201–204
    preventive care management in, 208–209
    vs. public health, 198–199
    quality improvement in, 199t, 225t–226t
    safety in, 199t, 226t–227t
    team-based interventions in, 205–207, 217t
    teamwork and collaboration in, 199t, 220t–223t
    value-based care and purchasing in, 213–214
    vs. wellness programs or disease management programs, 200
Population identification, 201–204
Population management, 199
Poverty
    and care of children, 37
    and health, 28–29
P4P (Pay-for-performance), 213–214, **324**
PPO (preferred provider organization), **324**
Practice-based population health (PBPH), **324**
Practice skills, community dimensions of, 108t–109t
Precertification, **324**
Pre-contemplation stage of change, 76
Predictive models in population health management, 210
Pre-encounter chart review, 94–95
Preferred provider organization (PPO), **324**
Preparation stage of change, 76
Prescription drug monitoring programs (PDMPs), 34, **324**
Presence, **324**
Prevention
    in population health management, 208–209
    primary, **325**

Index

secondary, **325**
in self-management support, 124
tertiary, **327**
Preventive care management in population health management, 208–209
Pre-visit chart review, 94–95, **324**
Primary care
defined, **324**
policy initiatives for care coordination in, 41–42
Primary Care Almanac (PCA), 8
Primary care coordination, health information technology in, 281
Primary care providers (PCPs)
behavioral and mental health services by, 33
defined, **324**
in population health management, 205–206, 207
Primary prevention, **325**
Privacy, 23
PRO(s) (patient-reported outcomes), 265
Problem-focused diagnosis, 140
Problem solving
in plan of care, 99
as self-management skill, 59, 127
Process indicators, nursing informatics and, 273–275
Productivity, **325**
Professional competencies in health care, 101
Professional organization advocacy, 45
Professional performance, standards of practice for advocacy in, 25–27
Professional practice evaluation, standards of practice for advocacy in, 26
Professional standards for telehealth nursing, 291
Project Re-Engineered Discharge (Project RED), 183–184, 241, **325**, 330
Provider order entries, computerized, 178
Provider Orders for Life-Sustaining Treatment (POLST), 84
Pruritus, self-management support for, 123
Psychological barriers to self-management, 124–125
Psychosocial status assessment in population health management, 211
Public health
big data and, 205
vs. population health management, 198–199
Public Health Nursing Competencies, 13t
Public policy development, advocacy and, 39–41

Q

Quality and Safety Education for Nurses (QSEN) competencies
and CCTM RN Model, 9–10, 13t
on nursing informatics, 267
on person-centered care, 138

Quality domains, 213
Quality improvement
in cross-setting communications and transitions, 188t–189t
defined, **325**
nursing informatics and, 272–275, 274t, 280t
nursing process and, 146t
in population health management, 199t, 225t–226t
Quality measures and outcomes, 103
Quality of care
impact of teamwork on, 171t
Medicare reimbursement and, 236
Quality of life in population health management, 211

R

RBRVS (resource-based relative value scale), **325**
RCA (root cause analysis), **325**
"Reaching level of solidarity," 83
"Reaching level of truthfulness," 83
"Reaching out," 82–83
"Red flags" in monitoring and measuring, 102–103
Re-Engineered Discharge (Project RED), 183–184, 241, **325**, 330
Reflective thinking
in nursing process, 138
in self-management support, 127
Refugee children, 38
Registries
defined, **317**
in population identification, 203
Regulatory standards for telehealth nursing, 291
Rehospitalizations, State Action on Avoidable, 184
Reimbursement and quality of care, 236
Reimbursement models, population health and, 212
Relationship with individuals and families
developing, 76–77
maintaining, 82–83
Relaxation in plan of care, 99
Reminders, 58
Remote patient monitoring
big data and, 205
defined, 325
in telehealth nursing, 289, 290, 311
"Removing mask of anonymity," 83
Report cards, **325**
Research and development
big data and, 205
standards of practice for advocacy in, 25–26
Research utilization, **325**

Note: Page numbers followed by t and f indicate tables and figures, respectively; those in **boldface** refer to glossary entries

Index

Resource(s)
   list of, 329–330
   and teamwork, 166
Resource-based relative value scale (RBRVS), **325**
Resource utilization
   standards of practice for advocacy in, 26
   in transition between acute and ambulatory care, 237
Resuscitation status, 84
Revenue, **325**
Risk assessment in population health management, 210
Risk diagnosis, 140
Risk management, **325**
Risk stratification, 95–97
   for chronic disease, 95, 96t
   defined, **325**
   in population identification, 203–204
Root cause analysis (RCA), **325**

S

Safety
   cultural, **318**
   health information technology and, 269–272, 277t–279t
   impact of teamwork on, 171t
   nursing process and, 147t
   in plan of care, 99
   in population health management, 199t, 226t–227t
   in transition between acute and ambulatory care, 245t
Safety and Assurance Factors for EHR Resiliences (SAFER), 270
Safety seats for children, 37
SBAR (Situation, Background, Assessment and Recommendation) tool, **325**
Scope and Standards of Practice for Registered Nurses in Care Coordination and Transition Management (AAACN), 23
Screening for social determinants of health in children, 29
SDOH (social determinants of health)
   and advocacy, 28–30
   defined, **326**
   in population health management, 211
Secondary prevention, **325**
Self-care, **325**
Self-determination, right to, 22
Self-efficacy
   defined, **325**
   in self-management support, 127
   support for, 78
Self-evaluation in self-management support, 128
Self-management, barriers to, 124–126
Self-management model, 78–82, 79f–81f
Self-management skills, 58–59
   support for development of, 126–129
Self-management support, 121–134
   case studies on, 134
   competency in, 121–122
   defined, **325**
   for diabetes, 129, 134
   health promotion and disease prevention in, 124
   knowledge, skills, and attitudes for, 130t–133t
   knowledge and understanding of chronic conditions in, 122–124
   methods for, 128–129
   outcome measure for, 133t
   skill development in, 125–128
   social and lifestyle adaptations in, 124–125
   for weight management, 134
Self-monitoring
   in plan of care, 99
   in self-management support, 127
Self-regulation in self-management support, 126
SES (socioeconomic status) and health, 28–29
Shared decision-making, 163
Shortness of breath, self-management support for, 123
Shots by STFM, 60, 331
Silent Generation, 53
Simply Sayin', 59, 331
Situation, Background, Assessment and Recommendation (SBAR) tool, **325**
Sleep disturbances, self-management support for, 123
Sleep goals in plan of care, 99
SMART goals, 140, **325**
SNOMED-CT (Systematized Nomenclature of Medicine–Clinical Terms), 273, **326**
Social adaptations in self-management support, 124–126
Social barriers to self-management, 125
Social determinants of health (SDOH)
   and advocacy, 28–30
   defined, **326**
   in population health management, 211
Social groups and education of individuals and families, 53
Social worker in population health management, 207
Socioeconomic status (SES) and health, 28–29
Solidarity, reaching level of, 83
Specialty care, transition to, 239
Stakeholders, 41
Standard(s), defined, **326**
Standards of practice
   advocacy and, 23–27
   in Clinical Practice domain, 23–25
   collaboration, teamwork and, 161–162

Index

defined, **326**
for organizational and professional performance, 25–27
State Action on Avoidable Rehospitalizations (STAAR), 184, 241–242
State practice acts, **326**
Strategic planning, **326**
Subjective data, 139
Subpopulation identification, 201–203, 217
Substance abuse, CAGE questionnaire on, 92
Supervision, **326**
Support structure, 76
Support systems, assessment of, 125
Surrogate decision-maker for health care, 83
Surveillance for social determinants of health in children, 29
Symptom management
　for chronic conditions, 122–123
　as self-management skill, 58
Synchronous interactions in telehealth nursing, 292
System(s), impact of team on, 171t
Systematized Nomenclature of Medicine–Clinical Terms (SNOMED-CT), 273, **326**
Systems level advocacy, 19, **326**

T

TCM (Transitional Care Model), 240
TCM (Transitional Care Management) Services in plan of care, 99–100
"Teach-back" method, 54, 56–57, **326**
Team(s), characteristics of high-performing, 163–165, 206
Team-based care, interprofessional, 101
Team-based interventions in population health management, 205–207, 217t
Team building
　in cross-setting communications and transitions, 186t–187t
　defined, **326**
Team development, 165, 168t
Team leadership, 164–165
Team members
　individuals and families as, 77
　in population health management, 207
Team roles, 165, 169t, 207
Team Strategies and Tools to Enhance Performance and Patient Safety (TeamSTEPPS) program, 163, 178, **326**
Teamwork, 159–173
　background of, 159–161
　barriers to, 165–166
　basic principles and values to guide, 160–161
　case studies on, 172–173
　vs. collaboration, 159–160
　communication and, 161, 165–166, 170t
　competency in, 159
　consultation and, 162
　coordination of care and, 161
　defined, **326**
　in education of individuals and families, 56
　environment and, 162
　ethics and, 162
　evaluation and, 162
　in health care, **326**
　impact on safety and quality of care of, 171t
　interprofessional, 101, 162–163
　key elements and evidence-based strategies for, 163–165
　knowledge, skills, and attitudes for, 113t–114t, 160, 168t–171t
　participation of CCTM RN as member or leader in, 166–167
　in population health management, 199t, 220t–223t
　and professional practice standards, 161–162
　resources and, 166
　in telehealth nursing, 294, 305t–306t
　in transition between acute and ambulatory care, 245t–246t
Technology
　and advocacy, 41
　information, 58
　wearable, 58, 266, **327**
Technology expertise in telehealth nursing, 294–295, 307t–308t
Technology Informatics Guiding Education Reform (TIGER), 267
Telehealth, defined, **326**
Telehealth nursing practice (telenursing), 58, 287–311
　case studies on, 309–311
　communication in, 292–294, 302t–304t
　competency in, 288
　defined, 288, **326**
　essential elements of, 291
　health portals in, 58, 268, 288, 310, **324**
　knowledge, skills, and attitudes for, 296t–308t
　mHealth in, 289–290
　mobile apps in, 289, 290–291
　overview of, 288
　principles of, 291–292, 298t–301t
　professional standards in, 287, 291, 296t–297t
　remote patient monitoring in, 289, 290, 311
　synchronous vs. asynchronous interactions in, 292
　teamwork and collaboration in, 294, 305t–306t
　technologies used in, 288
　technology expertise in, 294–295, 307t–308t
　triage in, 291–292, 298t–301t, **327**
　video conferencing in, 288–289, 309

Note: Page numbers followed by t and f indicate tables and figures, respectively; those in **boldface** refer to glossary entries

Index

Telemedicine, **326**
Telemonitoring, **326**
Telephone nursing, **327**
Telephone triage, 291–292, 298t–301t, **327**
Telepresenter, 288–289
Terminology, standardized nursing, 145, 145f
Tertiary prevention, **327**
The Joint Commission (TJC), **321**
TIC (trauma-informed care), 30, 36
TIGER (Technology Informatics Guiding Education Reform), 267
Tolerance to opioids, 59
Transitional acute care coordination, health information technology in, 282
Transitional care
    core features of, 3
    defined, 3, 176, 235, **327**
    vs. transition management, 3
Transitional Care Management (TCM) Services in plan of care, 99–100
Transitional Care Model (TCM), 240
Transition management
    application of evidence-based tools for, 243
    case studies on, 248–261
    defined, 3, **327**
    engagement of individual, family, and interprofessional team during, 242–243
    evidence-based models for, 239–242
    knowledge, skills, and attitude for, 244t–247t
    opportunities for, 237–239
    standards guiding, 236–237
    vs. transitional care, 3
Transition models, evidence-based, 239–242
Transition(s) of care. See Care transitions
Transitions Coach, 241
Translational research, **327**
Transtheoretical Model of Change, 76, **327**
Trauma, children's response to, 29, 36
Trauma-informed care (TIC), 30, 36
Treat-to-target, 141, 141f
Triage, telehealth, 291–292, 298t–301t, **327**
TriCare, **327**
Triple Aim, 42, 206
"True negotiation of care," 83
Truthfulness, reaching level of, 83

U

UCR (usual, customary, and reasonable), **327**
Universal Discharge Checklist, 179, 252t–253t, 259t–260t
Universal precautions approach
    to education of individuals and families, 53–54
    to health literacy, 31

Up-to-Date for Patients and Caregivers, 59, 331
Urinary incontinence, self-management support for, 123
U.S. Preventive Services Task Force (USPSTF), 94–95, **327**
Usual, customary, and reasonable (UCR), **327**
Utilitarianism, **327**
Utilization management, **327**

V

VA (Veterans Administration), telehealth monitoring by, 289
Value(s), for interprofessional practice, 110t
Value-based health care in population health management, 213–214
Value modifier, 6
Variable costs, 327
Veracity, **327**
Veterans, behavioral health services for, 46
Veterans Administration (VA), telehealth monitoring by, 289
Veterans Health Administration (VHA), telehealth monitoring by, 289
Video conferencing, 288–289, 309, **327**
Virtual home visit, 289
Visit planning, 94–95
Visual impairment, telehealth nursing with, 293–294

W

Wearable technology, 58, 266, **327**
WebMD for iPad, 60, 331
Websites, reliability of, 57
Weight management
    in plan of care, 99
    self-management support for, 134
Well-being in population health management, 211
Wellness programs, population health management vs., 200
Withdrawal from opioids, 59
Wizdy Pets, 60, 331

Y

Young adult care, transition from pediatric to, 239

Z

Zarit Burden Interview, **327**, 330